Applied Theories in
Occupational Therapy
A Practical Approach

Applied Theories in
Occupational Therapy
A Practical Approach

Marilyn B. Cole, MS, OTR/L, FAOTA

Roseanna Tufano, LMFT, OTR/L

Department of Occupational Therapy
Quinnipiac University
Hamden, Connecticut

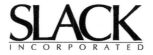

SLACK
INCORPORATED

Published by: SLACK Incorporated
                  6900 Grove Road
                  Thorofare, NJ 08086 USA
                  Telephone: 856-848-1000
                  Fax: 856-853-5991
                  www.slackbooks.com

Contact SLACK Incorporated for more information about other books in this field or about the availability of our books from distributors outside the United States.

Library of Congress Cataloging-in-Publication Data

Cole, Marilyn B., 1945-
  Applied theories in occupational therapy : a practical approach / Marilyn B. Cole, Roseanna Tufano.
     p. ; cm.
  Includes bibliographical references and index.
  ISBN-13: 978-1-55642-573-8 (alk. paper)
  ISBN-10: 1-55642-573-2 (alk. paper)
  1. Occupational therapy--Philosophy. I. Tufano, Roseanna. II. Title.
  [DNLM: 1. Occupational Therapy. 2. Models, Theoretical. 3. Occupational Health Services. 4. Occupational Health.
WB 555 C689a 2008]

RM735.C633 2008
615.8'515--dc22
                          2007043630

Printed in the United States of America.

Last digit is print number: 20 19 18 17 16 15 14 13

DEDICATIONS

To my students, clients, and colleagues, and my family, children, and parents, who have collectively taught me more about occupational therapy, and about life, than words could ever express.

— M. C.

To my family—my origin and my ongoing inspiration. With particular gratitude to my mother, Angela, who watches over me from above.

— R. T.

CONTENTS

CONTENTS

SECTION II: OCCUPATION-BASED MODELS

SECTION III: FRAMES OF REFERENCE

Applied Theroies in Occupational Therapy: A Pratical Guide Instructor's Manual is also available from SLACK Incorporated. Don't miss this important companion to this book. To obtain the Instructor's Manual, please visit http://www.efacultylounge.com.

ABOUT THE AUTHORS

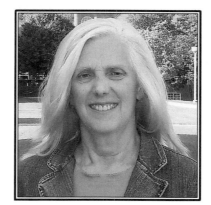

Marilyn B. (Marli) Cole, MS, OTR/L, FAOTA, is an occupational therapy Professor Emerita at Quinnipiac University in Hamden, Connecticut. She is the author of *Group Dynamics in Occupational Therapy*, now in its third edition (SLACK Incorporated, 2005). A graduate of University of Pennsylvania, she practiced for 16 years in mental health, pediatrics, and geriatrics. She holds an advanced certification in Sensory Integration and has published chapters on theory application, client-centered groups, occupational therapy (OT) interventions in retirement, volunteering, and end-of-life issues, theories of aging, and theory development in OT. As an educator, she has taught courses in therapeutic use of self, group leadership, frames of reference, psychopathology, geriatrics, sensory integration, group dynamics, evaluation, intervention, health conditions, problem-based learning, and research. As a fieldwork I coordinator, she has developed student experiences in hospital and community mental health, geriatrics, wellness, and prevention in the United States, England, Costa Rica, and Australia. Research interests and journal publications include mental health assessment, group size and engagement, time mastery, therapeutic relationships, civic engagement, and OT interventions for the Third Age (retirement). At home in Connecticut or in Freeport, Bahamas, Marli and her husband, Martin Schiraldi, enjoy traveling, cruising, skiing, sailing, and scuba diving.

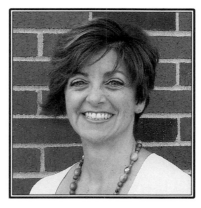

Roseanna Tufano, LMFT, OTR/L, is an Assistant Professor in Occupational Therapy at Quinnipiac University as well as the Academic Coordinator for the department. Her interests and expertise are within the practice of mental health, where she has practiced for over 25 years among varied levels of care. As an educator, she has taught courses in OT theory application, psychopathology, group dynamics, psychosocial adaptation to physical disorders, and mental health interventions. She has published several chapters on related topics and has lectured and consulted to both professional and consumer-oriented audiences. With her advanced clinical degree in Marriage and Family Therapy, Roseanna joins her husband Lou in a private practice called "Enduring Families" aimed to support individuals and families to endure meaningful roles. Likewise, she is very active in serving students within the Quinnipiac University community and was given the "Outstanding Faculty Award" by the Student Government Association in both 1999 and 2003. Among her most memorable endeavors at Quinnipiac, she delivered the "Freshman Address" at the University Convocation where her daughter, Carissa, sat among the incoming class of 2006. She enjoys traveling and spending family time with her husband; children, Carissa and Brett; and dog, Armani.

PREFACE

What's Theory Got to Do With It?

Many students (and practitioners) tend to tune out whenever we talk about theory. Occupational therapists are practical by nature and consider themselves involved in the real world of practice. Theory is for academic types—researchers need to know about theory. Practitioners need assessment tools (short ones, if possible); practitioners need techniques that work, intervention strategies for solving real problems, and short documentation forms. We know. We've been there too.

The idea for this book began around 5 years ago. We had been teaching theory courses for about 10 years, and we had never found one comprehensive textbook on occupational therapy (OT) theory that beginning students could understand. We are great believers in the notion that theory guides practice and have always carried this torch within our OT department, our professional relationships, and among our students. We have patiently watched our OT profession struggle with its identity and have been confused by the resurgence of labels that have been associated with theory and occupation. In fact, we have found that in recent years, it has only gotten worse. There are approaches, frames of reference, models of practice, conceptual foundations, umbrella theories, occupational performance models, meta-theories, grand theories, paradigms, philosophies, and bodies of knowledge. Theory itself involves concepts, constructs, postulates, propositions, principles, hypotheses, arguments, and assumptions. Just a quick glance at the latest OT textbooks tells us that even the most esteemed scholars and writers in our profession don't agree on the meaning of these terms. Sometimes it makes us want to scream. And we're the professors!

But of course we know how important theory is and how basic it is to what occupational therapists do. We are simply trying to find a way to make theory simple and alive, not confusing, irrelevant, or overwhelming, to our students. This has always been our dream, our persistent mission, and our albatross. So now, we have written our own book about it.

What Is Applied Theory?

Applied theory is the outcome of applied research, intended to address problems of practical interest to occupational therapists. Many levels of theory exist in our profession, and there is much confusion about what to call them. For the sake of simplicity, we are calling them all applied theories.

While attempting to make things simple, we also realize that the theoretical advances that have occurred in OT are not simple at all. For occupational therapists in the trenches, the gap between theory and practice may never have been wider. Many have resisted the use of the new American Occupational Therapy Association (AOTA) OT Practice Framework, questioned why we needed yet another occupational performance model, and turned a blind eye to the researchers who have challenged our traditional practice methods by citing contradictory evidence. What's theory got to do with it? For the sake of these skeptics, we'd like to take it one logical step at a time.

1. Occupational therapists in the 1970s could not agree on what they had in common.

2. Occupational therapists in different specialty areas (psychiatry, physical disabilities, pediatrics, etc.) used different frames of reference. In the 1980s, we discovered that this concrete level of applied theory did not help to unify the profession. Something more was needed.

3. We stopped looking for a common frame of reference and began to study what all of them had in common. This led to a broader, more general level of theory, which focused on occupation. (The trends and evolution of OT theory reviewed in Chapter 1 trace this process in greater detail.)

While moving to broader theories of occupation seems simple and logical in retrospect, its implications are quite complex. Hooper (2006) explains it as an epistemological transformation, or a shift in way we define knowledge and in the methods by which we acquire knowledge. The mid-century reductionistic approach led occupational therapists to develop and research many specific techniques, such as sensory integration for the treatment of children with learning disability, biomechanical strategies for the treatment of hand injury, and cognitive rehabilitation for the treatment of traumatic brain injury. These applied theories, while useful and valid, represented fragments of occupation developed in isolation of each other. (Chapter 2 discusses more fully the influences of the medical model and the profession's move toward a client-centered model.) Broader theories of occupation, such as the model of human occupation (Kielhofner & Burke, 1980) and subsequent occupation-based models, served the purpose of defining the interconnections among the fragments or components of occupation. Furthermore, the application of general system theory and dynamic systems theories (discussed in Chapter 3), influenced the newer occupation-based models in synthesizing much of the specific knowledge developed earlier within the multiple dimensions of occupation (Hooper, 2006).

It is a relief to learn that occupation-based models are not going to replace all of the collected wisdom of OT's more traditional frames of reference. However, as practitioners, occupational therapists will be expected to use specific techniques within the context of the broader occupation-based models, and this requires an understanding on both levels. In fact, OT students and practitioners need to develop an appreciation of the all levels of theory as necessary within our new paradigm of client-centered, holistic, and systems-oriented OT practice.

Evolution of Occupational Therapy Theory

We begin this text with a presentation of eight current trends in the field based on a content analysis of the past 20 years of Slagle lectures, which have been given by the OT profession's most esteemed scholars and leaders. Next, reviewing the conceptual history of OT from its founding in the United States gives a perspective on how far our profession has come and why various applied theories have developed along the way. We examine the influence of the medical model, the client-centered model, and the impact of systems theories in science and health care, which have profoundly affected the past and recent growth in the OT profession.

Without this background, new students and graduates cannot possibly appreciate the enormity of what has occurred. Over the past 25 to 30 years, we have witnessed the elevation of OT from an "allied medical profession" to a profession in its own right complete with its own body of knowledge and research, its unique theories of occupation, and, with a masters degree entry level, the community of scholars needed to continue the quest for prominence as a profession.

Reilly's (1962) famous Slagle lecture at an OT conference reopened our eyes, ears, and hearts to appreciating the reality that nothing is ever what is seems. Persons cannot be treated in a vacuum. Our clients are influenced by many factors, often unseen, and their behaviors make sense to them. So, Chapter 3 highlights general system theory and its contributory role in redefining our understanding of occupation, context, disability, and health.

In Chapter 4, we attempt to sort out the different levels of applied theory, their definitions, and the different ways each guides our practice. We limit our discussion to three levels: paradigm, occupation-based models, and frames of reference. Chapter 5 discusses how OT can impact and restore health and well-being within local and global communities and within the continuum of disability and wellness. The OT Practice Framework (AOTA, 2002) is integrated throughout the book, with particular attention in Chapters 2, 4, and 21. The authors recognize this document as a useful guideline to the application of all levels of theory of practice.

Section II reviews five currently used occupation-based models, and Section III reviews nine frames of reference. None of these chapters is intended to be comprehensive, and students are directed to original sources for further information. We focus on application by structuring these consistently, giving specific guidelines as examples, and providing cases and learning exercises to help students understand how to apply each in both disability and wellness practice areas.

References

American Occupational Therapy Association. (2002). The occupational therapy association practice framework: Domain and process. *American Journal of Occupational Therapy, 56*, 609–639.

Hooper, B. (2006). Epistemological transformations in occupational therapy: Educational implications and challenges. *Occupational Therapy Journal of Research, 26*, 15–24.

Kielhofner, G., & Burke, J. (1980). A model of human occupation, part I: Conceptual framework and content. *American Journal of Occupational Therapy, 34*, 572–581.

Reilly, M. (1962). Occupational therapy can be one of the great ideas of 20th century medicine. *American Journal of Occupational Therapy, 16*, 1–9.

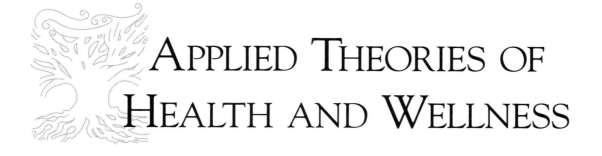

Section I

APPLIED THEORIES OF HEALTH AND WELLNESS

Section I's purpose is to provide a perspective on where the profession of occupational therapy (OT) fits in the broader spectrum of health care, wellness, and community services.

__Chapter 1__ begins with current trends within the profession that have been derived from the past 20 years of Slagle lectures. A content analysis of these lectures uses the combined wisdom of many of the profession's top leaders and scholars to predict some future directions to help guide our students as they prepare to enter this dynamic and ever-changing field (Cole, 2003). These trends tell us that the basic guiding premises and theories behind the profession as a whole have shifted to one that is holistic, client-centered, and systems-oriented. Chapter 1 continues with a historical perspective, a review of OT's founding concepts, earlier paradigm shifts, and the evolution of theory in the context of other historical events in our nation's history.

__Chapter 2__ focuses on the two main models of health care within which occupational therapists currently practice: the medical model and the client-centered or community model. The philosophical and theoretical assumptions of each are discussed and compared. We include a global perspective of health care in reviewing the World Health Organization's (WHO's) International Classification of Function (ICF), Disability, and Health (WHO, 2001) with a focus on the theoretical implications for OT practice. We then look at the models of OT in the United States, the OT Practice Framework (AOTA, 2002) and the Canadian Model of Occupational Performance (CMOP) (Law & Mills, 1998), within the backdrop of recent changes in the paradigm of health care generally.

__Chapter 3__ looks closer at two major theoretical trends in the new paradigm of OT: holism and the systems perspective. Systems theory has changed the face of both basic and applied sciences in the 21st century and has called into question many of the concepts inherent in OT's more traditional frames of reference and models of practice. By understanding systems theory, we see more clearly how the holistic trend in health care changes our view of the patient or client to one who both embodies (client factors) and interacts with (contexts) multiple systems, all of which impact occupational performance, engagement in activities, and participation in life.

__Chapter 4__ discusses the organization of knowledge within the OT profession. As our knowledge base continues to build, a recog-

nition of the different levels of theory and the need to differentiate concepts from inside and outside the profession take on greater importance. We use a combination of sources in describing the relationships among philosophy, paradigm, overarching theories, model of practice, and frames of reference. We propose three basic levels of theory for the OT profession:

- *Paradigm (philosophy, code of ethics, values, core concepts), and the OT Practice Framework (AOTA, 2002).*

- *Occupation-based models (focusing on the interaction of person, environment, and occupation)*

- *Frames of reference (focusing on specific areas within OT's domain).*

While all of these levels represent applied theories, we hope to clarify the differences and describe how each is appropriately applied in OT practice.

__Chapter 5__ reviews some of the current trends of health care that include well-being, health promotion and prevention, and a focus on public health. As health delivery moves toward community-based practice, it is important to recognize and understand the different models of service within which OT will need to interact. New roles for OT in community settings will need to be identified, defined, or created by our practitioners, students, and new graduates as the profession moves farther from the shadow of the medical model. Community as a concept is presented in both a local and a global perspective as themes of social justice, political advocacy, and inclusion continue to shape OT practice.

REFERENCES

American Occupational Therapy Association. (2002). *Occupational therapy practice framework: Domain and process.* American Journal of Occupational Therapy, 56, 609–639.

Cole, M. (2003, June 8). Trends from the Slagle lectures: 1986-2001. Paper presentation. Washington, DC: American Occupational Therapy Association Annual Conference & Expo.

Law, M., & Mills, J. (1998). Client-centered occupational therapy. In M. Law (Ed.), *Client-centered occupational therapy.* Thorofare, NJ: SLACK Incorporated.

World Health Organization. (2001). *International classification of functioning, disability, and health.* Geneva: Author.

Chapter 1

Occupational Therapy's Broadening Horizons

"Occupational therapy could be one of the great ideas of twentieth century medicine."

– MARY REILLY (1962, P. 1)

The purpose of this chapter is to define the broad theoretical basis of the profession of occupational therapy (OT), taking into account a number of recent trends and changes. First, we will review the major new theoretical trends within our profession, as defined by leaders in the field. Second, we will review the founding principles of our profession that have endured over time. The paradigm shifts will be outlined, showing how and why our profession has changed and grown since its beginnings. Third, we will trace the theoretical history of OT, highlighting the contexts for development of new theories and how they are currently affecting our practice. This review will give the beginning student a foundation to understand the potential usefulness of the many models of practice and frames of reference being published, taught, and applied in today's practice.

Eight Major Trends

Eleanor Clarke Slagle was perhaps the best-known founder of the profession of OT. The lecture award given each year by the American Occupational Therapy Association (AOTA) in her name is the highest scholarly honor awarded in our profession. DeBeer (1987) observed that the central themes and issues of concern to the profession are reflected in these lectures. In the mid-1980s, DeBeer observed, "occupational therapy appears to be in an era of specialization" (p. 527). She used content analysis of the previous 30 years of Slagle lectures to identify common themes and trends in the profession. The following eight themes represent the continuation of this process and were derived from themes of Slagle lectures from 1986 to 2001 (Cole, 2003). Their content has centered around three major areas: theory, philosophy, and research. As such, these lectures provide a good foundation upon which to re-evaluate the theoretical perspective of the profession and to make some predictions about its future direction. Where appropriate, other theorists are cited to further substantiate these trends.

1. Moving Away From the Medical Model

Occupation is, quite simply, what humans do. People have been doing things since the dawn of creation, so occupation is not a new concept. According to this broad definition, the things we do day-to-day, week-to-week, and year-to-year are all occupations. Occupation has never been a uniquely medical concept. Rather, it is a part of the fabric of life itself.

The founders of OT, nearly a century ago, built our profession upon the healing power of occupation, thus forming a link between medical practice and OT. For most of the 20th century, occupational therapists have practiced within the bounds of the medical model, working in hospitals and health care-based community programs and guided by doctors' referral. The current health care system, in its effort to contain health care costs, has temporarily swept OT along on its wave of cutbacks and brought our link with the medical model into question (Christiansen, 1999; Clark, 1993; Nelson, 1996). Furthermore, this link is being challenged by occupational scientists, who envision a broader role for those specializing in the knowledge of human occupation (Clark, 1993; Zemke, 2004).

OT's move to a community model began as early as the 1960s, but this move was not continuous. Specialization into various areas of practice complicated the picture during the 1970s and 1980s. Pediatric specialists moved away from hospitals and into public schools. Hand therapists moved into private practice, still bound by doctor's referral. Mental health specialists stayed behind in hospitals or day treatment centers where blanket reimbursement covered OT services. Many physical management specialists moved away from hospitals into outpatient rehabilitation centers or home care. Geriatric specialists increased their ranks in skilled nursing facilities, enduring and adapting to declining Medicare coverage.

Clearly, the trend toward the community model continues. Patients are now called clients. Unlike patients, who are passive recipients of treatment, clients make an informed choice about who will treat them and how. Never has it been more important to communicate the value of OT services to our clients directly. Our role has expanded from merely therapist to educator, collaborator, and advocate. OT practice within the community rejects medical diagnosis as a guide to practice and adopts the World Health Organization's (WHO) system of classification based on function, compensation, adaptation, and inclusion (2001).

2. Moving Toward a Holistic Approach

Reductionism and holism are opposites. The medical model is a good example of a reductionistic approach. In reductionism's view, man is like a machine. When it breaks down, the doctor identifies the part that is broken (diagnosis) and fixes it (prescription). In the holistic view, man is a living organism that cannot be separated into parts. Physical, psychological, social, and spiritual aspects are not viewed or treated separately but as one interdependent whole: the whole person. In OT, the reductionistic approach became problematic in the early 1980s when so many divergent specialty areas within the profession made it impossible to articulate a unified professional identity. Awareness of this identity crisis began the current movement toward generalist practice in which function and occupational adaptation rather than disability become the focus of intervention (Schultz & Schkade, 1992). Some vestiges of OT's identity problem still remain. For example, there is still a tendency to separate physical and psychological issues in our clients. However, current thinking compels occupational therapists to address both together, regardless of the presenting diagnosis. Peloquin (2005b) discusses the dichotomy of affect and cognition: "Most will agree that the forces behind science—curiosity, motivation, a desire to know—seem as much affective as intellectual. Only when the best of artistry and science coexist can practitioners extend the profession's ethos more broadly into" the world (p. 103). The "art and science" of OT are merging as the pendulum swings toward a holistic approach.

3. Expanding the Definition of Occupation

Not so long ago, the term *occupation* was thought to be interchangeable with the word *activity*. Since occupation was so often misunderstood, why not call occupational therapists "activities therapists"? A review of the founding principles of our profession put an end to this debate. Breines (1995) writes, "At the outset of the profession, the term occupation was deliberately selected because of both its ambiguity and its comprehensiveness" (p. 458). Nelson (1996) states, "The use of occupation as a therapeutic method is the essence of the profession of occupational therapy" (p. 11).

He further advocates "occupation, not the A word" because "the term activity lacks the connotation of intentionality. The term activity denotes motion, for example, volcanic activity, molecular activity, and gastric activity, not occupation, which is replete with meaning and purpose" (p. 22).

Trombly (1995) explored the use of occupation as both means and end, "as a treatment end goal and as means to remediate impairments. In both dimensions, meaningfulness and purposefulness are key therapeutic qualities. Purposefulness is hypothesized to organize behavior and meaningfulness to motivate performance" (p. 960).

Christiansen (1999) proposes the most basic and comprehensive view of occupation to date: "occupation as identity" (p. 547). He views occupation as "the principal means through which people develop and express their personal identities." In simple terms, we are what we do. This definition breaks away from the boundaries of health care in that "the ultimate goal of occupational therapy services is well-being, not health" (p. 547). This view of occupation expands the role of OT not only into areas of wellness and prevention but, potentially, all aspects of life: education, industry, politics, organizations, and beyond.

4. Understanding Cognition, Sensation, and Neuroscience

The last two decades have ushered in phenomenal advancements in brain research. Technology for observing brain activity has demonstrated, without a doubt, that the brain acts globally (evidence supporting the holistic perspective) and is capable of enormous plasticity (in adapting and compensating for lost functions). A number of theorists have integrated new brain research with OT approaches. Allen (1987) used cognitive responses while engaged in activity to devise an accurate method for analyzing activities and for measuring the stages of cognitive disability.

Dunn (2001) studied sensory processing patterns in the context of neuroscience and social science and presented research applying this with various disorders. Her sensory processing model gives insight to the nature of sensory processing across the life span and implies specific strategies for intervention.

Farber (1989) hypothesizes, "In-depth knowledge of the neurosciences serves as a common denominator that can enhance our ability to interpret all aspects of human behavior" (p. 637). She uses three compelling examples. First, research shows that lifestyle has a profound effect on the immune system. This implies that the occupations we choose have implications for our overall health and our ability to recover and heal. Second, current research shows an organic basis for psychopathology. This provides further evidence of the connection between mental and physical illness and supports OT's holistic approach. Third, the plasticity of the brain may be observed as the central nervous system reorganizes and establishes new pathways for function during recovery from traumatic brain injury. Farber shows that a heightened understanding of neurological processes can provide evidence to guide OT interventions in many areas of practice.

5. Embracing Occupational Science

Occupational science has been defined as the study of the form, function, and meaning of human occupation. It emerged as a new academic discipline in 1989 at the University of Southern California, where Elizabeth Yerxa is credited with its founding (Yerxa, Clark, Frank, et al., 1989). The contribution of occupational science to the profession of OT has been the source of much theoretical controversy. Clark (1993) presented an example of occupational science in action by using occupational story making with an elderly stroke victim to rebuild a meaningful life. She suggests that occupational therapists use occupational science as a guide to clinical reasoning. Although not a Slagle lecturer, Ann Wilcock similarly promoted occupational science by establishing the first *Journal of Occupational Science* in Australia. Wilcock (2001a) emphasizes that occupational science is not a frame of reference or a model of practice. She describes occupation as a "synthesis of doing, being, and becoming" (p. 413). In her view, occupation is carried out at family, community, national, international, and individual levels. Science is defined by Wilcock as "knowledge gathered by systematic and rigorous study" (p. 413). The three stated objectives of the National Society for the Promotion of Occupational Therapy in 1917 (Constitution of the National Society for the Promotion of Occupational Therapy, Inc., 1917, p. 1, as cited in Wilcock, 2001b) in the United States were: "(1) the advancement of occupation as a therapeutic measure, (2) the study of the effect of occupation upon the human being, and (3) the scientific dispensation of this knowledge" (p. 1). Wilcock points out that the first was accomplished with the foundation of OT. Forgotten for most of the 20th century, the second and third objectives have now re-emerged as occupational science. Mosey (1993) argues that occupational science and OT should remain separate, each with its own body of knowledge and research methodology. The consensus today concurs with both Wilcock and Mosey that occupational science can inform traditional practice but should remain a separate academic discipline.

6. Building an Evidence-Based Practice

Holm (2000) declared in her Slagle lecture a "mandate for the new millennium: evidenced-based practice" (p. 575). Evidence refers to research studies showing the effectiveness of OT techniques. This mandate provides the profession with its latest buzzwords. Evidence-based practice has been viewed as a wake-up call to clinicians and academicians alike, compelling them to read and become familiar with published research in the field. Holm points out the need for occupational therapists to use research to justify what they do and how they do it. Occupational therapists need to provide evidence to both clients and reimbursement sources that OT really works.

Twenty years ago, Reed (1986) warned the profession that "researchers need to provide more information as to why certain media and methods become a part of our tool kit" (p. 604). Reed observed that occupational therapists often select or discard certain media and methods for reasons other than research, such as culture, politics, and economics. Henderson (1988) discussed the need for theory development, particularly in the area of OT technology. Technology defines that part of the profession's knowledge that "tells us how to use purposeful activity to help our patients reach independent function" (p. 568). All three categories of OT knowledge—philosophy, science, and technology—are important, but technology is the area most in need of research.

Out of 12 Slagle lectures over the past 15 years, three lectures (25%)* focus on the need for continued research both now and in the future, showing this to be a major trend.

7. Human Adaptation in the Context of Culture and Community

Adaptation has long held a central place in the OT intervention process. As one looks at the sequence of the Slagle lectures from 1986 to 2005, the frequency of referral to context in its various forms increases. Allen, Fine, Clark, Grady, Nelson, Christiansen, Dunn, and Zemke all discuss one or more of the contexts of the environments within which a person performs an occupation. Allen (1987) emphasizes the adaptation of the environment as a critical role for occupational therapists when assisting clients and their caregivers in managing cognitive disabilities. Grady (1994) promotes the value of "inclusion of all persons into the community they choose and into the world community at large" (p. 300). Only when occupations lead to desired roles in culture and society can they be considered by the client to be therapeutic (Clark, 1993). Zemke (2004) explores temporal (time) and spatial (physical) contexts as they affect everyday activities, comparing familiar places and routine tasks with well-established neural pathways of the human brain. The AOTA (2002) Practice Framework defines seven contexts to consider: cultural, physical, social, personal, spiritual, temporal, and virtual (p. 623). These contexts are described more fully in Chapter 3. Internationally, the WHO defines both internal and external determinants of function and disability, giving recognition to the influence of context on both occupational performance and its role in health and well being (2001). Our 2005 Slagle lecturer, Suzanne Peloquin (2005a, 2005b), has turned our attention back to the art of OT, delineating four elements of artistry in practice: 1) the capacity to establish rapport, 2) the enactment of empathy, 3) the act of getting others to know and use their potential,

---

This statistic comes from Cole's 2003 content analysis.

and 4) the act of helping others to become participants in a community of others.

8. Putting the Client First

The trend toward client-centered practice influences a broad range of health care disciplines both here and abroad. While acknowledged by most American OT leaders, this trend began outside the United States. In the 1980s, the Canadian Association of Occupational Therapists (CAOT), together with the Canadian Department of National Health and Welfare (1983), defined the principles of client-centered practice for OT. These are based on the works of Carl Rogers (1961), Abraham Maslow, (1970) and other humanistic psychotherapists and include an individualized approach to persons with health conditions or other problems for which they need assistance. The occupational therapist collaborates with the client as an equal partner and takes on the role of an enabler (Matheson, 1998). A clear departure from the medical model is evident because the client seeks out professional services as needed and directs his or her own progression toward fulfillment, self-knowledge, growth, and self-actualization through occupational engagement and mastery (Hagedorn, 2001). The Canadian model and the client-centered approach are further described in Chapter 2.

While client-centered practice has been mentioned and supported by several Slagle lecturers (Clark, Fisher, Fine, Grady, Nelson, & Christiansen), an analysis of the abstracts does not mention the term *client*. Apparently, the American OT theorists prefer the terms *person* or *human*. In spite of this, the AOTA (2002) Practice Framework uses the term *client* consistently and specifies that during evaluation, information should be gathered using a "client-centered approach" (p. 616), and OT intervention should be "based on the client's priorities" (p. 617). The more common themes of the Slagle lectures referring to the client or person are the concepts of culture, values, meaning, preference, and choice. Spirituality (Trombly, 1995; Clark, 1993), resilience (Fine, 1990; Peloquin, 2005a), adaptation (Fine, 1990; Grady, 1994), and identity (Christiansen, 1999) all focus on the subjectivity of occupation from the client's perspective.

The reasoning process proposed by Fisher (1998) in her Slagle lecture suggests a client-centered approach beginning with the development of therapeutic rapport, together with "establish(ing) client-centered performance context" and "identify(ing) strengths and problems of occupational performance" (p. 515). The Occupational Therapy Intervention Process Model (OTIPM) Fisher proposed reflects the trend toward top-down approaches that begin with the client's occupational priorities.

Summary

These eight trends, supported by the themes found by content analysis of the past 16 Slagle lectures, have helped us to understand the many theoretical and pragmatic changes faced by occupational therapists today (Table 1-1). These lectures confirm that our professional paradigm has shifted from one of fragmentation and extremes of specialization found by DeBeer in the mid 1980s, to one almost directly the opposite. The current paradigm is holistic, client-centered, and systems-oriented. It moves our profession away from the reductionism of the medical model and into the community. By necessity, the definition of the *patient* or *client* has expanded to include the many contexts in which the person responds to demands for occupational performance. In doing so, OT has broadened its horizons beyond the scope of disability to a world of wellness and prevention. Occupational therapists have moved beyond the walls of hospitals, clinics, schools, and nursing homes; many have entered the realms of home care, community centers, industries, and corporations. Some practitioners have entered positions in the insurance industry, influencing the criteria for third-party payment and governmental regulation. Our leaders seem to be predicting that occupational therapists of the future will be better informed (research), working in a broader spectrum of practice, building stronger ties with clients, and well positioned to influence the building of the inclusive community envisioned by Grady. We will promote a better defined and more prominent role for occupation in the lives of all we serve.

THE EVOLUTION OF OCCUPATIONAL THERAPY

Although the healing powers of occupation were not unknown prior to 1900, we will begin there in tracing the theoretical roots that led to the official "founding" of OT as a profession in 1917. Many influences paved the way for the founding of the OT profession.

Arts and Crafts Movement

The *arts and crafts movement* came about as a reaction against the industrial revolution that was occurring in Europe and the United States at the turn of the century. The movement filled the need to recognize the skilled craftsmen and craftswomen that were being replaced by machines and factories by preserving the tools of their trades and providing training in their use. The Guildhall in London and the Hull House in Chicago are examples of establishments that housed the preservation of handcrafts and offered instruction in weaving, woodworking, basketry, printing, and many others. Under the influence of several founders, including George Barton, Susan Tracy, and Eleanor Clarke Slagle, crafts became a central focus of the early OT practice.

Table 1-1			
Slagle Lectures and Themes, 1986 to 2005			
Year	**Lecturer**	**Topic**	**Themes**
1986	Kathlyn Reed	Tools of practice: Heritage or baggage	Therapy, practice, theory, person/culture
1987	Claudia Allen	Activity: Occupational therapy's treatment method	Therapy, occupation, function, theory
1988	Anne Henderson	Occupational therapy knowledge: From practice to theory	Practice, theory, function, research
1989	Shereen Farber	Neuroscience and occupational therapy: Vital connections	Neuroscience, function, theory, practice
1990	Susan Fine	Resilience and human adaptability: Who rises above adversity?	Person/culture, theory, occupation
1991	Not given		
1992	Not given		
1993	Florence Clark	Occupation embedded in a real life: Interweaving occupational science and occupational therapy	Occupation, research, person/culture, practice
1994	Ann Grady	Building inclusive community: A challenge for occupational therapy	Context, theory, person/culture, function
1995	Catherine Trombly	Occupation: Purposefulness and meaningfulness as therapeutic mechanisms	Occupation, theory, person/culture
1996	David Nelson	Why the profession of occupational therapy will flourish in the 21st century	Occupation, theory, practice
1997	Not given		
1998	Anne Fisher	Uniting practice and theory in an occupational framework	Practice, theory, occupation
1999	Charles Christiansen	Defining lives: Occupation as identity	Person/culture, occupation, theory
2000	Margo Holm	Our mandate for the new millennium: Evidence-based practice	Research, practice, therapy
2001	Winnie Dunn	The sensations of everyday life: Empirical, theoretical and pragmatic considerations	Neuroscience, theory, practice, research
2002	Not Given		
2003	Charlotte Royeen	Chaotic occupational therapy: collective wisdom for a complex profession	Theory, person/culture, theory, practice
2004	Ruth Zemke	Time, space, and the kaleidoscopes of occupation	Context, theory, occupation, person/culture
2005	Suzanne Peloquin	Embracing our ethos, reclaiming our heart	Practice, person/culture, theory

Theme choices are occupation, therapy, person/culture, function, context, neuroscience, practice, theory, and research.

Humanistic Philosophy and Moral Treatment

Humanistic philosophy, predominant in the 19th century, viewed all men as equal and governed by natural universal laws. Therefore, society at large had a moral obligation to help "invalids" (both mental and physical) to return to the mainstream of life (Kielhofner, 2004). This view became the basis for *moral treatment* in the early 20th century, recognizing that people with disabilities have a right to engage in the tasks and events of everyday life in order to become more physically functional and to restore a sense of well being. Occupation, in the humanistic view, is morally uplifting. According to humanism, disease is seen more as a disorganization of life habits that has forced individuals to be idle. *Idleness* is the absence of occupation. Adolph

Meyer described a holistic view of patients as "pulsating with the rhythm of rest and activity" (1921, p. 83). In the original paradigm of occupation, daily activities were used to structure time and to recreate a normal pattern of work, play, and rest within a supportive environment.

Mental Hygiene

The *mental hygiene* movement in particular viewed the negative effects of idleness as the precursor of morbid introspection, a common symptom of mental illness. This might be recognized today as the hallucinations and delusions that often accompany psychosis such as schizophrenia or manic depressive disorder. In several state mental hospitals (New York, Michigan, Illinois), Eleanor Clarke Slagle, among others, devised a schedule of daily activity for inpatients in a cheerful and supportive environment as the logical antidote. This aspect of OT is based on common sense, not science. In particular, the female founders—Slagle, Tracy, and Johnson—set up institutional treatment and training programs within which the occupations of work, leisure, and self care were of primary focus. These occupations have also been called *activities of daily living (ADL)*. Tasks were graded to fit the patient's capabilities, and environments provided both physical and social support for engagement in activities of many types, including crafts, grounds keeping, productive work, and participation in group recreational activities. Dunton, one of the OT founders, identified "craftsmanship and sportsmanship" as the two primary lessons to be learned by patients during mental and physical convalescence through engagement in occupation.

Pragmatism in Education, Health, and Social Reform

Pragmatism was a dominant educational philosophy at the time of OT's formation (Reed, 2006, personal communication). Originally based on the developmental and relational theories of Darwin and Hegel at the turn of the century, pragmatism views knowledge as the result of active experience in the world. In other words, theories that have value and usefulness in everyday life are adaptive and will survive, while those that do not stand the test of practical application will be forgotten. Pragmatism is a holistic approach linking theory and practice as interdependent concepts—an idea that has somehow been forgotten in most recent accounts of the history of OT (Breines, 1987). The Hull House, which sought to preserve arts and crafts and provided instruction in skilled craftsmanship at the University of Chicago, is an example of the importance of outreach to the community. The Hull House was a place where academicians, such as Adolph Meyer, William Dunton, and John Dewey, conducted study while others, such as Jane Addams and Eleanor Clarke Slagle, served to meet the social and health needs of the community; as such, it was "a center where philosophy and practicality met" (Breines, 1987, p. 523). Estelle Breines has identified eight concepts from the philosophy of pragmatism that are compatible with some of the newer theories being applied in today's practice. Table 1-2 presents examples of some of the core concepts of pragmatism that apply to OT practice today.

Functional and Vocational Re-Education

Two of the OT founders, Barton and Kidner, were architects. Barton's main contribution involved providing a structure for the organization of OT, and he brought a devotion to the healing power of arts and crafts, which he demonstrated in his own OT workshop at Consolation House. This was a model for the curative workshops and rehabilitation centers emerging in later decades. Kidner specialized in the design of hospitals, asylums, and sanitariums, therefore contributing ideas of how to "engineer" or structure the physical environment in support of functional re-education through engagement in work or leisure activities. As such, he made a significant contribution to the use of occupation in the treatment of chronic illness, including vocational retraining of soldiers returning from World War I (WWI) in both Canada and the United States. Thus, in the paradigm of occupation, the influence of multiple contexts in the performance of occupations is recognized.

Medicine and Medical Ethics

Kielhofner (2004) describes the medical discipline as opposed to the paradigm of occupation from the beginning. Two founders, Barton and Dunton, acknowledged the scientific promise of OT as a cure for illness, therefore promoting its link with medicine. However, increasingly, the medical community placed pressure on OT professionals to provide scientific evidence for their methods, a trend that eventually led to the mid-century paradigm shift toward reductionism.

Occupational Therapy Is Founded in 1917

Some claim the term *occupational therapy* was coined by George Barton in 1914 (Hagedorn, 2001) as a way to describe the healing potential of occupations, which Mr. Barton discovered when he overcame his own disability (tuberculosis, amputation, paralysis) by engaging in the occupations of carpentry and gardening (Licht, 1967; Quiroga, 1995). According to other sources, William Dunton, a medical doctor, coined the term in a 1911 publication (Kielhofner, 2004; Quiroga, 1995).

Barton invited the seven original founders of the National Association for the Promotion of Occupational Therapy to gather at Consolation House (a workshop for convalescents) in Clifford Springs, New York, including himself, Isabel Newton, William Dunton, Thomas Kidner, Susan Johnson, Susan Tracy, and Eleanor Clarke Slagle (Figure 1-1).

Table 1-2

Pragmatic Concepts in Today's Occupational Therapy Practice

Core Themes of Pragmatism in OT*

- Time and space, mind and body are unified in active occupation.

- Active participation structures development for the individual and for society.

- Human development moves from ego to exo-centricity and consensuality, replicating evolution.

- All elements of performance influence one another because of the interactive nature of all systems.

- The subjective nature of human beings is reflected in their performance and must be respected.

- The uniqueness of individuals is counterbalanced by their relationship with their community.

- Science and philosophy must be united to understand and enhance human occupation

- Grading activity along evolutional and developmental sequences enhances learning and performance and, therefore, health.

Examples in 21st Century OT Theory and Practice

- The motor learning approach focuses on a meaningful task to re-establish the motor skills and neural connections necessary for skilled movement.

- Children learn new skills when presented with challenges in their environment (spatiotemporal adaptation, sensory integration frames).

- Children develop an identity by moving beyond the self to an awareness of others and by taking on a variety of roles in their community.

- Occupation-based models reflect the dynamic interaction of person, environment, and occupational performance.

- Client-centered practice focuses on the unique culture, preferences, and priorities of each individual.

- The MOHO focuses on re-establishing order within the human open system so that clients can find meaningful roles in society.

- Occupational science studies human occupation and develops or tests the validity of theories occupational therapists apply in practice.

- Life-span developmental theories provide guidelines for the transitions and life tasks of early, middle, and older adulthood.

*Adapted from Breines, E. (1987). Pragmatism as a foundation for occupational therapy curricula. American Journal of Occupational Therapy, 41, 524.

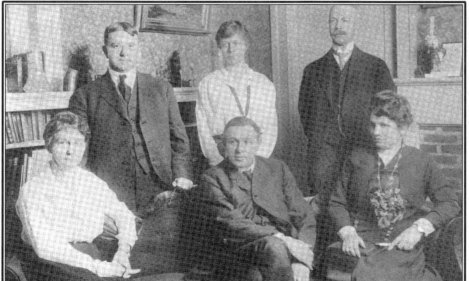

Figure 1-1. Founders of Occupational Therapy. (Back row, left to right: William Dunton, Isabel Newton, Thomas Kidner. Front row, left to right: Susan Johnson, Barton, Eleanor Clarke Slagle. Susan Tracy was invited but not present). (Reprinted with permission from *American Journal of Occupational Therapy*. (1967, September-October). Front cover.)

George Barton

George Barton's (1871 to 1923) association with OT has been described as "watching a comet" (Quiroga, 1995). He crusaded untiringly for OT to be recognized, organized the original national association, and became its first president. However, after marrying Isabel Newton, then secretary of Consolation House, he resigned as President in order to treat his own ailments using OT. Barton died in 1923.

William Rush Dunton

William Rush Dunton (1868 to 1950+), a medical doctor (MD) educated at the University of Pennsylvania specializing in psychiatry, provided OT with its initial connection to medicine. Dr. Dunton acknowledged the multidisciplinary nature of the profession, drawing also from social science, mental hygiene, vocational education, and recreation as well as medicine. Dunton took over the presidency of the AOTA after Barton left and established the profession's first journal, which he continued to edit until the 1950s. Dunton wrote several books about OT, the first in 1911, titled *Occupational Therapy, A Manual for Nurses*. Another book, *Reconstruction Therapy*, published in 1919, outlined the use of crafts and other occupations in restoring productive functioning to wounded soldiers. Dunton's publications were widely read and did much to spread the word about OT throughout the medical community.

Thomas Kidner

Thomas Kidner (1866 to 1932), born and educated in England, emigrated to Canada in 1900 where he was appointed Vocational Secretary of the Canadian military hospitals. He contributed knowledge about the vocational retraining of war veterans using graded occupations and adapted environments. He served as president of the AOTA from 1923 to 1928, and he later offered his vision for the scope, organization, and characteristics of OT services, which emphasized individualized treatment and patient preparation for productive roles in society. Although not a doctor himself, Kidner's positions as architect of rehabilitation facilities and curative workshops helped to align OT practice with that of medicine.

Eleanor Clarke Slagle

Eleanor Clarke Slagle (1871 to 1942) began her training in music but soon turned her attention to philanthropy and the mental hygiene movement. At the Hull House in Chicago, she was a contemporary of Jane Addams, enrolling in craft classes there as early as 1911, and later returned as an instructor. Her interest in care of the disabled stemmed from having been a family caregiver (for father, brother, and nephew). Slagle worked with Dr. Dunton as well as psychiatrist Adolph Meyer at Johns Hopkins and developed her own OT technique of *habit training*, which she established at several state hospitals (New York, Michigan, and Illinois), and eventually instructed staff members in mental hospitals nationwide. Mrs. Slagle served the AOTA as its President from 1919 to 1920 and for many additional years as Secretary and Treasurer, always standing firmly for the promotion of OT as a profession. As a leader for OT, Eleanor Clarke Slagle has been said to have "a presence that commanded admiration and respect" (Licht, 1967, p. 271). In her later years, she worked to establish educational standards for OT education programs and worked with the American Medical Association (AMA) to develop guidelines and to establish a national registry for qualified practitioners. The AOTA, in 1955, created an annual lectureship in memory of Eleanor Clarke Slagle, which continues to be the profession's highest honor.

Susan Tracy

Susan Tracy (1878 to 1928), a nurse from Massachusetts, first organized OT classes for nurses in 1906 in the Boston area and later in New York and Chicago. Her textbook, *Invalid Occupations*, published in 1910, continued to be widely used until the 1940s. Tracy created an OT program at the Adams Nervine Asylum, which catered to patients with *neurasthenia*, a newly identified disorder characterized by morbid anxiety, unexplained fatigue, irrational fears, sleep and appetite abnormalities, and compulsive sexual behaviors (but not insanity). Neurasthenia was among a group of chronic disorders said to result from the stresses of industrialization during the early 1900s. As the OT founder who did not attend its initial meeting, Tracy may have conceived her role as more practical than theoretical.

Susan Johnson

Susan Johnson (1876 to 1932), also a nurse, taught OT at Columbia University in New York. An educator and craftswoman, Johnson was active in women's philanthropy and reform and expanded the scope of OT in the treatment of physical and chronic illness. According to Quiroga (1995), the female founders were not in agreement about the position of OT as a free-standing profession. Tracy and Johnson, both nurses by background, remained committed to education and service in the field but left the leadership positions to their male counterparts.

Herbert J. Hall

Herbert J. Hall (1870 to 1923), although not present at the initial meeting in 1917, has been described as a "near founder" because of his significant contributions to the establishment of OT as a new profession (Peloquin, 1991). Hall, a graduate of Harvard Medical School and contemporary of Dr. Dunton, described artistic crafts as a "work cure" for patients with chronic medical and psychiatric disorders at his crafts workshops at Devereau Mansion in Marblehead, Massachusetts. He served as president of the AOTA from 1920 to 1923. With craftswoman Mertice Buck, Hall published *The Work of Our Hands*, promoting the benefits of OT, such as instilling initiative and interest, improving concentration and endurance, and providing a sense of pride and accomplishment while learning new

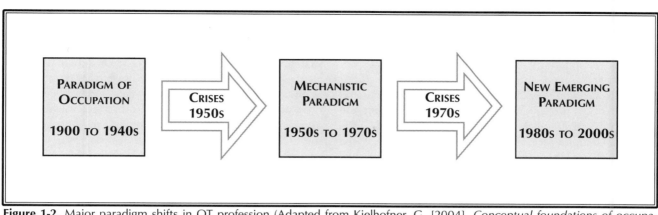

Figure 1-2. Major paradigm shifts in OT profession (Adapted from Kielhofner, G. [2004]. *Conceptual foundations of occupational therapy* [3rd ed.]. Philadelphia: FA Davis.)

skills and trades that prepared patients to re-enter the "work-a-day world" (Hall & Buck, 1915). As such, Hall envisioned OT as "beyond diversion" and "essential to a full recovery" (Quiroga, 1995).

The Paradigm of Occupation: Summary

The concepts derived from the founders define the original paradigm of the OT profession. The main organizing principle was first articulated by Dunton (1919): occupation is as necessary to human life as food and drink. The central role of occupation in human life provides the basis for both the beginning paradigm and the one emerging today. In fact, we might say that we have returned to our roots or come full circle, beginning again where we started as a profession.

PARADIGM SHIFTS IN 20TH-CENTURY OCCUPATIONAL THERAPY

In reviewing the first 60 years of OT, Kielhofner and Burke (1977) traced the theoretical shifts in perspective since the beginning of the century. They identified some major changes in our professional paradigm. A *paradigm* represents the knowledge base, values, and worldview upon which occupational therapists can agree through shared experience and that provide a basis for OT practice. These authors identified two major paradigm shifts: from the original paradigm of occupation (1900 to 1940s), to the mechanistic paradigm aligned with the medical model (1950s to 1970s), and again to the *new emerging paradigm* (1980s onward), involving a return to occupation as the primary focus for the profession. Figure 1-2 visually describes these major paradigm shifts.

Kuhn (1970) observed that when new problems emerge that cannot be solved under the old paradigm, a scientific revolution produces a new worldview. The original concepts, values, and worldview upon which the OT profession was founded is called the *paradigm of occupation* (Kielhofner & Burke, 1977). The first shift occurred in the late 1940s and 1950s, when the profession came under pressure from medicine to provide scientific evidence for its practice. This resulted in a shift to a *mechanistic paradigm* that was consistent with the medical model. Occupational therapists in the mid-20th century adopted a biomedical worldview, valuing scientific evidence and following the laws of cause and effect governing anatomy, physiology, and human development. The medical model views man as a machine to which health can be restored by accurately identifying the broken parts (diagnosis) and fixing them (prescription). The medical model is further defined in Chapter 2.

A second crisis happened to OT's practice within the medical model. The profession's development became excessively caught up in the scientific movement of the mid-20th century, and by the 1970s, so many OT specializations existed that we could no longer see the forest through the trees. Psychiatric OT, physical disabilities OT, pediatrics, hand therapy, geriatric OT, and school-based OT are some of the many specializations of the 1970s. In the 1980s, managed care began using these narrow and limited definitions of OT's role in rehabilitation as a basis of reimbursement, creating a huge problem with the old paradigm. A broader definition of OT's domain of concern was clearly needed for our profession to remain relevant and valued in the new millennium.

THEORETICAL HISTORY OF OCCUPATIONAL THERAPY

In the next section, we will briefly examine each decade, noting the health care trends, historical context, and specific theories in OT that emerged and prevailed in each. Each era/decade from 1900 to 2000 is outlined in Table 1-3. In a project done for the AOTA Representative Assembly, the members of an Ad Hoc Committee on Historical Foundations identified nine themes that contributed to the foundations of OT: 1) economics, 2) education, 3) health and medicine, 4) philosophy, 5) politics and government, 6) professions, 7) psychology, 8) religion and spirituality, and 9) social movements (Kathlyn Reed, 2006, personal communication). The findings (Part 1) of the Historical Foundations committee are due to be published in *Occupational Therapy Practice* in April of 2006. For a visual perspective of the roots and theoretical history of OT during the 20th century, see Figure 1-3.

The 1920s: Habit Training and Reconstruction

Most people associate the "roaring '20s" with a booming post-WWI economy; a preoccupation with music, dance, fashion, and style; as well as an optimistic outlook that ended abruptly with the stock market crash of 1929. In the realm of health care, United States society put its faith in medicine and science to provide remedies for everything from insanity to chronic disease. Between 1917 and 1920, the number of hospitals in the United States more than doubled, and occupational therapists became a part of the medical services offered there. This decade saw a rapid growth in training programs for occupational therapists and a vast increase in our numbers.

Eleanor Clarke Slagle, working with psychiatrist Adolph Meyer, developed the habit training approach, which offered a full schedule of ordinary daily activities including crafts, work tasks, and group recreations in order to promote both mental and physical health for patients institutionalized for mental illness. Meyer and Slagle both viewed "habit training" as a holistic approach using the principles of humanistic philosophy (Meyer, 1921). Hall contributed to this theory in his view of crafts as a means of restoring "authentic living" to persons with disabilities (1916).

The "Reconstructionist Movement" also began holistically. For soldiers returning from war, broken bodies had to be "reconstructed," a task that included physical reconditioning through occupations such as handcrafts and manual labor and the mental incentives provided by their wives and sweethearts who were taught to encourage the men in their lives "not to lose hope" (Quiroga, 1995). Reconstruction also extended to those factory workers who fell victim to industrial accidents, common in a time when productivity took precedence over safety in the workplace. The overall goal of rehabilitation involved retraining, re-educating, and restoring physical and mental functions that enabled persons with disability to re-enter the work force. However, occupational reconstruction aides quickly learned that as "therapists" working in health care settings under a doctor's supervision, they were both more highly respected and better paid. By the end of the decade, OT was clearly identified as a health care profession, working hand in hand with medical practitioners.

The biomechanical approach began during the industrial revolution. Efficiency experts studied human movements, endurance, fatigue, and other effects on the body as an attempt to make factory workers more efficient and their output more productive. The biomechanical model, using scientific evidence from time and motion studies in the 1920s, became the basis for activity analysis in OT and, applied to ADL, has become the preferred frame of reference for the treatment of physical disabilities—a trend that continues to the present.

The 1930s: Biomechanical and Behavior Modification Frames of Reference

In the 1930s, the scientific movement continued through the use of adapted crafts such as weighted sanders for woodworking and floor looms with weights attached to provide muscle training while performing the steps of the handcraft. During the economic depression of the 1930s, occupational therapists continued to work in convalescent hospitals, sanatoriums, or retreats, where patients with chronic mental illness or incurable diseases such as tuberculosis and polio sometimes stayed for several years. People with other incurable conditions, such as mental retardation or developmental disabilities, were also institutionalized. These institutions provided the most scientific and modern treatment available at that time, and occupational therapists considered themselves fortunate to be a part of such highly respected medical care.

Behaviorists such as Watson, Skinner, and Pavlov became well known in the 1930s. These early learning theorists used the scientific method to study human behavior, making breakthrough discoveries about how people learn and why they behave as they do. Behavior modification was first used as a therapeutic approach in institutions to reinforce desirable behaviors while using negative reinforcement to extinguish undesirable behaviors.

Psychoanalytic theorists such as Freud, Jung, and Erikson also published during the 1930s, but their therapeutic application became more commonly known in later decades.

The 1940s: Vocational Training, Activity Analysis, and Rehabilitation Models

World War II (WWII) brought the focus of health care back to vocational rehabilitation and the need to retrain returning soldiers with a variety of disabilities for occupations suitable for the home front. Several changes in social policy had occurred since WWI, including the New Deal (providing social security income for persons with disabilities) and the GI Bill (providing funding for vocational

Table 1-3

History of Occupational Therapy Theory: Socioeconomic and Political Influences

Years	OT Theories and Theorists	Historical Events	Health Care Trends
1900s and 1910s	Paradigm of Occupation created by founders and others; Occupational Therapy founded in 1917; Training of reconstruction aides	Industrial Revolution; WWI; Time and motion studies; Women's right to vote	Many immigrants in "insane asylums"; Humanitarian influence; "Work Cure" replaced "Rest Cure" for chronic illness
1920s	Eleanor Clarke Slagle: Habit training, arts and crafts, biomechanical; Adolph Meyer: Philosophy of OT	Post WWI: Age of inventions; Booming economy; Silent movies and radio	Long-term institutionalization for chronic health conditions
1930s	National registration for occupational therapists began; B. F. Skinner, behaviorism; Behavior modification; Biomechanical FOR prominent	The Great Depression, prohibition, and growth of organized crime	Pre-WWII, political unrest regarding poverty and unemployment
1940s	Advances in physical rehabilitation; Psychoanalysis prominent in mental health settings	WWII; the Holocaust; Golden age of jazz; Color movies and television; Baby boom begins	Vocational rehabilitation movement; Retraining of returning soldiers
1950s	Curative workshop: Helen Willard and Claire Spackman; Bobaths NDT; WFOT founded in 1952	Communism rise; Cold War begins; Advent of Rock and Roll	Antipsychotic medications; Neurological breakthroughs; Vaccines developed for polio and other diseases
1960s	Group dynamics; Fidler's task-oriented approach; Mosey's Three Frames (psychoanalytic, acquisitional, and developmental); Llorens' Growth and development; Motor Control approaches.	Social consciousness regarding civil rights; Sexual revolution; Vietnam war protests; 1964: baby boom ends	Widespread deinstitutionalization; Shift to community programs and agencies (but without sufficient funding)
1970s	Sensory integration, A. Jean Ayres; Lorna Jean King, Growth of cognitive behaviorism; Llorens' Ego adaptive and Growth and development approaches	Energy shortage; Runaway inflation	OT in school systems; Education of children with disabilities.
1980s	MOHO; Allen's Cognitive Disabilities; Toglia and Abreu; Cognitive Perceptual Approach	Fall of communism; End of Cold War	OBRA provides standards of care and cost containment
1990s	Motor Learning; Trombly's Task-oriented approach; Toglia's Multi-contextual approach; Schkade and Shultz, Occupational adaptation; Law and Baptiste's Client-centered approach; Dunn's Ecology of Human Performance	Desert Storm Growth of computer and communication technology; World Wide Web; Booming economy	DRG's criteria limits health care costs, growth of HMO's (managed care)
2000s	The OT Practice Framework; WHO's ICF; Systems Approaches	Recession; Terrorism (9/11); War in Iraq; Katrina and other natural disasters	Growth of community-based programs, wellness programs, and family-centered care

WWI = World War I, WWII = World War II, WFOT = World Federation of Occupational Therapists, OBRA = Omnibus Budget Reconciliation Act, DRG = Diagnostic Related Group, HMO = health maintenance organization, FOR = frame of reference, NDT = neurodevelopmental therapy, ICF = International Classification of Function, MOHO = Model of Human Occupation.

Adapted in part from Reed, K. L. (2005). An annotated history of the concepts used in occupational therapy. In C. Christiansen & C. Baum (Eds.), Occupational therapy: performance, participation, and well-being (pp. 567–626). Thorofare, NJ: SLACK Incorporated.

Figure 1-3. OT theory tree. (Created by Marilyn B. Cole. Reprinted with permission.) (*Note:* We would like to acknowledge Dr. Reed for reviewing the drawing and for suggesting changes that make it a more accurate metaphor.)

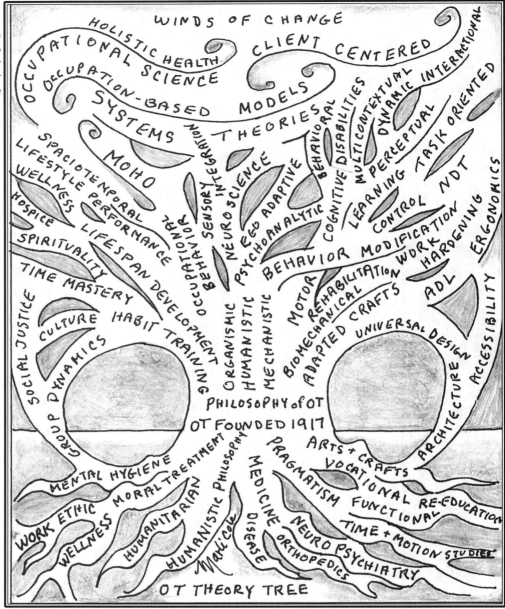

retraining), which facilitated the payment for OT services in physical rehabilitation and prevocational training programs. The vocational training programs extended to both physical and mental health settings, which often led to supervised work placements within the hospital itself. For others with special needs, *sheltered workshops* were set up where persons with disability could earn modest wages by doing contract work in an adapted and carefully supervised environment.

Kinetic Model

The kinetic model, published by Sidney Licht in 1947, provided a scientific basis for the analysis of activities using a *biomechanical* frame of reference. Claire Spackman interpreted this model for treating patients with physical injuries in the first edition of *Occupational Therapy*, which she edited with Helen Willard in 1947.

Rehabilitation Model

The rehabilitation model was further developed in OT curative workshops such as the one Spackman directed in Philadelphia, which focused on the analysis of tasks, their adaptation to facilitate continued function in ADL, and the use of compensatory techniques such as the fabrication and use of adaptive equipment to support continued functioning in work, leisure, and self-care activities (Spackman, 1947a, 1947b). Ultimately, the goal of OT was to return restored patients to competitive employment and independent community living.

The 1950s: Psychoanalytic Frames and Sensory Motor Frames Emerge

Developments in the field of medicine, such as the widespread use of major tranquilizers like Thorazine for schizophrenia and mood stabilizers like Librium for manic-depressive illness, now enhanced the patients' ability to respond to OT. In this decade, the psychoanalytic frame of reference became prominent, and for OT, craft activities were thought to have diagnostic attributes, symbolically revealing the previously unknown primary processes of the unconscious mind (Azima & Azima, 1959). Occupational therapists worked side by side with psychiatrists in helping patients to reveal and openly discuss their fixations and unconscious conflicts and hopefully to resolve them. Object relations theory, an outgrowth of Freudian psychoanalysis, led to an emphasis in OT on the "use of self as a therapeutic tool" (West, 1959, p. 26). Psychoanalytic and object relations concepts were further interpreted for OT by Gail and Jay Fidler (Fidler & Fidler, 1954, 1963) as part of the communication process with patients in mental health settings.

Breakthroughs in the field of neurology can be seen in the work of Margaret Rood, a researcher trained in both occupational and physical therapy. Rood developed many techniques for facilitating reflex and voluntary movement for persons with various forms of paralysis. Her sensorimotor therapy model, published in 1954, served as a basis for many others, notably A. Jean Ayres' (1963) work in perceptual motor development (later called sensory integration), Mary Fiorentino's reflex development model (1961, 1974), and Berta and Karel Bobath's neurodevelopmental therapy (NDT), originating during the 1950s in England although not prevalent until later decades in the United States (Bobath, 1972).

The 1960s: Social Reform

In the United States, the 1960s could be called a decade of social reform. Authority was questioned on every front, from the religious and ethical codes regarding sexuality to the wisdom of the United States government in drafting young men to fight in the Vietnam War. Public protest demonstrations became a common event on the nightly news, dealing with many issues including civil rights, racial integration, recognition of diverse lifestyles, and the rights of minorities. In the wave of protests, institutions such as prisons and mental hospitals were characterized as havens of antiquated authority systems and the rampant abuse of power. Goffman (1961), in his book *Asylums: Essays on the Social Situation of Mental Patients and Other Inmates*, exposed the many negative influences of institutions, including their reinforcement of sick behaviors and forced conformity. The public view of institutions had changed, and political and economic forces now called for their downsizing and eventual closing.

The early 1960s saw a massive deinstitutionalization movement, motivated by great strides in the use of medication to prevent (Salk vaccine), cure (antibiotics), or manage (phenothiazines in psychiatry) many formerly chronic and debilitating health conditions. The focus of OT in both mental and physical health care settings became the pressing need for patients to acquire skills for independent living in anticipation of their move to the community.

Many disabled individuals, having been hospitalized for long periods, also needed to be "resocialized," giving rise to the use of group treatment in OT. West (1959) points out that while occupational therapists have "traditionally worked with numbers of patients in 'groups,' by and large [their] treatment has not utilized the principles of group process and group dynamics" (West, 1959, p. 43). Building on this growing awareness of the importance of group treatment, the study of group dynamics and group leadership was added to the OT educational curriculum. In health care settings, OT groups became a means of learning social skills, including communication, cooperation, and mutual respect for the rights of one another. Gail Fidler first published her task-oriented group model in 1969 as an example of occupational therapists' use of groups in current practice: Fidler's "Task-Oriented Groups as a Context for Treatment," demonstrating the use of group tasks to help persons with schizophrenia to learn ego-skills. Mosey's 1970 publication of "developmental groups," describing five levels of group interaction skills, further defined OT's use of the dynamics of groups in treatment.

The passage of Medicare and Medicaid legislation in the mid-1960s was an attempt to make health care services available to all citizens. The Community Mental Health Act of 1963 called for the provision of mental health services at a variety of levels, including inpatient, outpatient, and day hospital programs; emergency services, consultation and educational programs; and established community mental health centers to facilitate the move from long-term hospitals to the community.

In mental health, a reformed organization within institutional treatment settings promoted OT as a component of the *therapeutic milieu*. This concept originated in England as an outgrowth of Edelson's (1964) therapeutic community approach to the treatment of mental illness. In this approach, patients and staff met together each day (community meeting) to discuss treatment goals; structure the day's educational, recreational, and vocational opportunities; encourage mutual responsibility for carrying out these goals; and to engage in group problem solving to address issues with living and working together toward recovery. An effort was made in the therapeutic milieu approach to equalize power between patients and therapists, to discourage the patient sick role, and instead, to encourage active participation in treatment, goal setting, and making therapeutic behavior change.

Other OT frames of references continued to emerge and were published throughout the 1970s, including Mary

Reilly's "occupational behavior" (1962) and A. Jean Ayres' "sensory integration" (1968), a trend that has continued to the present.

The 1970s: Identity Crisis, Decade of Frames of Reference

The 1970s found OT as a profession in a state of crisis. By the late 1960s, a split between OT specialists in psychiatry and physical disabilities was identified, with offshoots in pediatric and geriatric OT and hand therapy specialties. This mobilized our national organization, AOTA, to search for common threads through symposiums that gathered contemporary OT leaders to identify and articulate the profession's frames of reference. Several prominent leaders did so. Mosey (1970) identified three frames of reference for mental health OT practice, *acquisitional* (based on behavioral or learning theory), *psychoanalytic* (object relations), and *developmental* (recapitulation of ontogenesis). Llorens (1970) described *facilitating growth and development* as an OT frame of reference based on a comprehensive review of then contemporary theories of human development, including Gesell, Erikson, Freud, and Ayres, among others.

Many other professional leaders published frames of reference during the 1970s, reflecting the broad diversity of OT practice. They included Mary Reilly's play model (1974), Ruth Brunyate Weimer's prevention model (1972), Anne Mosey's activity therapy (1973) and bio-psycho-social (1974) models, Gail and Jay Fidlers' doing and becoming (1978), Gary Kielhofner's temporal adaptation (1977), and Lorna Jean King's individual adaptation model (1978) using sensory integration with adults.

At the conclusion of the 1970s, the AOTA had established the Representative Assembly and had made an attempt to unify practice through publication of the "Uniform Terminology" document in 1979. However, more turmoil lay ahead for the OT profession.

The 1980s: Standardized Assessments and Clinical Reasoning

Four problems in the OT profession shaped this decade: accountability, a manpower shortage, a lack of a unified theoretical base, and a lack of research to validate OT practice.

Political and economic trends greatly influenced the theoretical developments in OT during the 1980s. Health care costs were skyrocketing, and both federal and private health care reimbursement sectors supported the legislation of cost cutting measures such as Medicare reform and the Omnibus Budget Reconciliation Act (OBRA) of 1987 (Evanofski, 2003). As managed care began to take hold, *accountability* became an issue for OT. New systems of reimbursement placed pressure on OT practitioners to provide evidence of the effectiveness of therapy and proof of their clients' progress toward functional goals. Occupational

therapists lacked standardized, valid, and reliable assessment tools, and their creation became a priority for the profession. From 1983 to 1984 the American Occupational Therapy Foundation (AOTF), which was established a few decades earlier, offered grants to OT researchers for the development of standardized assessment tools for measuring occupational performance.

The manpower shortage signified society's unmet need for what OT could provide. One reason for the increased demand occurred as a result of the passage of Public Law 94-142, which called for the education of handicapped children within the public schools. Occupational therapists could help children with a wide variety of disabilities to adapt to mainstream classrooms where they could interact with nondisabled children. Another political incentive was OT's movement toward state licensure, which identified registered occupational therapists (OTRs) and certified OT assistants (COTAs) as qualified providers of occupation-based services in a variety of areas, including acute hospitals, sub-acute rehabilitation, skilled nursing facilities, and mental health services. State licensure was perceived as mutually protective for both providers and consumers because it prevented nonqualified personnel from being hired at lower pay to provide these services. State licensure for OT currently exists in nearly every state in the United States.

Throughout the 1980s, the proliferation of frames of reference, theories, and models in OT continued. Those with responsibility for teaching occupational theory found it difficult to keep up with the many new theoretical approaches being published, not only in the *American Journal of Occupational Therapy*, but also in the *Occupational Therapy Journal of Research*, the *Occupational Therapy in Mental Health Journal*, and other interdisciplinary journals. Some of the frames of reference include Gilfoyle and Grady's (1981) *spatiotemporal adaptation* in pediatrics, Mildred Ross's (Ross & Burdick, 1981) *sensory integration groups* for adults, Howe and Briggs' (1982) ecological systems model, the Client-Centered Task Force in Canada (Townsend, 1998), Abreu and Toglia's *cognitive perceptual rehabilitation* (1987), Allen's cognitive disabilities frame (1982, 1987), and Reed's *personal adaptation model* (1980).

In addition to these frames, many of which we still use today, three more fundamental theoretical developments occurred in the 1980s: 1) Kielhofner and Burke's Model of Human Occupation (MOHO) (Kielhofner, 1980a, 1980b; Kielhofner & Burke, 1980; Kielhofner, Burke, & Igi, 1980), the first of the occupation-based models published in various forms throughout the decade; 2) the emergence of clinical reasoning as a form of inquiry (Mattingly, 1989; Mattingly & Fleming, 1994; Rogers, 1983); and 3) the birth of occupational science (Yerxa et al., 1989).

Just prior to the 1980s, some scholars began to suggest what we now recognize as the paradigm shift away from the mechanistic, reductionistic, biomedical view of health care and occupation and toward a holistic, organismic, and client-centered perspective. Kielhofner and Burke (1977) published an article reviewing the conceptual history of OT and proposing a new paradigm, the MOHO. Their approach departed from most earlier efforts in that it seemed to look backwards rather than forwards and to call for the profession to reclaim the original concepts of the OT founders. A resurgence of interest in the history of OT ensued, and many publications either reviewed or republished writings from the 1920s and earlier (Serrett, 1985; Kielhofner & Burke, 1980; Barris, Kielhofner, & Watts, 1988). Furthermore, MOHO differed from the other frames of reference in OT in another important way. While its scope was broad enough to envelop the entire human open system with all of its mental and physical components and subsystems (rather than addressing any specific age group or area of disability), MOHO's focus sought to better understand and explain the one thing that is both unique and common to all of OT practice—human occupation.

Another original approach was the emergence of clinical reasoning. Joan Rogers (1983) introduced the concept in her Slagle lecture to the profession, followed by a collaborative study of the clinical reasoning process of OT (Mattingly, 1989; Mattingly & Fleming, 1994; Mattingly & Gillette, 1991), which was funded jointly by the AOTA and AOTF. The collaboration between Cheryl Mattingly, an anthropologist, and Maureen Fleming, an occupational therapist and educator, focused attention on the thinking process that expert occupational therapists use during treatment and interactions with clients. Using naturalistic or qualitative methodology, this research resulted in the identification of three distinct lines of reasoning occupational therapists typically use in their work, which Mattingly and Fleming call "the three track mind" (1994, p. 119):

- *Procedural reasoning:* addressing the client's functional limitations through the specific assessment and intervention techniques appropriate for that area of disability in order to remediate, adapt, or compensate for lost occupational abilities

- *Interactive reasoning:* collaborating with the client to encourage, coach, problem-solve, and promote active engagement in occupation. This part of the reasoning process focuses on therapist–client communication, emotions, and motivational issues of occupational performance.

- *Conditional reasoning:* connecting with the client in his or her own culture and world in order to create meaningful occupational experiences. This line of reasoning may not always be conscious but involves OT's therapeutic use of self in order to convey empathy with a nonjudgmental, culturally sensitive approach in order to visualize how clients see themselves both now and in the future.

The findings of the clinical reasoning study identify those parts of OT practice (interactive and conditional)

that went "underground" in order to adhere to the scientific objectivity of the biomedical model. These reasoning tracks more closely resembled the client-centered approach, demonstrating that occupational therapists had retained the ideals of earlier years despite their lack of importance in medical settings. This research transcended the tools and techniques of practice and helped to define the broadening parameters of our role as occupational therapists today.

The third theoretical achievement of the 1980s for OT was the birth of *occupational science*. Occupational science was defined by Elizabeth Yerxa (Yerxa et al., 1989) at the University of Southern California, not as an applied science but as an academic discipline that is the focus of doctoral research. The difference is as follows: OT applies theory in order to use it for a practical purpose, such as enabling the performance of self-care tasks for persons with different types of disability; occupational science, as an academic discipline, is not concerned with practicality or usefulness. It is a purer form of study that seeks a better understanding of the form, function, and meaning of occupation for its own sake. For example, an occupational scientist might explore all of the parameters of a specific occupation, such as preparing a cup of tea. The social, cultural, temporal, and physical aspects of making a cup of tea can increase our understanding of how occupations affect our own lives, and this knowledge can help us to use other occupations to enhance our own lives and those of others (Hannam, 1997). Occupation has meaning for its own sake without concern for how it will be applied. As Mosey (1993) suggests, there is a clear distinction between the basic science of occupation and the applied science of OT, and each has a different purpose and methods for theoretical development.

The efforts by the AOTA to unify the profession by creating a common language and defining our practice came to fruition in 1989 with the publication of *Uniform Terminology for Occupational Therapy, Second Edition*. This document was updated from the original 1979 version by a task force that began its work in 1983. By then, the uniform terminology had been extensively used in AOTA's official documents, and its definition of the scope of OT practice served as a guideline for the accreditation of OT educational programs. Its application in practice was facilitated by the use of a grid that defined the intersection of occupational performance areas and performance components (Dunn & McGourty, 1989). For example, a child's sensory awareness (a performance component) could be addressed by occupational therapists during self-care, play, and classroom activities (performance areas). This process clarified OT's role in health care by always addressing and reporting OT interventions in the context of occupations. This set the stage for the development of occupational performance models during the next decade.

The 1990s: Growth of Occupational Performance Models, Decade of the Brain

The monumental theoretical changes that began in the 1980s seemed chaotic to many practitioners and educators. Scholars argued about how to organize the many levels of theory being presented and published, describing them variously as models, paradigms, and frames of reference. Occupational therapists in diverse areas of practice united around the concept of occupation, and most of the occupation-based models described in Section II were introduced in the 1990s. These included the following:

- Person–Environment–Occupational–Performance Model (Christiansen & Baum, 1991)
- Occupational Adaptation Model (Schkade & Shultz, 1992)
- Ecology of Human Performance (Dunn, Brown, & McGuigan, 1994)
- Model of Occupational Functioning (Trombly, 1995)
- Person–Environment–Occupation Model (Law et al., 1996)
- Canadian Model of Occupational Performance (CAOT, 1997)

Meanwhile, Kielhofner and others continued to update the MOHO, incorporating many new concepts regarding the interactions of person, environment, and occupation. The AOTA began the revision of *Uniform Terminology* using occupation-based ideas to develop the OT Practice Framework that was accepted and published in 2002.

Significant frames of reference that developed during the 1990s are Joan Toglia's multicontextual approach to cognitive rehabilitation (1991), Betty Abreu's *quadraphonic approach* (Abreu, 1998; Abreu & Hinojosa, 1992), and Mathiowetz and Bass Haugen's contemporary task-oriented model of motor learning (1994). These applied theories further developed throughout the decade, incorporating many new developments in neuroscience and brain research.

On the research front, large numbers of masters and doctoral level OT students published research studies validating the effectiveness of OT, which served to raise the level of recognition for the profession within the medical community and elsewhere. A prime example of this trend is the Well Elderly Study (Clark, et al., 1997), a highly respected randomized controlled trial that demonstrated the effectiveness of OT prevention for independent-living older adults. This study was published in the *Journal of the American Medical Association* with follow-up studies appearing in the *American Journal of Occupational Therapy* and other professional publications.

The 1990s saw the climax of the crisis predicted by scholars of the 1980s. The OT job market grew dramatically in the early 1990s, creating the need to educate more students to fill the positions. The passing of the Americans with Disabilities Act in 1990 contributed to this trend. Many new educational programs began, and with news of the job market and salaries hitting new heights, the number of students attracted to the field grew exponentially. But by the end of the decade, the job market fell as quickly as it had risen. Managed care and cost cutting legislative measures for medical services generally have been blamed for the decline in OT positions, but this "crisis" applied mainly to occupational therapists who worked within the medical model.

One reason for the late 1990s decline in students entering the OT profession was Resolution J, passed by AOTA's Representative Assembly, mandating the profession's move to a master's degree entry level. This meant that students could no longer qualify to take the national certification exam with only a 4-year bachelor's degree. They would need 5 academic years plus another half year of fieldwork, a more costly endeavor, to become a qualified OTR. The thinking behind the decision was to raise the level of professionalism for OT to that of related health care disciplines such as physical therapy and speech/language therapists. The move to entry-level masters together with the decrease in jobs precipitated a dramatic decrease in students majoring in OT, and many of the educational programs opened earlier in the decade were closed. We now understand that the decrease was only temporary and that more jobs are materializing in the community sector. However, for many OT practitioners and educators, the end of the 1990s truly felt like a crisis that meant the end of OT practice as we knew it.

Occupational Therapy in the 21st Century

We began this chapter with trends that will likely affect the future of OT practice, and these continue through the first decade of the new millennium. In 2001, we saw the WHO's revision of its classification system (WHO, 2001), which contains many parallels with the OT Practice Framework (AOTA, 2002) and paves the way for OT practice within the community. Student enrollment has increased steadily, accompanied by increases in the job market.

The next chapter will elaborate on the similarities and differences in the medical model and the client-centered model, and their relationships with WHO's International Classification of Functioning (ICF) and AOTA's Practice Framework.

LEARNING ACTIVITY

History of Theory

Guideline: 5 pages, 1-inch margins, single spaced, 1 page per decade

Class exercise or individual paper: Choose 5 decades in the 20th century and answer the following questions for each:

1. What are the major historical events effecting the United States during this decade? Identify and describe at least three.

2. Describe the socio-political climate during this decade. Who were the presidents, and what political party was in power? What was happening with the economy? How did the socio-political trends of this decade effect health care in the United States?

3. Describe the lifestyle of the middle class during this decade. If you were an occupational therapist, what would a typical patient/client be like?

4. What OT theories emerged or prevailed during this decade? How did the historical events and socio-political trends of the times help to shape practice?

5. If you were an occupational therapist during this decade, where would you choose to be practicing and why?

REFERENCES

Abreu, B. (1998). The quadraphonic approach: Holistic rehabilitation for brain injury. In N. Katz (Ed.), *Cognition and occupation in rehabilitation: Cognitive models for intervention in occupational therapy* (pp. 51–98). Bethesda, MD: American Occupational Therapy Association.

Abreu, B., & Hinojosa, J. (1992). Process approach for cognitive perceptual and postural control dysfunction for adults with brain injury. In N. Katz (Ed.), *Cognitive rehabilitation: Models for intervention in occupational therapy.* Stoneham, MA: Butterworth-Heinemann.

Abreu, B., & Toglia, J. (1987). Cognitive rehabilitation: A model for occupational therapy. *American Journal of Occupational Therapy, 41,* 439–448.

Allen, C. K. (1982). Independence through activity: The practice of occupational therapy (psychiatry). *American Journal of Occupational Therapy, 36,* 731–739.

Allen, C. K. (1987). Activity: Occupational therapy's treatment method. *American Journal of Occupational Therapy, 41,* 563–575.

American Occupational Therapy Association. (1979). Uniform terminology for reporting occupational therapy services. *Occupational Therapy News, 35*(11), 1–8.

American Occupational Therapy Association. (1989). Uniform terminology for reporting OT services (2nd ed.). *American Journal of Occupational therapy, 43,* 808–815.

American Occupational Therapy Association. (2002). Occupational therapy practice framework: Domain and process. *American Journal of Occupational Therapy, 56,* 609–639.

Ayres, A. J. (1963). The development of perceptual-motor abilities: A theoretical basis for the treatment of dysfunction. (Eleanor Clarke Slagle Lecture). *American Journal of Occupational Therapy, 17,* 221–225.

Ayres, A. J. (1968). Sensory integrative processes and neurophysiological learning disabilities. In J. Helmuth (Ed.), *Learning Disorders* (vol. 3, pp. 41–58). Seattle, WA: Special Child Publications.

Azima, H., & Azima, F. (1959). Outline of a dynamic theory of occupational therapy. *American Journal of Occupational Therapy, 13,* 1-7.

Barris, R., Kielhofner, G., & Watts, J. H. (1988). *Bodies of knowledge in psychosocial practice.* Thorofare, NJ: SLACK Incorporated.

Breines, E. (1987). Pragmatism as a foundation for occupational therapy curricula. *American Journal of Occupational Therapy, 41,* 522–525.

Breines, E. (1995). Understanding occupation as the founders did. *British Journal of Occupational Therapy, 58,* 458–460.

Bobath, B. (1972). The Neurodevelopmental approach to treatment. In P. Pearson (Ed.), *Physical therapy in developmental disabilities.* Springfield, IL: Charles Thomas.

Canadian Department of National Health and Welfare and the Canadian Occupational Therapy Association (1983). *Guidelines for the client-centred practice of occupational therapy.* Ottawa, ON: Minister of Supply and Services, Canada, Catalog #H39-33/1983E.

Canadian Association of Occupational Therapists (1997). *Enabling occupation: An occupational therapy perspective.* Ottawa, ON: CAOT Publications ACE.

Christiansen, C. H. (1999). Defining lives: Occupation as identity, an essay on competence, coherence, and the creation of meaning. *American Journal of Occupational Therapy, 53,* 547–558.

Christiansen, C. H., & Baum, C. M (Eds.). (1991). *Occupational therapy: Overcoming human performance deficits.* Thorofare, NJ: SLACK Incorporated.

Clark, F. (1993). Occupation embedded in a real life: Interweaving occupational science and occupational therapy. *American Journal of Occupational Therapy, 47,* 1067–1077.

Clark, C., Azen, S., Zemke, R., Jackson, J., Carlson, M., Mandel, D., et al. (1997). Occupational therapy for independent-living older adults: A randomized controlled trial. *Journal of the American Medical Association, 278,* 1321–1326.

Cole, M. (2003). Trends from the Slagle lectures: 1986–2001. Paper presentation # 215 at the American Occupational Therapy Association Annual Conference & Expo. June 8, 2003, Washington, DC.

DeBeer, F. (1987). Major themes in occupational therapy: A content analysis of the Eleanor Clarke Slagle lectures 1955-1985. *American Journal of Occupational Therapy, 41*(8), 527–531.

Dunn, W. (2001). The sensations of everyday life: Empirical, theoretical, pragmatic considerations. *American Journal of Occupational Therapy, 55,* 608–620.

Dunn, W., Brown, C. & McGuigan, A. (1994). The ecology of human performance: A framework for considering the effect of context, *American Journal of Occupational Therapy, 48,* 595–607.

Dunn, W. & McGourty, L. (1989). Application of uniform terminology to practice. *American Journal of Occupational Therapy, 43,* 817–831.

Dunton, W. (1919). *Reconstruction therapy.* Philadelphia: Saunders.

Edelson, M. (1964). *Ego psychology: Group dynamics and the therapeutic community.* New York: Grune & Stratton.

Evanofski, M. (2003). Occupational therapy reimbursement, regulation, and the evolving scope of practice. In E. Crepeau, E. Cohn, & B. Boyt Schell (Eds.), *Willard & Spackman's Occupational Therapy (*10th ed., pp. 887–905). Philadelphia, PA: Lippincott Williams and Wilkins.

Farber, S. D. (1989). Neuroscience and occupational therapy: Vital connections. *American Journal of Occupational Therapy, 43,* 637–645.

Fidler, G. (1969). The task-oriented group as a context for treatment. *American Journal of Occupational Therapy, 23,* 43–48.

Fidler, G., & Fidler, J. (1954). *Occupational therapy: A communication process in psychiatry.* New York: Macmillan.

Fidler, G., & Fidler, J. (1963). *Occupational therapy: A communication process in psychiatry* (2nd ed.). New York: Macmillan.

Fidler, G., & Fidler, J. (1978). Doing and becoming: Purposeful action and self-actualization. *American Journal of Occupational Therapy, 32,* 305–310.

Fine, S. B. (1990). Resilience and human adaptability: Who rises above adversity? *American Journal of Occupational Therapy, 44,* 493–503.

Fiorentino, M. (1961, 1974) in Padilla, R. (Ed.). (2005). *A professional legacy: The Eleanor Clarke Slagle lectures in occupational therapy 1955–2004* (2nd ed.). Bethesda, MD: American Occupational Therapy Association, Inc.

Fisher, A. G. (1998). Uniting practice and theory in an occupational framework. *American Journal of Occupational Therapy, 52,* 509–520.

Goffman, E. (1961). *Asylums: Essays on the social situation of mental patients and other inmates.* New York: Doubleday, Inc.

Grady, A. P. (1994). Building inclusive community: A challenge for occupational therapy. *American Journal of Occupational Therapy, 48,* 300–310.

Hagedorn, R. (2001). *Foundations for practice in occupational therapy* (3rd ed.). London: Churchill Livingstone.

Hall, H. J., & Buck, M. (1915). *The work of our hands: A study of occupations for invalids.* New York: Moffat, Yard & Co.

Hall, H. (1916). *Handicrafts for the handicapped.* Concord, MA: Rumford Press.

Hannam, D. (1997). More than a cup of tea: Meaning construction in an everyday occupation. *Journal of Occupational Science, Australia, 4,* 69–74.

Henderson, A. (1988). Occupational therapy knowledge: From practice to theory. *American Journal of Occupational Therapy, 42,* 567–576.

Holm, M. B. (2000). Our mandate for the new millennium: Evidence-based practice. *American Journal of Occupational Therapy, 54,* 575–585.

Howe, M. C., & Briggs, A. K. (1982). Ecological systems models for occupational therapy. *American Journal of Occupational Therapy, 36,* 322–327.

Kielhofner, G. (1977). Temporal adaptation: A conceptual framework for occupational therapy. *American Journal of Occupational Therapy, 31,* 235–242.

Kielhofner, G. (1980a). A model of human occupation, Part 2: Ontogenesis from the perspective of temporal adaptation. *American Journal of Occupational Therapy, 34,* 657–663.

Kielhofner, G. (1980b). A model of human occupation, Part 3: Benign and vicious cycles. *American Journal of Occupational Therapy, 34,* 731–737.

Kielhofner, G. (2004). *Conceptual foundations of occupational therapy* (3rd ed.). Philadelphia: FA Davis.

Kielhofner, G., & Burke, J. (1977). Occupational therapy after 60 years: An account of changing identity and knowledge. *American Journal of Occupational Therapy, 31,* 675–689.

Kielhofner, G., & Burke, J. (1980). A model of human occupation, Part 1: Conceptual framework and content. *American Journal of Occupational Therapy, 34,* 572–581.

Kielhofner, G., Burke, J., & Igi, C. (1980). A model of human occupation, Part 4: Assessment and intervention. *American Journal of Occupational Therapy, 34,* 777–788.

King, L. J. (1978). Toward a science of adaptive responses. *American Journal of Occupational Therapy, 32,* 429–437.

Kuhn, T. (1970). *The structure of scientific revolutions* (2nd ed.). Chicago: University of Chicago Press.

Law, M., Cooper, B., Strong, S., Stewart, D., Rigby, P., & Letts, L. (1996). The Person–Environment–Occupational Model: A transactive approach to occupational performance. *Canadian Journal of Occupational Therapy, 63*(1), 9–23.

Licht, S. (1967). The founding and founders of the American Occupational Therapy Association. *American Journal of Occupational Therapy, 21,* 269–277.

Llorens, L. (1970). Facilitating growth and development: the promise of occupational therapy. *American Journal of Occupational Therapy, 24,* 93–101.

Maslow, A. (1970). *Motivation and personality* (Revised ed.). New York: Harper & Row.

Matheson, L. N. (1998). Engaging the person in the process: Planning together for occupational therapy intervention (pp. 107–122). In M. Law (Ed.). *Client-centered occupational therapy.* Thorofare, NJ: SLACK Incorporated.

Mathiowetz, V., & Bass Haugen, J. (1994). Motor behavior research: Implications for therapeutic approaches to central nervous system dysfunction. *American Journal of Occupational Therapy, 48,* 733–745.

Mattingly, C., & Fleming, M. (1994). *Clinical reasoning: Forms of inquiry in a therapeutic practice.* Philadelphia: FA Davis.

Mattingly, C., & Gillette, N. (1991). Anthropology, occupational therapy, and action research. *American Journal of Occupational Therapy, 45,* 972–978.

Mattingly, C. (1989). Thinking with stories: Story and experience in a clinical practice. Unpublished doctoral dissertation. Cambridge, MA: Massachusetts Institute of Technology

Meyer, A. (1921, 1983). The philosophy of occupational therapy. *Occupational Therapy in Mental Health, 2,* 79–87.

Mosey, A. (1970). *Three frames of reference for mental health.* Thorofare, NJ: SLACK Incorporated.

Mosey, A. (1973). *Activities therapy.* New York: Raven Press.

Mosey, A. (1974). An alternative: The biopsychosocial model. *American Journal of Occupational Therapy, 28,* 137–140.

Mosey, A. (1993). Partition of occupational science and occupational therapy: Sorting out some issues. *American Journal of Occupational Therapy, 47,* 751–754.

Nelson, D. L. (1996). Why the profession of occupational therapy will flourish in the 21st century. *American Journal of Occupational Therapy, 51,* 11–24.

Peloquin, S. M. (1991). Looking back: Occupational therapy service, Individual and collective understandings of the founders (Part 2). *American Journal of Occupational Therapy, 45,* 733–744.

Peloquin, S. M. (2005a). The art of occupational therapy: Engaging hearts in practice. In F. Kronenberg, S. Algado, & N. Pollard (Eds.), *Occupational Therapy Without Borders* (pp. 99–109). New York: Elsevier, Churchill & Livingstone.

Peloquin, S. M. (2005b). Embracing our ethos, reclaiming our heart. *American Journal of Occupational Therapy, 59,* 611–625.

Quiroga, V. A. (1995). *Occupational therapy: The first 30 years 1900–1930.* Bethesda, MD: American Occupational Therapy Association, Inc.

Reed, K. L. (1986). Tools of practice: Heritage or baggage? *American Journal of Occupational Therapy, 40,* 597–605.

Reed, K. L. (2005). An annotated history of the concepts used in occupational therapy. In C. Christiansen & C. Baum (Eds.), *Occupational therapy: performance, participation, and well-being* (pp. 567–626). Thorofare, NJ: SLACK Incorporated.

Reed, K., & Sanderson, S. (1980). *Concepts of occupational therapy.* Baltimore, MD: Williams & Wilkins.

Reed, K., & Sanderson, S. (1992). *Concepts of occupational therapy* (3rd ed.). Baltimore, MD: Williams & Wilkins.

Reilly, M. (1962). The Eleanor Clarke Slagle: Occupational therapy can be one of the great ideas of 20th century medicine. *American Journal of Occupational Therapy, 16,* 1–9.

Reilly, M. (1974). *Play as exploratory learning.* Beverly Hills, CA: Sage.

Rogers, C. (1961). *On becoming a person: a therapist's view of psychotherapy.* Boston, MA: Houghton Mifflin Company.

Rogers, J. (1983). Eleanor Clarke Slagle Lecture: Clinical reasoning: The ethics, science, and art. *American Journal of Occupational Therapy, 9,* 601–616.

Rood, M. (1954). Neurophysiological reactions as a basis for physical therapy. *Physical Therapy Review, 34,* 444–449.

Ross, M., & Burdick, D. (1981). *Sensory integration: A training manual for therapists and teachers for regressed, psychiatric, and geriatric patient groups.* Thorofare, NJ: SLACK Incorporated.

Schkade, J., & Schultz, S. (1992). Occupational adaptation: Toward a holistic approach for contemporary practice, Part 1. *American Journal of Occupational Therapy, 46,* 829–837.

Schultz, S., & Schkade, J. (1992). Occupational adaptation: Toward a holistic approach for contemporary practice, Part 2. *American Journal of Occupational Therapy, 46,* 917–925.

Serrett, K. D. (1985). *Philosophical and historical roots of occupational therapy.* New York: Haworth Press.

Spackman, C. (1947). Occupational therapy for the restoration of physical function. In H. Willard & C. Spackman (Eds.), *Occupational Therapy.* (3rd ed., pp. 231–233). Philadelphia: Lippincott.

Spackman, C. (1947). Occupational therapy for the restoration of physical function. In H. Willard & C. Spackman (Eds.), *Occupational Therapy.* (3rd ed., pp. 167–225, 1963). Philadelphia: Lippincott.

Toglia, J. (1991). Generalization of treatment: A multicontextual approach to cognitive-perceptual impairment in the brain-injured adult. *American Journal of Occupational Therapy, 45,* 505–516.

Townsend, E. (1998). Client-centered occupational therapy: The Canadian experience. In M. Law (Ed.), *Client-centered occupational therapy.* Thorofare, NJ: SLACK Incorporated.

Trombly, C. A. (1995). Occupation: Purposefulness and meaningfulness as therapeutic mechanisms. *American Journal of Occupational Therapy, 49,* 960–972.

Weimer, R. B. (1972). Some concepts of prevention as an aspect of community health. *American Journal of Occupational Therapy, 26,* 1–9.

West, W. (1959). *Changing concepts and practice in psychiatric occupational therapy.* Dubuque, IA: Wm. C. Brown Book Company.

Wilcock, A. (2001a). *An occupational perspective of health.* Thorofare, NJ: SLACK Incorporated.

Wilcock, A. (2001b). Occupational science: the key to broadening horizons. *British journal of Occupational Therapy, 64,* 412–417.

World Health Organization. (2001). *International classification of function, disability, and health.* Geneva: Author.

Yerxa, E. J., Clark, F., Frank, G., Jackson, J., Parham, D., Pierce, D., et al. (1989). An introduction to occupational science: A foundation for occupational therapy in the 21st century. *Occupational Therapy in Health Care, 6,* 1–17.

Zemke, R. (2004). Time, space, and the kaleidoscopes of occupation. *American Journal of Occupational Therapy, 58,* 608–620.

Chapter 2

APPLIED MODELS OF HEALTH CARE IN OCCUPATIONAL THERAPY PRACTICE

"The profession of occupational therapy will flourish because occupation, its core, is so basic to human health yet so flexible, depending on the needs of the individual human being."

– DAVID NELSON (1997, P. 11)

This chapter will review the prevailing models of health care and occupational therapy (OT), including the medical model, the World Health Organization (WHO) model (WHO, 2001), the client-centered practice model, and the American Occupational Therapy Association's (AOTA's) OT Practice Framework (AOTA, 2002). These provide a further context for understanding the changes that are occurring in the OT profession both nationally and globally and how they will affect the theories we develop and apply now and in the future.

MEDICAL MODEL

What would you do if you had a high fever? Perhaps you would take your own temperature and note other symptoms (e.g., fatigue, headache) that you might recognize as a head cold or this year's version of the flu. Maybe you would take aspirin or an over-the-counter cold remedy. But eventually, if the fever persisted, you would end up in a doctor's office. There, the doctor might check other signs such as blood pressure, listen to your breathing with a stethoscope, and maybe have a look at your ears for signs of inflammation. By the time your feet hit the examination room floor, you would probably have a diagnosis, some general instructions on how to manage the symptoms, and at least one prescription to be filled at the drugstore on the way home.

Now suppose you fell off a ladder and broke your ankle. Hopefully you would be able to reach your cell phone to call 911 or be taken in someone's car to the nearest hospital or clinic. As soon as you enter a medical clinic or hospital, you become a *patient*, or recipient of medically based services offered at that facility. Considering your inability to walk, the Emergency Room personnel may meet you at the door with a wheelchair or a gurney (mobile bed), and you will probably be placed in a *treatment room* or space separated by a curtain for privacy. Depending on the urgency of your condition, you will wait to be seen by a *doctor, nurse practitioner,* or *physician's assistant.* Of course, someone from admissions will ask you for identifying data (name, address, age, etc.) and for evidence of *medical insurance.* You can probably visualize what happens after that. In fact, most of us take the medical model for granted; it is so much a part of our culture and lifestyle.

There are thousands of diseases, illnesses, injuries, and syndromes listed and described in medical textbooks and journals, each with a unique name. *Medical diagnosis* is the process of analyzing a patient's signs and symptoms, and *reducing* the problem to a specific, narrowly defined cause. Hence, the medical model is often described as *reductionistic.* Once the doctor names the disease—pneumonia, for example—he or she can then apply what is known about that illness in order to *prescribe a treatment*—for example, antibiotic medication, bed rest, maintenance of a sterile environment, increased fluid intake, or other specific instructions leading to a *cure.* The patient, a passive recipient of treatment, complies with the doctor's instructions in order to get well, feel better, and restore health. This describes the unique terminology of the medical model as we know it. The process has remained the same for at least the past century and is likely to continue well into the next one.

Occupational Therapy and the Medical Model

OT has been associated with the medical model from its beginnings. Early in the 20th century, humanism influenced the practice of medicine by promoting a holistic approach that encouraged experimentation with many new and creative treatment methods. Without this openness, the central role of occupation in the restoration and maintenance of health, which inspired the birth of our profession, may never have become known. However, by the 1930s, the scientific movement had gathered sufficient strength to shape medicine and OT practice in ways that allowed both to benefit from the rapidly growing body of scientific research that was developing.

The medical model of health care came into existence because of the conditions of the times. In the 1930s and 1940s, many diseases were on the rise, such as tuberculosis and polio, for which there was no cure. Scientific research led to an understanding of how bacteria spreads disease and what measures could be taken to prevent it. Medicine applied the scientific method to develop medications and vaccines to prevent or cure many of the diseases of the mid-20th century. OT struggled to keep up with the advances in medicine and adopted practice methods for remediation, adaptation, and compensation. *Remediation* involved the use of occupations to restore the ability to function. For example, in persons with depression or anxiety disorders, OT worked side by side with medicine in order to hasten recovery. Occupational therapists developed *adaptations* to the task and environment in order to enable occupational functioning despite the limitations brought on by illness or injury. In using *compensatory strategies*, occupational therapists took over where medicine left off. For example, splinting, adaptive equipment, and more recently, robotics and computer-assisted technology are used by occupational therapists to enable activities of daily living (ADL) for persons with partial paralysis from polio, a stroke, or a spinal cord injury, for which no further improvement could be gained with other medical treatment.

For most of the 20th century, occupational therapists worked in hospitals, nursing homes, rehabilitation centers, day hospitals, and outpatient clinics under the auspices of the medical model. Occupational therapists became a part of the health care teams that offered a multidisciplinary approach to the treatment of illness and disease. As such, OT often required a doctor's prescription in order to be paid for by Medicare or other health insurance, and this requirement remains written into many states' OT licensure laws even today. In the 21st century, our profession appears to be in the midst of a transition, and changes in public policy will be needed in order to fully adopt a broader paradigm of occupation and to become truly client-centered.

Characteristics of the Traditional Medical Model

Characteristics of the *traditional* medical model are described by Kielhofner (2004) as reductionistic, mechanistic, and scientific. The scientific method requires that a research problem be narrowly defined in order to study it more rigorously. For example, the action of a muscle is broken down into nerves, circulation, molecules, cells, and the nutrients such as fat, protein, and carbohydrates that make up the cells so that each component can be studied in detail. Much of our scientific knowledge of the physical world has been developed through careful examination of the relationships among component parts. Medicine used the scientific method in the development of biochemistry,

anatomy, physiology, genetics, pharmacology, nutrition, and bioengineering (Kielhofner, 2004). This method of study encouraged the belief, prevalent in medical practice and research, that the human body operates like a complex machine. As such, "the task of medicine was conceived as repairing breakdowns in the machine" (Capra, 1982; Kielhofner, 2004, p. 231), thus restoring a state of health, normalcy, and homeostasis. In the traditional medical model, health is defined as the absence of disease (e.g., no more pain); norms are based on vast collections of clinical data (e.g., a body temperature of 98.6 degrees) and homeostasis, or a balance of physical and mental health (e.g., patient can be discharged from medical care and resume previous life activities).

OT theories that were developed within the medical model have been identified by Kielhofner (2004) as behavioral, psychoanalytic, and sensory integration. We would add cognitive disabilities, biomechanical, motor control theories, and any other approaches that were developed for the treatment of specific disabilities. These OT frames of reference focus on components of performance, and as such, are not occupation-based. However, the concepts within these frames of reference have been, or can be, validated by research using the scientific method. Therefore, while some of these frames of reference have been criticized for their reductionistic focus, they have produced many reliable and valid assessment tools and provide the basis for a multitude of clinical strategies and techniques that have recognized positive outcomes. We predict that their usefulness will re-emerge as tools to be applied during the evaluation, intervention, and outcomes phases of the OT process outlined in the OT Practice Framework.

Pros and Cons of the Medical Model

Critics of the medical model have emphasized its reductionism and its mechanistic view of the human body. In fact, the paradigm shift in the OT profession occurred largely because the medical model had backed OT into a proverbial corner, limiting its scope to only those practices that directly affected "symptoms" or restricted independent functioning in ADL. When I (M. Cole) consulted for a large state mental health facility about 10 years ago, I found very few occupational therapists on staff, and those that remained focused exclusively on ADL skill building for clients who would soon be relocated to community settings. My role as a consultant was to educate the staff concerning standardized assessment tools that could be used to measure progress in self care and social skills and to help them determine client readiness for community placement. Soon after my consultancy ended, the entire facility was closed, leaving many severely disabled clients without needed health services.

This experience demonstrates how the reductionistic pressures of the scientific method, fueled by the cost reduction measures for all medical services during the 1990s, had rendered the medical model grossly inadequate to meet the needs of clients with ongoing mental or physical health conditions. Everywhere in society, signs of this inadequacy abound. Many formerly institutionalized mental health clients now live among the homeless or have entered our already overcrowded prison system. Working people are either losing their health insurance or facing higher prices for far less coverage. Prescription drugs, advertised as cures for everything from arthritis and high blood pressure to insomnia, appear to have replaced the need for hands-on therapy, at least in the eyes of today's television watching population.

Reimbursement systems that follow the guidelines of the medical model have reduced access and limited the ways clients can use OT services. Most occupational therapists are aware that neither Medicare nor private health insurance will pay for health services rendered only to "maintain" function for our clients. Progress must be continually demonstrated through the use of valid and reliable assessment tools, mostly products of research studies using the scientific method. The medical model has convinced third-party payers that *health* should be defined as the absence of disease. The client-centered model being adopted by OT and others goes further to include well-being, quality of life, and the client's continued ability to engage in meaningful activities and to participate in life (AOTA, 2002; WHO, 2001).

Yet, without the medical model, many of the scientific advances of the 20th century would not have been possible. Under the guidance of the medical model, OT was able to take advantage of the knowledge developed in the areas of psychiatry, biomechanics, behaviorism, and neurophysiology in the earlier years, which led to some of the most widely used applied theories in OT today.

Examples are sensory integration, neurodevelopmental therapy (NDT), biomechanical rehabilitation, motor learning, dynamic interactional, and cognitive behavioral approaches in OT. The scientific method was used in designing research studies to test these applied theories and to develop reliable and valid assessment tools. Assessments also serve as evidence for administrators or managers of health service agencies, rehabilitation centers, and school-based services that the methods occupational therapists use have been and continue to be effective. Furthermore, despite the profession's move away from the medical model, many occupational therapists still practice in medical-based settings.

Another advantage of the medical model is the prestige it has brought to OT over the years as an allied health profession. Educational programs for OT were jointly accredited by the American Medical Association (AMA) from the days of Eleanor Clarke Slagle until quite recently, requiring OT students to take classes in anatomy, physiology, neurology, and physical and mental health conditions. This medical preparation has influenced public recognition for OT professionals as equals with other professions such as physical therapy and encouraged our continued national certification and state licensure, setting us apart from less "scientific" professions.

The medical model, furthermore, gives us a common language with which to communicate with other professionals as more occupational therapists collaborate with treatment teams when providing health care services. Until the sociopolitical systems catch up with the paradigm shift to client-centered practice, occupational therapists will need to maintain relationships with members of the current system of health care delivery, which still relies heavily on the medical model.

CLIENT-CENTERED MODEL

Client-centered practice is the basic therapy model for the OT Practice Framework (AOTA, 2002). (See Table 2-1 for a comparison of medical model and client-centered model terminology.) However, the concepts behind it are not new. Client-centered concepts were inherent in the movement toward a community-based model of practice in the 1960s when large numbers of patients with ongoing health conditions moved out of institutions. It was thought that individuals with disabilities needed opportunities to practice utilizing community resources in order to learn to function independently in their own communities (Scaffa, 2001; Watanabe, 1967). Attributes of the community model at that time included the clients taking on more responsibility for their own treatment and a subsequent change in the occupational therapist's role from healer to supporter, enabler, and advocate. However, toward the latter part of the 20th century, there was much trepidation among occupational therapists about moving away from the traditional medical model. In 1984, Mary Reilly warned the profession to carefully examine the implications of *patient* and *client*. In a time when reimbursement for OT services relied almost exclusively on the medical model, she feared that a move to client-centered practice would greatly jeopardize access to OT services for those who needed it most—the chronically ill. She writes, "The shift to a client system represents, perhaps, a desperate strategy to survive under the awesome pressure of the self-interest of medicine" (Reilly, 1984, p. 406). She continues, "the good news is that historical OT contains the wit, wisdom, and technology to construct a golden parachute that would bail the service out of hospitals and into the community" (Reilly, 1984, p. 406). Reilly was again true to her prophetic nature. Twenty years later, occupational therapists have finally begun to make the transition to a community-based, client-centered practice.

Foundational Concepts of Client-Centered Practice

The work of Carl Rogers, a humanistic psychologist and psychotherapist, forms the basis for the current client-centered approach. During the 1950s, he called his therapeutic approach client-centered therapy (Rogers, 1951; Law & Mills, 1998). Rogers believed that the best way to

Table 2-1
Comparison of Medical Model and Client-Centered Model Terminology

Medical Model	**Client-Centered Model**
Patient: passive recipient of treatment. Implies a sick role and a lack or participation or responsibility, requires compliance with doctor's orders.	*Client:* actively seeks assistance from medical and other professionals or experts, shifts responsibility for solving health problems onto the client
Health: absence of disease	*Health:* mental and physical fitness and a sense of well-being
Disease: illness or injury affecting	*Health condition:* any circumstance that interferes with full participation in life
Diagnosis: identification of disease through analysis of signs, symptoms, and syndromes which allow the doctor to predict the course of illness and to prescribe remedies	*Disability:* experienced by the person, sometimes determined by the person's experience of illness; that which prevents the person from participating in life
Prescription: medications or specific techniques or instructions intended to cure disease and/or manage symptoms	*Enablement:* sharing expertise that empowers the client to set reasonable goals and make informed choices regarding interventions to remove barriers to participation in life
Objective methods of study are based on experimental research, data gathering, and norms.	Subjective methods of study based on qualitative research, looking at each individual's culture, perceptions, and situation.
Outcome is measured by objective measures applied by the medical professional.	Outcome includes both objective measures and client satisfaction with results.
Treatment: specific medical or surgical procedures prescribed by a doctor or specialist in order to heal or cure a disease	*Intervention:* procedures and strategies created by collaboration between client and professional, to overcome barriers to occupational performance
Occupational therapist applies expertise to focus on using activities to relieve symptoms, to adapt task demands, or to compensate for disability. Rehabilitation ends when the patient has met functional goals established by the therapist and/or medical treatment team.	Occupational therapist collaborates with client to identify occupational problems and priorities, set goals, and enable client participation through supporting skill development and taking preventive actions and/or through adaptation of tasks and environments.

understand an individual client was by using the client's own "self view" or personal frame of reference. The attainment and drive to reach self actualization is believed to be the motivating factor that inspires each person to change. Rogers also stressed that the most significant components to an effective therapeutic relationship include a therapist's ability to show genuineness, acceptance, and empathy coupled with the client's ability to perceive these expressions generated by a therapist. In the 1970s and 1980s, Rogers' therapeutic approach not only impacted the psychotherapy world but also influenced education, industry, and politics that were particularly focused on efforts for world peace. Rogers eventually decided to change the name of his approach to person-centered therapy as a way to reflect the broadening application and universality of this perspective. The focus within this therapeutic style centers on the growth of the individual person, not in solving the problem. Person-centered therapy is a process of self discovery and exploration that is facilitated by a therapist (Corey, 1994).

A second well-known proponent of the humanistic philosophy was Abraham Maslow, who focused much of his research on the nature of the self-actualizing person. He is known for establishing the theory of hierarchy of needs, which states that man is internally and externally driven by various forces to satisfy his needs and reach a sense of self-fulfillment. Like Rogers, Maslow believed that people are basically trustworthy, self-protecting, and self-governing. Individuals may resort to unhealthy tendencies because their more fundamental needs, such as physical and safety needs, are not being met. Satisfying needs is healthy; withholding or restricting is not. The highest level of achievement is "self-actualization" or the capacity to be all that one can be. Persons who are self-actualized can appreciate knowledge, peace, aesthetics, and spirituality (Maslow, 1970). Maslow's concept of self-actualization closely relates to the issues of quality of life and well-being so often mentioned in current OT models.

Client-centeredness first appeared in the OT literature during the 1980s to 1990s as a model designed by the Canadian Association of Occupational Therapy (CAOT). Canadian occupational therapists interpreted many of the humanistic principles of Rogers and Maslow in ways that served as guidelines for their application in practice. For

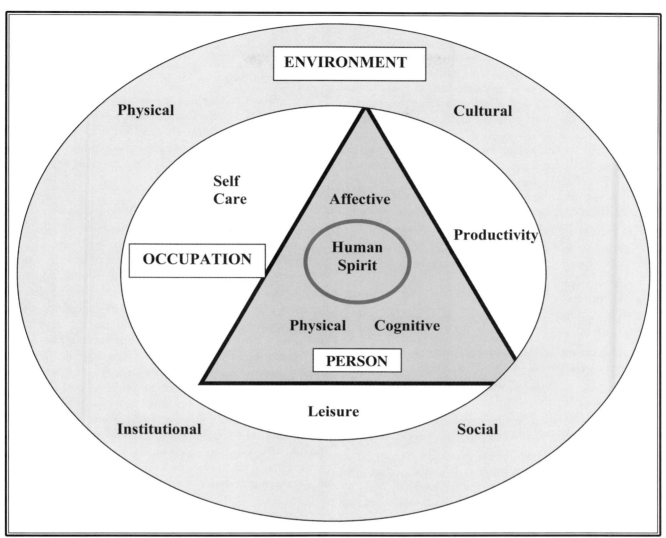

Figure 2-1. Client-centered model. (Adapted with permission from Canadian Occupational Therapy Association. [1998]. *Canadian occupational performance measure* [3rd ed.]. Ottawa, CA: Author.)

this reason, it makes sense to review the Canadian model here, rather than in Section II (Figure 2-1).

Client-Centered Practice and the Canadian Model

Client-centered practice, as defined by the CAOT (CAOT, 1997), follows the Canadian Model of Occupational Performance (CMOP), which illustrates how occupational performance evolves from the interactions among the person, the environment, and the occupation itself. According to Kielhofner, the "most important contribution of this model [CMOP] to explaining therapy has been discussion of the nature and process of the client-centered model" (2004, p. 99).

The Person

The person includes physical, cognitive, and affective components bound together by a central core of being,

which is spirituality. Physical factors include strength and energy, flexibility, range of motion, endurance, and pain. Cognition includes things like thinking, reasoning, memory, perception, communication, and motor planning. These cognitive processes are essential in learning and adapting to new circumstances when performing occupations. The affective component includes feelings and attitudes and affects a person's motivation, self-concept, and relationships with others. Occupational science tells us that "what we do is who we are." In other words, the activities we engage in and the occupations we choose, help define who we are. This view of the person confirms the central role of occupation in defining a person's identity. According to Christiansen (1999), "occupations are more than movements strung together, more than simply doing something. They are opportunities to express the self, to create an identity" (p. 552).

Human Spirituality

One of the unique features of Canadian model of client-centered practice is the central role of the human spirit in self-identity, self-direction, and occupational choice. Spirituality is defined as "a pervasive life force, manifestation of a higher self, source of will and self-determination, and a sense of meaning, purpose, and connectedness that people experience in the context of their environment" (CAOT, 1997, p. 182). Human spirituality may also be defined as the experience of meaning (Urbanowski & Vargo, 1994). This broad definition includes religious faith as well as the meaning of everyday activities and the symbolic significance of occupations as a part of one's culture.

Key points:
- Empathy and reflective listening clarify the experience of meaning related to illness and recovery.
- Human spirit is at the center of bio-psycho-social functioning.
- What we "do" reflects who we are (occupational science).
- Real meaning exists in performance of ordinary everyday activities (Meyer, 1921, 1983).
- Meaning is explored through the therapeutic relationship.
- Each crisis has a "nuclear problem" (Dixon, 1987): one that threatens something the person considers essential for a meaningful life.
- OT must identify "nuclear tasks": things that need doing to resolve the crisis (restore "everyday life")
- OT gives "opportunities" rather than "prescriptions" (Meyer, 1921).
- Collaboration and respect for client choices are essential in maintaining motivation, enabling occupation, and restoring function (Clark, 1993; Rosenfeld, 1997).

The Environment

The environment in the CMOP is composed of physical, social, cultural, and institutional elements. These are the contexts in which clients perform occupations. Examples of physical environments are home, classroom, workplace, or natural environments like the outdoors. Social environments include family, coworkers, and community organizations. Cultural environments may overlap with social and include religious, ethnic, and political factors, which can affect the opportunities for, and barriers to, participation in life. Institutional environments include the political and social systems that afford opportunities and provide rules and limits to one's occupations. Obeying laws and observing the rights of others are examples of the influence of political and social systems on a person's behavior.

The OT Practice Framework (AOTA, 2002) includes the additional contexts of personal (age, gender, socioeconomic, and educational status), spiritual (fundamental life orientation), temporal (time of year, stages of life, duration), and virtual (e-mail, telephone, television, and radio) (AOTA, 2002, p. 623).

Occupation

Occupation is the third component of the CMOP. The categories of occupation include self-care, productivity, and leisure. These are defined to include most ADL, home, work, and community activities, recreation, and socialization. All of the tasks people do are potentially the focus of OT services.

Occupational Performance

Occupational performance results from the interaction of all three components: person, environment, and occupation. The occupational therapist's unique role is one of *enabling occupation*. The client-centered approach emphasizes that occupational performance is best defined by each individual based on his or her experience rather than therapist observation. The client's perception of his or her own occupational performance determines the degree of satisfaction. For this reason, occupational therapists need to communicate and collaborate with the client when setting goals according to client priorities and designing interventions that have meaning for the client both personally and within his culture or social group. To accomplish this, therapeutic engagement with the client is the primary task in OT. Goal accomplishment in therapy and client satisfaction with the outcome both rely on the quality of the therapeutic relationship.

Forming a Collaborative Partnership With the Client

The methods used by occupational therapists to form therapeutic relationships are based on the principles of Carl Rogers (1961), Abraham Maslow (1968), and other humanists. These include therapeutic use of self, respect, genuineness, nonjudgmental acceptance, and a nondirective style of communication. These principles all facilitate the process of self-actualization within the client. Let us look more closely at these key methods to establishing a therapeutic and collaborative alliance with clients by briefly defining each principle.

- *Respect:* an attitude in which the occupational therapist views the client as an equal partner in establishing goals and priorities and designing interventions. This involves listening and empathizing with the client while he tells his life story and refraining from premature advice-giving. Respecting the client means having faith in his ability to understand and to reason out solutions to problems. Occupational therapist's offer help by facilitating and guiding the client through the process of self-understanding and action planning.

- *Genuineness:* treating the client as a person worthy of our respect. When we respond to clients in ways that show our humanity, they are encouraged to put their trust in us as therapists. Occupational therapist's need to develop skill in engaging in genuine interactions while maintaining a focus on the client. Therapists strategically learn to use their own emotional responses as a guide in giving the client helpful feedback.

- *Nonjudgmental acceptance:* Carl Rogers used this term to identify the therapist's responsibility to set aside any possible biases about the client based on appearance, social, cultural, or any other factors that may lead to possible misconceptions. The therapist must accept the client as he or she is, without exception. This means that as therapists, we must be willing to look inward and examine our personal responses to clients, a process that leads to the development of *therapeutic use of self.*

- *Nondirective style:* Rogers perfected the art of nondirective therapy by using prompts and open questions that encouraged the client to establish the direction of therapy. He asked questions that clients could not answer with "yes" or "no," but would compel clients to explain, describe, or elaborate on their problem relationships or life issues. Occupational therapists do this when interviewing the client for the first time, giving the client a free choice of topics to discuss, issues to explore, and occupational priorities on which to focus in therapy. The COPM is an OT assessment tool that incorporates these concepts, asking clients to identify occupational problems and to rank their priorities.

- *Self-actualization:* the highest level of achievement at the peak of Abraham Maslow's pyramid, or hierarchy of needs. According to Maslow, people have an innate desire to be the best they can be—to achieve their human potential. In his hierarchy, Maslow outlines five levels of basic human needs, moving from 1) basic physiological needs like food and shelter, to 2) safety (both emotional and physical), to 3) belonging and love which serves as support and guidance for further growth, to 4) self-esteem or confidence building for effective occupational performance, to 5) self-actualization, representing the highest level of human achievement, which can be measured only in terms of life satisfaction for the individual person.

Six Principles of Client-Centered Practice

In various publications about client-centered practice, the following six principles are identified for OT practice (Law & Mills, 1998).

1. Client Autonomy and Choice

The therapist enters the therapeutic relationship under the assumption that the client has the right to direct his or her own therapy. This concept stems from Maslow's belief that people are intrinsically motivated to improve their condition in life. Maslow called this natural desire to move up toward the peak of his hierarchy of needs the "formative tendency" (Maslow, 1968). Persons are internally motivated to continue striving for perfection, achievement, and a sense of well-being. In OT, illness and disability can be seen as barriers to self-actualization. However, the true impact of illness or disability on one's occupations lies in the perception of the client.

The first step in client-centered practice is to listen to the client and to gain a clear understanding of his or her culture, values, and beliefs. In doing so, the therapist is able to respect the choices clients make and the contexts within which their occupational priorities are established.

When clients set their own goals and choose therapeutic tasks that hold the most meaning for them, they are naturally motivated to put forth their best effort. This is one of the main advantages of the client-centered approach.

2. Respect for Diversity

Rogers recommends the therapist develop an attitude of unconditional positive regard. This means refraining from making value judgments about the client's character based on our own standards and viewpoint. Rogers proposed that clients deserve the benefit of every doubt, just because they are human. Human beings, by definition, are worthy and capable of doing good and overcoming bad. It is more than putting a good spin on unfortunate circumstances. It means cultivating a genuine positive and supportive view of the client and communicating genuine concern and caring. Clients come from many diverse backgrounds, and their social roles and relationships within their own world have a powerful effect on the way they experience illness, therapy, and the process of recovery.

3. Therapeutic Partnership and Shared Responsibility

This collaborative partnership implies that both therapist and client come to the table as equals, each with his or her own expertise. The occupational therapist brings expertise about the theories and techniques of practice and the knowledge base of the profession, while the client brings expertise regarding his own illness or disability as a lived experience. The key ingredient of a successful partnership is the establishment of a trusting relationship based on understanding, empathy, and mutual respect.

This principle of client-centered practice might be the most difficult one to apply, because as health professionals, occupational therapists have traditionally played a more powerful role. In order to be truly client-centered, it is necessary to give up some power and to equalize the balance of control so that clients feel confident in making good decisions for themselves.

4. Enablement and Empowerment

This principle refers to the occupational therapist's role in promoting client participation in all aspects of OT services. In addressing occupational issues and problems, the client and therapist might brainstorm together to determine the best way for the client to perform a task. When clients' occupational issues are unclear, the occupational therapist employs therapeutic use of self to assist them in sorting out their occupational goals and priorities. Occupational therapists also educate the clients by suggesting alternatives and sharing their vision of what is possible. It may be necessary to assist the client in deciding among intervention approaches by weighing the potential benefits and risks of each alternative.

Enabling Occupation

Enabling occupation means using our OT knowledge, skills, and techniques to assist the client in doing something he or she wants to do. This is very different from a traditional rehabilitation model, in which the therapist chooses an appropriate task and adapts it for the client. The therapist uses professional expertise in both approaches, but the difference lies in how goals are set, and who gets to choose the occupations to be addressed. In a rehabilitation model, the therapist makes the choice. In a client-centered model, the therapist and client make the choices together.

Empowerment

Empowerment often means letting go of control and trusting the client to carry out a plan of action. Clients, too, may expect more direction from us than they actually need. We might empower clients by helping them to structure their daily activities so that goals can be more easily met. For example, when exercises need to be incorporated into a clients' daily routine, clients might initially need to write down a plan for specific movement sequences and the time and place where these will occur. We might provide a system for clients to keep track of their own progress using a check sheet and to build in a system of self-reinforcement. Occupational therapists will need to expand their knowledge of self-management techniques in order to enable clients to self-direct their application of therapeutic strategies. Establishing groups might be one way to assist clients in staying motivated by supporting and encouraging one another when client goals are similar.

5. Contextual Congruence: Recognizing Environmental Conditions and Demands

Contexts are external or environmental considerations that influence the performance of an activity or occupation. They might be circumstances, social expectations or obligations, or physical or economic factors. Congruence means agreement. In the performance of a task, contextual congruence means that the external features of the environment fit, encourage, or facilitate the performance. For example, Mary might need to clean her house, but when she is working on a writing deadline and coming home late every night, she is too tired to start cleaning. The occupation of house cleaning is not contextually congruent for her at this point in time. It is temporarily not her priority and does not fit with her lifestyle or needs. If Mary were a client, she would need help to organize her work in order to do it more efficiently and to meet her deadline. If her therapist could help her do that, then she would consider the intervention to be contextually congruent, helping her with the occupation she considers to be most important and meaningful *right now*.

Therapeutic recommendations in the medical model have often been ignored by clients because the specific conditions faced within their physical and social environments have not been considered. For example, we might ask the mother of a learning disabled child to provide an hour of outdoor play after school each day. When the mother does not comply, we might assume a lack of motivation or an uncooperative attitude. What might be the environmental conditions and demands that create barriers in this case? What would be an alternate explanation for this mother not following the occupational therapist's recommendations?

6. Accessibility and Flexibility

Many clients have situations and circumstances that do not fit the "typical" interventions. The client-centered therapist approaches each client as an individual with a unique experience of a health condition and a different configuration of contextual factors that influence his or her problems with occupational performance. Occupational performance is an experienced phenomenon rather than an observed phenomenon (Law & Mills, 1998, p.4). Therefore, the client's awareness and ability to communicate his or her perceptions is key to our understanding of the occupational problems encountered. As occupational therapists, we need to know more than what we can see the client doing or not doing; we need to understand the problem from the client's perspective. When and how we offer intervention and the ways we communicate with clients will need to change as clients themselves change or as their situations and circumstances change. For example, a female high school teacher with a hip replacement has different occupational issues as she moves from hospital, to rehabilitation center, to her home, and then back to work. Each environment and circumstance presents different demands, issues, and problems. The therapist is required to think outside the proverbial box in assisting clients in a more flexible fashion.

Summary of Canadian Model of Occupational Performance

The client-centered aspects of the CMOP contribute greatly to our understanding of what is meant by client-centered practice. Additionally, Canada has demonstrated its usefulness in making the transition to community-based OT, a difficult transition for occupational therapists in the United States because of the differences in public policy regarding health care (further described in Chapter 5).

Function and dysfunction in the CMOP are attributed to the nature of the person-environment-occupation balance. Changes in any part of the system can cause problems with occupational performance. Motivation is considered to be intrinsic and is facilitated by clients' participation in identifying meaningful goals and occupational priorities. The model is not explicit in detailing a rationale for the therapeutic process (McColl & Pranger, 1994). Therefore, it is necessary to apply other models or frames of reference within the course of intervention. The primary method of therapeutic change is the therapist's therapeutic use of self, which establishes a collaborative partnership to enable the client by doing "with clients instead of to or for them" (Polatajko, 1992). Interventions include "facilitating, guiding, coaching, prompting, listening, reflecting, encouraging, or otherwise collaborating with people so that individuals, groups, agencies, or organizations have the means and opportunity to participate in shaping their own lives" (Law et al., 1997, p. 50). This process is guided by the six basic principles of client-centered practice listed previously.

Some concepts from the client-centered practice model are embedded in two important documents published in this decade, the International Classification of Functioning (ICF) (WHO, 2001) and the OT Practice Framework (AOTA, 2002). Next, we will review each of these models.

INTERNATIONAL CLASSIFICATION OF FUNCTIONING MODEL

The WHO made significant revisions to its classification system, which reflect the shift to a holistic and systems perspective of global health care. The ICF Model encompasses all aspects of human health and some health-relevant components of well-being, and its intent is as a companion classification system for the *International Classification of Disease*, 10th Edition (ICD-10), which classifies all known diseases, both mental and physical. The stated purposes of ICF are as follows:

- To provide a scientific basis for studying health and health determinants
- To establish a common language
- To allow comparison across countries, disciplines, and time
- To provide systematic coding for purposes of record keeping and research

Holistic Perspective

The initial publication was titled International Classification of Impairments, Disabilities, and Handicaps (ICIDH) (WHO, 1980). Each of these terms has been replaced to reflect the shift to a holistic perspective:

- Handicap is changed to "participation restriction."
- Disability is changed to "activity limitation."
- Impairment is changed to "health condition," an umbrella term for not only disease, disorder, injury, and trauma, but also conditions such as pregnancy, aging, stress, congenital anomaly, and genetic predisposition.

In its 2001 revision, WHO seeks to broaden the horizons of health-related research, service provision, and policy making beyond the constraints of the medical model. It states, "there is a widely held misunderstanding that ICF is only about people with disability; in fact, it is about all people" (WHO, 2001, p. 7).

Systems Orientation

ICF perceives a person's functioning and/or disability as a "dynamic interaction" between a health condition and contextual factors. Contextual factors are those external factors, "features of the physical, social, and attitudinal world," which facilitate or hinder participation (WHO, 2001, p. 8). Accordingly, ICF is divided into two parts. The first lists the components of human functioning and disability, including both body systems and structures and activities and participation, denoting both an individual and a societal perspective. The systems of the human body and the activities represented closely resemble OT's domain of concern according to the OT Practice Framework (AOTA, 2002).

The second half of ICF lists and classifies contexts in the following categories:

- *Products and technology*: includes foods, consumable goods, money, and the systems for distributing these, as well as objects and tools for other systems such as education, sports and recreation, and the practice of religion
- *Natural and human-made environments*: includes land and water, climate, population, light, noise, vibration, natural events such as an earthquake or tsunami, human-made events such as war, and time-related changes such as seasons
- *Support and relationships*: includes immediate and extended family, friends, acquaintances, authority figures, subordinates, care providers, domesticated animals, strangers, health care providers, and other professionals
- *Attitudes*: includes individual and societal views, biases, and stigmas, as well as norms, practices, and ideologies
- *Services, systems, and policies*: includes a vast range of systems such as economic, educational, media, transportation, housing, utilities, communication, legal systems, labor and employment, political, and civil

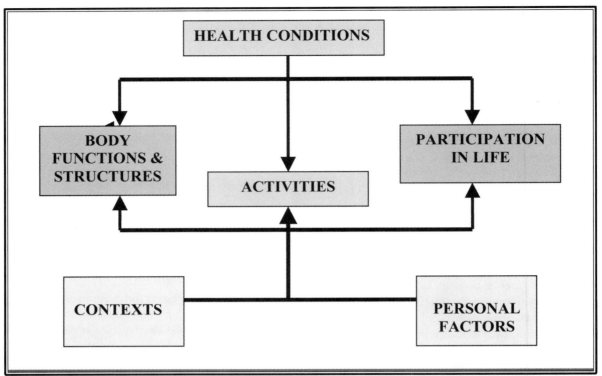

Figure 2-2. ICF Model of Functioning and Disability. (Reprinted with permission from World Health Organization. [2001]. *International classification of functioning, disability, and health.* Geneva: Author.)

protection systems. This category includes the system of health care as well as general social support.

The inclusion of so many external or environmental factors reflects the systems view of occupational performance—that it is a product of the interaction among the person, the task, and the environment. The basic language of ICF is compatible with that of OT in this regard, stating that "improvement of participation (can be encouraged) by removing or mitigating societal hindrances and encouraging the provision of social supports and facilitators" (WHO, 2001, p. 6). The model of functioning and disability also describes the interaction of ICF components in a diagram (Figure 2-2).

International Classification of Functioning's Medical and Social Models

ICF claims to reflect an integration of the medical and social models by using a bio-psycho-social approach. The medical model views disability as a problem of the person created by disease or trauma and requiring the services of a health care professional, such as medication, surgery, or rehabilitation. In the social view, disability is a socially created problem, and its management requires some form of social action. By combining aspects of both, ICF remains neutral regarding the required responses to problems that it classifies.

Impact on Occupational Therapy

The language of the ICF has an uncanny resemblance to the OT Practice Framework as well as several occupation-based models that have emerged in recent years. Authors of the Framework intentionally used some of ICF's language "in order to create more obvious links with terminology outside the profession" (AOTA, 2002, p. 637). The fact that the ICF Model recognizes activities as the main determinant of disability places occupational therapists in an ideal position to play a part in the evaluation and intervention. Furthermore, ICF's expanded definition of health, the expectation of "participation" in life, and the central role of "context" as a facilitator or barrier to participation, have obvious parallels in AOTA's Framework document (2002).

Other definitions also reflect the tendency toward a subjective view of occupation, and the interaction of personal and contextual factors as determents of ability or disability. For example, ICF makes a distinction between the performance and capacity to perform an activity. The performance of an activity is described as a "lived experience" (p. 15), such as an occupation performed in one's natural context. Capacity refers to the person's potential ability to perform an activity, which may be assessed within optimal or standard conditions. The difference between the potential (capacity) and actual (performance) might suggest ways in which the environmental conditions could be altered to improve occupational performance.

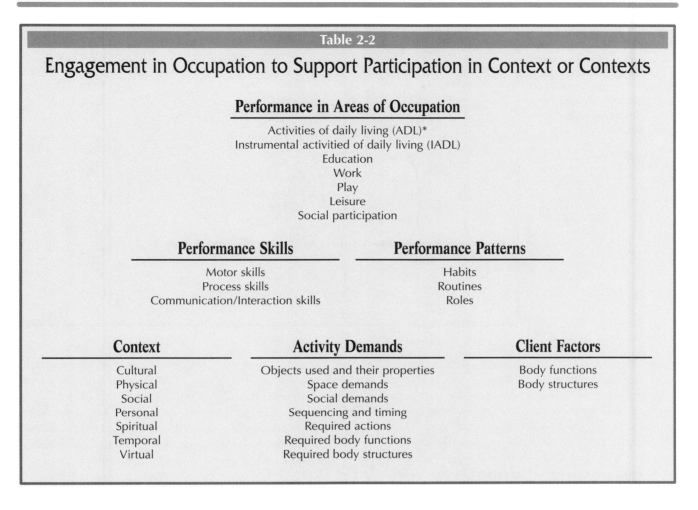

Table 2-2

Engagement in Occupation to Support Participation in Context or Contexts

Performance in Areas of Occupation

Activities of daily living (ADL)*
Instrumental activitied of daily living (IADL)
Education
Work
Play
Leisure
Social participation

Performance Skills	Performance Patterns
Motor skills	Habits
Process skills	Routines
Communication/Interaction skills	Roles

Context	Activity Demands	Client Factors
Cultural	Objects used and their properties	Body functions
Physical	Space demands	Body structures
Social	Social demands	
Personal	Sequencing and timing	
Spiritual	Required actions	
Temporal	Required body functions	
Virtual	Required body structures	

AMERICAN OCCUPATIONAL THERAPY PRACTICE FRAMEWORK

The OT Practice Framework, adopted by the AOTA in 2002, serves as a tool to guide occupational therapists across all possible domains of practice. It is different from the Canadian Model in that it does not define the relationships among person, environment, and occupation, but rather, outlines the scope and nature of practice. Because of its broad nature, the Framework does not identify specific OT theoretical approaches but, rather, allows for each therapist to choose the occupation-based models and frames of reference that best fit the client and the practice setting. However, while some OT educators claim that the Framework is not theory-based at all, in the opinion of these authors, the document reflects many theoretical shifts in perspective that are consistent with occupation-based models published in the 1990s, such as Kielhofner's Model of Human Occupation (MOHO) (2004), Christiansen and Baum's Person-Environment-Occupation-Performance (1997; 2005), and Dunn, Brown, and McGuigan's Ecology of Human Performance (1994) models. Recent reviewers acknowledge the Framework's reflection of the philosophical and practice beliefs of the profession. They state, "the

Framework suggests that only OT theories should be used to develop practice guidelines" (Gutman, Mortera, Hinojosa, & Kramer, 2007, p. 120). The specific suggestions these authors raise for revision of the Framework document will be discussed in Chapter 4.

The OT Practice Framework consists of two parts, Domain and Process. The Domain lists six categories of engagement in occupation that encompass all of the areas with which occupational therapists are concerned. The categories include performance areas of occupation, performance skills, performance patterns, contexts, activity demands, and client factors. When compared with the *Uniform Terminology, Second Edition* (1989), containing only three occupational performance areas (work, leisure, and ADL) and a very long list of occupational performance components, this broad array of factors pertaining to the person, the activity, and the environment highlights the profession's continuing shift away from the medical model. The AOTA Practice Framework Domain is outlined in Table 2-2.

The Framework Collaborative Process Model (Figure 2-3) illustrates the way occupational therapists deliver services in collaboration with clients. The client-practitioner relationship determines the flow of evaluation, intervention, and outcome. Because this model must work for all possible

Figure 2-3. Framework Collaborative Process Model. (Adapted with permission from American Occupational Therapy Association. [2002]. *Occupational therapy practice framework.* Bethesda, MD: Author.)

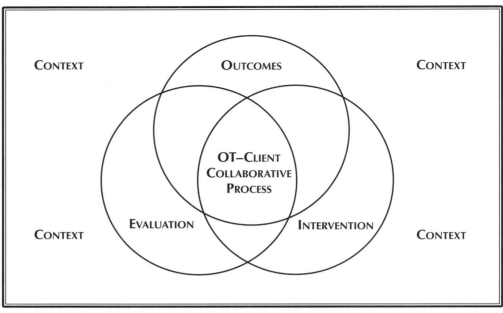

applications of OT across age spans and function-disability continuums, the Framework Process does not reflect specific frames of reference, assessments, or techniques. The occupational therapist applies specific occupation-based models (see Section II) and frames of reference (see Section III) as appropriate or needed throughout the process.

A model may be defined as a standard or example for imitation or comparison (Webster's Dictionary, 1981). The Framework Collaborative Process Model provides the profession with an example of how practice applies the theories that currently predominate science and medicine. It draws upon client-centered theory in placing the therapist–client collaboration at the center of service delivery, suggesting that the flow of evaluation, intervention, and outcome will be guided by the therapeutic relationship. It draws upon dynamical systems theory in its reflection of a nonlinear process, without a specific beginning or end. Contexts surrounding the entire therapist–client partnership have a dynamic interrelationship with client occupations, creating both facilitators and barriers to performance. A focus on occupation continues throughout the collaborative process, reflecting a holistic, top-down approach to client evaluation, intervention, and outcome. This embedded top-down approach was recently acknowledged by Gutman et al. (2007) as one in which "therapists are directed to use the occupational profile as the first step in the evaluation process" (p. 121). As such, the Framework draws upon all of the occupation-based models set forth by OT scholars near the end of the 20th century, reverting to the tradition Mary Reilly's occupational behavior theory of earlier years.

Using the Framework Model, OT professionals have no choice but to begin the service delivery process by exploring the client's occupations, their relationship to life roles, and their significance both individually and within preferred social groups (a top-down approach). It is no longer acceptable to address components of performance, such as movement, sensation, or cognition, in isolation (a bottom-up approach). Components are inseparable from engagement in tasks or activities clients view as essential to their identity, their sense of purpose, and their continued participation in whatever life situations and social roles they choose.

AOTA's decision to provide an occupation-based, rather than practice-based, model for the profession represents a fairly bold move, especially considering the persistence of medically focused reimbursement systems in the United States. Many OT practitioners struggle daily with the discrepancies between the Framework language and guidelines and the constraints of medical- or diagnosis-related documentation and reimbursement guidelines that tend to rely on the measurement of components rather than the occupational performance, satisfaction, development, and/or well-being of the individual. Perhaps the revisions suggested by Gutman et al. (2007) will result in the Framework's acknowledgment of the validity of multiple approaches that also consider the demands of a variety of practice settings.

Similarities With the Client-Centered Model

The "client-centered approach is used throughout the framework" (p. 615), and humanistic concepts are evident in the definitions of "collaborative relationship," "engagement in occupation," and "therapeutic use of self" (AOTA, 2002). The process of the Framework is described as dynamic and interactive in nature, reflecting its systems orientation. Contexts and the expanded definition of occupational performance to include the interaction of personal and environmental components are important features of both models.

Similarities with the Canadian Model may be seen in the evaluation, intervention, and outcome phases of therapy. The Canadian Model proposes the use of a "profile" of the client's occupations and issues, using a flexible and nonjudgmental format such as informal interview, which is similar to the occupational profile phase of the Framework. The intervention phase features the client–practitioner relationship as the guiding factor, which is similar to the Canadian view. The occupational performance outcome includes not only objective measurement of performance or result, but also client satisfaction with the outcome. This shift in emphasis from the measurement of function alone to the subjective judgment of the results by the client, implies that a reflective discussion of the effectiveness of therapy occurs not only at the end of treatment but all throughout the process.

Similarities in Occupational Therapy Evaluation Process

While neither system incorporates specific theories, strategies, or techniques, the Canadian Model has its own assessment tool, the COPM. This tool provides a good example and guideline for the Framework's occupational profile. Originally published in 1991, the COPM uses a semi-structured interview format to determine the occupational issues and problems from the client's perspective. Within this format, clients are asked to list their occupation problem areas, rate their own performance on a 10-point scale, and then prioritize by selecting the five areas that hold the highest importance for them. The assessment is intended for all ages and disability areas and can include caregivers, family members, teachers, and others associated with the client.

Theoretical Differences Between the CMOP and the OT Practice Framework

Some differences can also be seen in the Canadian view of the environment, which include four components (physical, cultural, social, and institutional) versus the Framework's seven contexts. The CMOP, which reflects the profession's paradigm in that country, defines the fundamental concepts of the person, occupation, and environment, and their relationship to one another (See Figure 2-1). In this regard, the CMOP may also be categorized as an *occupation-based model*, similar to those presented in Section II.* The OT Practice Framework, while acknowledging the importance of person, environment, and occupation, does not describe any specific relationship among them, leaving American occupational therapists free to choose from the multiple occupation-based models for their practice. Five of the most prominent occupation-based models are described in Section II.

LEARNING ACTIVITIES

Medical Model

1. Describe the last time you visited a doctor's office. What was the sequence of events that occurred beginning with setting up the appointment? Give all relevant details.

2. What was the medical problem that brought you there? Write a few sentences describing your signs and symptoms. How did you communicate these to the doctor?

3. How did this "medical problem" affect your ability to function in normal daily activities? Give two specific examples.

4. How well do you think the doctor's visit took care of your problem? What instructions did you get? What follow-up behaviors were expected of you as the patient? How satisfied were you with the outcome? Please explain.

5. How did your experience compare with the medical model described in this text? What was similar and what was different?

Client-Centered Model

1. Choose one of the following health conditions for the purpose of this exercise:
   o A broken wrist
   o A severe asthma condition
   o Chronic pain in your lower back
   o Social phobia (fear of public speaking, socializing)

2. Look up the diagnosis on the internet or in your textbooks, and write a paragraph describing it in medical terms. How is this condition typically treated within the medical model?

3. Discuss how this health condition might impact the tasks, activities, and occupations of your own life. Describe five problems with engagement in occupations that would likely cause you the most difficulty, and prioritize them according to their importance for you.

4. Assume you are seeking expert advice as client. Identify three "experts" you would choose, and write one paragraph on each, including a) how you would describe or present your problem to them, b) what information you would ask them to provide, and

---

The CMOP will not be repeated in Section II but may also be considered an occupation-based model and may be included in the analysis assignment in Chapter 11.

c) how you would define your relationship with this "professional" from a client's perspective.

Defining the Human Spirit

1. *Definition.* How would you define the human spirit for yourself? Your definition can include any of the following: philosophy of life, core values or beliefs, guidance from a higher power, your purpose in life, your life's work, what motivates you, words you live by, your lifetime goals, or what might be the "nucleus" of life for you.

2. *Life occupations.* Write a few paragraphs describing some of the activities, occupations, or tasks that you perceive as enacting or enhancing your life's purpose or work. What three activities would you choose as the most meaningful for you and how are they related to your spiritual self?

3. *Application in OT.* How might your understanding of the human spirit help you in your work with clients. What is the importance of the spiritual dimension in the client-centered practice model?

REFERENCES

American Occupational Therapy Association. (2002). *Occupational therapy practice framework.* Bethesda, MD: Author.

Canadian Occupational Therapy Association. (1997). *Canadian occupational performance measure* (3rd ed.). Ottawa, CA: Author.

Capra, F. (1982). *The turning point: Society and the rising culture.* New York: Simon & Schuster.

Christiansen, C. H. (1999). Defining lives: Occupation as identity: An essay on competence, coherence, and the creation of meaning. *American Journal of Occupational Therapy, 53,* 547–558.

Christiansen, C., & Baum, C. (1997). *Occupational therapy: Enabling function and well-being.* Thorofare, NJ: SLACK Incorporated.

Christiansen, C., & Baum, C. (2005). Person-Environment-Occupation-Performance: An occupation based framework for practice. In C. Christiansen & C. Baum (Eds.), *Occupational therapy: Performance, participation, and well-being* (pp. 242–266). Thorofare, NJ: SLACK Incorporated.

Clark, F. (1993). Occupation embedded in a real life: Interweaving occupational science and occupational therapy. *American Journal of Occupational Therapy, 47*(12),1067–1077.

Corey, G. (1994). *Theory and practice of group counseling* (4th ed.). Pacific Grove, CA: Brooks/Cole Publishing.

Dixon, S. (1987). *Working with people in crisis* (2nd ed.). St. Louis: Mosby.

Dunn, W., Brown, C., & McGuigan, A. (1994). The ecology of human performance: A framework for considering the effect of context. *American Journal of Occupational Therapy, 48,* 595–607.

Gutman, S. A., Mortera, M. H., Hinojosa, J., & Kramer, P. (2007). The issue is: Revision of the Occupational Therapy Practice Framework. *American Journal of Occupational Therapy, 61,* 119–126.

Kielhofner, G. (2004). *Conceptual foundations of occupational therapy* (3rd ed.). Philadelphia: FA Davis.

Law, M., & Mills, J. (1998). Client-centered occupational therapy. In M. Law (Ed.), *Client-centered occupational therapy.* Thorofare, NJ: SLACK Incorporated.

Law, M., Cooper, B., Strong, Stewart, D., Rigby, P., & Letts, L. (1997). A theoretical context for the practice of occupational therapy. In C. Christiansen & C. Baum (Eds.), *Occupational therapy: Achieving human performance needs in daily living* (2nd ed.). Thorofare, NJ: SLACK Incorporated.

Maslow, A. H. (1968). *Toward a psychology of being.* (Revised ed.). New York, NY: Van Nostrand Reinhold.

McColl, M., & Pranger, T. (1994). Theory and practice in the occupational therapy guidelines for client-centered practice. *Canadian Journal of Occupational Therapy, 61,* 250–259.

Meyer, A. (1921, 1983). The philosophy of occupational therapy. *Occupational Therapy in Mental Health, 2,* 79–87. Original 192

Nelson, D. (1997). Why the profession of occupational therapy will flourish in the 21st century. 1996 Eleanor Clarke Slagle lecture. *American Journal of Occupational Therapy, 51,* 11–24.

Polatajko, H. (1992). Naming and framing occupational therapy: A lecture dedicated to the life of Nancy B. *Canadian Journal of Occupational Therapy, 59,* 189–200.

Reilly, M. (1984). The issue is: The importance of the client versus patient issue for occupational therapy. *American Journal of Occupational Therapy, 38,* 404–406.

Rogers, C. (1961). *On becoming a person.* Boston: Houghton Mifflin.

Rogers, C. (1951). *Client-centered therapy.* Boston: Houghton-Mifflin.

Rosenfeld, M. (1997). Theory and practice in evaluation and treatment. In R. Rosenfeld (Ed.), *Motivational strategies in geriatric rehabilitation.* Bethesda, MD: American Occupational Therapy Association.

Scaffa, M. (2001). Community-based practice: Occupation-in-context. In M. Scaffa (Ed.), *Occupational therapy in community based practice settings* (pp. 3–18). Philadelphia, PA: FA Davis.

Urbanowski, R., & Vargo, J. (1994). Spirituality, daily practice, and the occupational performance model. *Canadian Journal of Occupational Therapy, 61,* 88–94.

Watanabe, S. G. (1967). The developing role of occupational therapy in psychiatric home service. *American Journal of Occupational Therapy, 21,* 353–356.

Webster's Dictionary. (1981). *Webster's new collegiate dictionary.* Springfield, MA: Merriam

World Health Organization. (1980). *International classification of impairment, disability, and handicap.* Geneva: Author

World Health Organization. (2001). *International classification of functioning, disability, and health.* Geneva: Author.

Chapter 3

APPLIED SYSTEMS THEORY
IN OCCUPATIONAL THERAPY

"The whole is more than the sum of its parts."

– ARISTOTLE

The purpose of this chapter is to define how systems theory has influenced occupational therapy (OT) practice. A description of the foundational concepts of general systems theory (von Bertalanffy, 1968, 1969) will initially be described to increase knowledge and provide a basic understanding for future application. Concepts from general systems theory may be found in the American Occupational Therapy Association (AOTA) OT Practice Framework (AOTA, 2002), the client-centered practice model (Law, Baptiste, Carswell, et al., 1998), and various other OT models including Model of Human Occupation (MOHO) (Kielhofner, 1978, 1980a, 1980b), Ecology of Human Performance (Dunn, Brown, & McGuigan, 1994), Occupational Adaptation (Schkade & Schultz, 1992; Schultz & Schkade, 1992), and Person-Environment-Occupation-Performance Model (Baum & Christiansen, 2005). This chapter will specifically look at how general systems theory is evident within the seven contexts of practice as defined in the OT Practice Framework. The reader will come to appreciate how a systems view offers occupational therapists a broad and holistic perspective for both health and disability awareness in practice today.

GENERAL SYSTEMS THEORY

Systems theory helps us to understand how things interact. Ludwig von Bertalanffy, a Hungarian biologist, founded the science of general systems theory (1968). This theory represented a paradigm shift in history, for von Bertalanffy reacted strongly to the reductionistic thinking of his day. While he had constructed his theory about systems as early as 1936, he hesitated to publicly present it until 1948. As with the introduction of any new theory, von Bertalanffy recognized that his thinking would be met with a good degree of skepticism. Therefore, he waited for the political climate to be more receptive to his different views. Until this point in time, scientists had tried to understand the human body by analyzing its parts or elements

(i.e., cells, organs, molecules, etc.). In effect, the human body was reduced into its component parts or units for scientific study, like one would view a machine. As previously described in both Chapters 1 and 2, this thinking is called reductionism and is defined as the idea that all phenomena can be reduced to scientific explanations. An example of this type of thinking in today's healthcare environment is the medical model.

In parallel fashion, history has revealed to us how the profession of OT has also undergone a much needed paradigm shift. Kielhofner was one of the first occupational therapists to identify how systems theory might positively influence practice. In Kielhofner's (1978) article, "General Systems Theory: Implications for Theory and Action in Occupational Therapy," he wrote that systems theory "… represents a new conceptual structuring of reality; it is an emerging paradigm of all science that will transform the former paradigm of reductionism" (p. 637). Two years later, Kielhofner and his colleagues published the MOHO (1980a, 1980b; Kielhoffner & Burke, 1880), a direct example of how systems theory could serve as a foundational framework for OT practice. The launching of MOHO was the profession's first attempt to promote a holistic perspective for treatment by an occupational therapist. Kielhofner offset the reductionistic thinking that had become so prevalent in OT practice and introduced the prospect of a broader conceptual model for practice. He stated that the "larger units of reality for occupational therapy under a systems framework are the human career, the social role, ecology, competency, and fitness for social participation" (Kielhofner, 1978, p. 638). The reductionistic approaches of OT did not embrace these areas of practice at all. However, the OT Practice Framework has embedded these components as a common standard of practice for today's health care world.

HOLISM

Von Bertalanffy opposed the idea of reductionism. In contrasting view to his colleagues at the time, his thinking focused on the relations between the parts that connect into a whole (von Bertalanffy, 1968) rather than the separate parts themselves. His systems theory included the view of holism, which is the antithesis of reductionism. Holism reflects the idea that entities cannot be explained nor understood from their separate parts or properties but only when regarded as an entire configuration. Holism offered an appreciation of human beings, focusing on their interdependency with one another and with the environment. One of the principles of general systems theory is that we can only understand the *whole* by regarding the links, interactions, and processes among the parts that make up the entire system. In effect, system's theorists expanded on the notion begun by Aristotle, who originally proposed a system view of life.

Within the profession of OT, a split occurred among practitioners in the late 1970s and 1980s. Kielhofner and his colleagues introduced the MOHO (1980a, 1980b) as a new wave of thinking and ultimately a contrasting view to practice. However, many occupational therapists continued to practice within the reductionistic paradigm of medicine rather than embracing this holistic model for conceptual thinking. Specializations in OT practice continued to be a popular trend. For example, it was common for occupational therapists to identify themselves as specialists in physical disability, mental health, pediatrics, geriatrics, and hands. While specialization enhanced the development of new modalities and technology in its respective areas, it also distracted us away from a holistic view of practice. The profession of OT eventually entered into an identity crisis as we found ourselves evolving further and further away from our professional roots (more fully described in Chapter 1). It was not until the 1990s that OT embarked on a mission of restoration and re-institution of the profession's holistic view of mankind and the value of occupation. This restoration process led to the emergence of new practice models that are discussed in Section II. Today's health care standards support that entry-level graduates from OT programs identify themselves as generalists among various practice domains rather than as specialists of one particular medical practice area.

CORE CONCEPTS OF SYSTEMS THEORY

Organismic biology and open systems thinking were two existing views that highly influenced von Bertalanffy in the development of general systems theory (Nichols, 1984). Organismic biology may be defined as the notion of organized wholes and the relationships among organs, cells, molecules, etc. rather than their separate parts. The

second construct to influence von Bertalanffy was the view of living organisms as open systems. This means that living organisms are influenced, exist, and are maintained by the following forces: 1) information or input that enters the system; 2) behaviors, thoughts, and reactions, called output, that result from internal processing of the input; and 3) feedback that comes from the environment about these behaviors, thoughts, reactions, and their consequences for other parts of the system.

An *open system* means that there is a constant interchange of information, energies, and materials with one's environment. An open system is constantly in motion and constantly changing. In other words, it is dynamic. Open systems are regulated by feedback, which can be positive or negative. A significant principle to the concept of open systems is the notion that any change in one part of a system will automatically alter the whole (Rapaport, 1986). This dynamic is often observed in family systems when one person becomes sick and everyone in the family is affected by that person's illness experience. The family typically experiences a period of imbalance as habits, routines, rituals, and interactive patterns are altered.

Von Bertalanffy believed that there are natural laws of organization governing systems on all levels of existence (von Bertalanffy, 1968). He attempted to unify science by suggesting that there are common principles amongst the various and different sciences (biology, psychology, physics, etc). Von Bertalanffy (1968) also believed that general system laws can be applied to any system of a particular type, irrespective of the particular properties of the systems and elements. Von Bertalanffy defined a *system* as follows:

1. A whole that functions as a whole by virtue of the interaction of its parts

2. An entity that is greater than the sum of its parts because it consists of 1) parts, 2) the way the parts act together, and 3) the qualities that emerge from these relationships

3. Anything physical, biological, psychological, sociological, or symbolic

4. An entity that can be static, mechanical, mechanically self-regulating, or organismically interactive with the environment

5. An entity with a hierarchy* to organize its complexity

A practitioner who provides interventions from a system perspective uses a different set of lenses to view the client than a practitioner who uses a reductionistic perspective such as the medical model. Let us look at each of the five principles of von Bertalanffy's system and directly apply it to how a health care practitioner may analyze a prospective client.

---

*In some applications of systems theory, a more dynamical interaction replaces the hierarchy. For example, in the human brain, a more flexible model of neural organization in which functions of control and coordination are distributed among many elements of the system rather than a single hierarchical level has been proposed (VanSant, 1991; Law, Missiuna, Pollock, & Stewart, 2005). More information about OT applications of dynamic systems theory will be discussed in subsequent chapters on motor learning (Chapter 19) and Toglia's dynamic interactional model (Chapter 15). The reader will also find more information about heterarchy in Chapter 7.

FIVE COMPONENTS OF SYSTEM THINKING: AN ILLUSTRATION

1. To illustrate the concept of the "whole" consisting of the interaction of its parts, let us use a typical system of health care. The "whole" can be exemplified by the Department of Mental Health and Addiction Services (DMHAS). The component parts of this system typically include inpatient services, outpatient services, addiction services, rehabilitation services, legal services, and social services, clubhouse models, and medical services including crisis intervention. The success of this health care system (whole) is dependent on the integration and synthesis of each component and its related service. It is common for a client to participate in multiple services at one time as a means to attain a long-term goal of healthy mental health functioning.

2. The mental health system is more that the sum of its parts, however. Two parts of DMHAS are 1) rehabilitation services, where one would typically find occupational therapists, and 2) medical services, managed by medical doctors and/or nurse practitioners. The manner in which these two parts interact will ultimately impact the client's level of care. For example, the client will have to make and keep appointments within each department and schedule times that do not overlap each other. A client will also hopefully integrate the benefits gained from each service to maintain an overall sense of well-being. The quality of care for a client is highly influenced by how well the services coordinate, complement, and integrate their various goals and objectives. Some of these outcome goals may be similar, while others are likely to be different. DMHAS, as a whole, has an overarching "mission statement" designed to represent and synthesize all of the purposes, values, and standards of each service. A client would likely report that he had a "good experience" if all of the related services met his expectations and he was able to reach his overall goals. However, if one service failed to meet the client's goals, he may perceive his entire experience as negative. Let us say that a client experiences major side effects with his medications (medical service) on a given day. This medication issue will likely affect his performance in rehab that day. For example, the client may refuse to participate in OT because he is not feeling "right" from his medication.

3. Practitioners and clients may directly or indirectly interface with multiple types of systems. Here are some examples to clarify the different types of systems identified by von Bertalanffy. The human body, in part, is composed of *biological* systems such as circulatory, digestive, neurological, and musculoskeletal. Practitioners and clients engage in various *societal groups* such as health care teams, families, church congregations, and health fitness clubs. *Mechanical* systems such as heating and air conditioning, a motor vehicle, or a computer make our lives more comfortable and manageable. Some of us also participate in a type of *symbolic* system that consists of an invisible bond or commitment among its members. Examples of symbolic systems include relief organizations (Red Cross), a community of scholars such as Ivy League, student clubs such as fraternities and sororities, and spiritual organizations such as the Knights of Columbus.

4. Systems have different qualities. A thermostat is an example of a mechanical self regulating system—once a certain temperature is set, the mechanism will initiate the controls to regulate heating and cooling to maintain that temperature. A mixture of chemicals in a sealed vial is an example of a closed system—there is no external source that can affect the process once it is sealed shut. For example, when a child shakes a snow globe, the particles move around making them look like "snow," but eventually they return to their original state—nothing has substantially changed. Human beings are open systems because we constantly interact with our environment, which in turn, affects our internal state of health and well-being. Occupation therapists directly apply this principle whenever we expect our clients to modify their behavior based on the positive and/or negative feedback that they receive from their environment.

5. There must be a hierarchy to create a sense of order within a system. A hierarchy is composed of separate levels or steps within a particular sequence. Each level is made up of various component parts. The levels interact in a particular order to create a designated outcome. The component parts of each level may be concrete (tangible) or symbolic (abstract); outcomes can also be visible or invisible in nature. A popular way to show a hierarchy is by pyramid design. Practitioners often refer to these depictions as a top-down or bottom-up approach. In a top-down approach, the highest level in a hierarchy will influence all the lower parts. An example of a top-down hierarchical approach is an organizational chart of a corporation that shows who is in charge on the highest level (chief executive officer) and who reports to whom in descending order. An example of a hierarchy that reflects a bottom-up approach is Maslow's hierarchy of needs theory. Maslow's pyramid demonstrates a set of levels depicting how persons seek to satisfy one set of needs before reaching the other. Beginning at the lowest level (physiological needs), a person will eventually achieve a sense of self-actualization (top tier) if they satisfy all of their needs in a progressive manner.

It is easier for practitioners to understand how a hierarchy works if the component parts are visible and concrete (i.e., like assembling the parts of a wheelchair). However, human beings consist of variables that we cannot always see (emotions). This does not mean that the variables do not exist. Within a family system, relationship levels are symbolic and, therefore, not overtly seen. The parent(s) in a family should be the executor(s), or top level of a hierarchy, whose task it is to create a sense of order for the family. Without a designated person or persons "in charge" to fulfill this role, chaos and confusion will emerge within the system. Families who have a faulty hierarchy structure become symptomatic.

For example, if a child acts like the head of his family and shares equal power with the parent(s), this child will eventually develop signs of stress over time from trying to fulfill a role that is not typical of him. An occupational therapist who works in pediatric home care may directly observe a child's disruption in occupations created by this role dysfunction.

HIERARCHY VERSUS HETERARCHY

A recent adaptation to the notion of hierarchy for OT practice has been brought to our attention by Kielhofner. Kelso and Tuller (1984) recognized a difference among the hierarchical nature of machines versus human systems. The internal parts of a living organism arrange themselves in "order" by cooperating together in a flexible and dynamic manner rather than in a fixed, predictable order. For example, within the human structure, body systems (circulatory, digestive, etc.), cognitive reasoning (decision making, concentration, etc.), and emotions (feelings) don't always interact in the same, predictable order every time. The situation at hand (context) may require that one component take the lead over another component. Could you imagine how difficult it would be if your body put you in a fight or flight mode every time you sat down to relax and read a book? Therefore, when the context (situation and environment) influences the order of sequence needed by internal systems to yield a certain response or outcome, this process is called adaptive. It would be appropriate for your body to react in fight or flight mode if the situation or context you were in consisted of danger. It would not be adaptive of your body to put you in fight or flight mode if you were in a situation that required relaxation such as going to sleep in your bed. The components within a living system function best if they can arrange themselves to fit the situation. This arrangement of order for living systems with its cooperative nature is called a heterarchy as opposed to a hierarchy.

Let us compare heterarchy and hierarchy. The major difference between these two principles is that hierarchies have fixed and predictable patterns that are predetermined while heterarchies have flexible and adaptable patterns to best suit the context or situation. The similarity between the two is that a sense of order must be established to avoid chaos. This sense of order is predetermined in hierarchy but not in heterarchy. In the earlier example of a hierarchy, it was discussed how an organizational chart demonstrated the principle of hierarchy (i.e., communication patterns are maintained at fixed levels that must occur in a specific order). Therefore, a technical worker (bottom level of the hierarchy) could not expect to report to the chief executive officer (top level of the hierarchy) because he would be breaking the rules of order for communication within that corporation. Instead, the technical worker will have to report to his supervisor/manager who is one level above him.

According to Kielhofner (2002), heterarchy is shown throughout human occupations: "When we consider any thought, emotion, or action, the parts of the human being and environment cooperate together according to local conditions created by what each element brings to the total dynamic" (p. 35). Living systems are open, flexible, and capable of an adaptive response, evident when adjustments are made to fit a desired outcome. Systems that are fixed or closed, evident when parts are lacking or incapable of reordering themselves to the desired outcome, will result in dysfunction or faulty operations.

Complex Systems and Chaos Theory

Complex systems theory, an outgrowth of general systems theory, is defined by Holland et al. (1990) as the new science of complexity that describes emergence, adaptation, and self-organization, all of general systems' principles. System dynamics is a method for understanding dynamic behavior of complex systems. This involves the identification of multifaceted interrelationships among system components, while recognizing that not all properties of the whole can be understood through analysis. Social dynamics in families and communities, and occupational performance within multiple and changing contexts, are examples of complex systems. In human systems, occupation can be viewed as dynamic for organizing multiple components within interrelated systems.

Chaos theory, another offshoot of systems theory, was defined by Royeen as dynamic systems or interwoven forces and motions of nonlinear systems (2003). She states that "even in cases of extreme disorder, what appears as chaos actually has an underlying order" (p. 613). Let us consider how chaos theory can be applied to a client who has dysfunctional daily living patterns. Occupational therapists would typically begin by assessing the person, the daily living occupations, and the environment wherein these activities take place. The outcome goal would likely be to restore a sense of healthy balance to this client's routines and habits in daily living. However, the intervention *process* of restoring a sense of balance to a person's life is extremely complex. If the practitioner attempts to intervene in a linear fashion by modifying person variables first, occupation variables secondly, and contextual variables third, the solution is unlikely to result in a therapeutic change. Unbeknownst to the practitioner, there is an interactive effect of the person, occupation, and environment variables that cannot be seen nor understood by isolating them one by one. The occupational therapist must first understand and analyze how these variables interactively led to chaotic behaviors by observing the "whole" process. Then the practitioner could begin to experiment with a different arrangement of this pattern by altering sequences (heterarchy) of the various components and modifying variables until a healthy balance is restored.

The term *chaos theory* was publicized by Lorenz (1980), a meteorologist who identified sensitivity to initial conditions, commonly known as the butterfly effect, as the variable that explains the unpredictable nature of weather conditions. What is true for weather predictions may also apply to the outcomes of our occupational interventions. Royeen suggests that chaos theory could possibly be used to unify divergent aspects of occupational science and OT (2003).

In summary, a practitioner who uses a holistic and systemic view of practice recognizes that a client is part of many systems (biological, family, social, etc.) that are dynamic and complex. A multitude of variables will have influence over his or her behavior. A client's present lifestyle and existence is an outcome based on a long and complex history including variables that are both visible and invisible to the observer. There exist many forms of input and feedback from a client's environment that have led to his or her occupational performance. From a system perspective, an OT practitioner would take the time to evaluate the client's habits, routines, and role behaviors by observing the whole process rather than breaking it down into separate isolated parts. There is not "one thing" that has created the presenting problem for a given client but rather a series of forces that have contributed to the client's present state of being. Feedback has both positive and negative influences on a person's behavior. Therapeutic change is a continuous process and not an event that happens at one point in time, such as one session or one therapy group. The client's "problem" will not be truly understood if one employs linear reasoning as an attempt to fit events and behaviors into the equation $A + B = C$ (cause and effect thinking). Client behaviors are viewed as a complex outcome of interactive variables that change over time.

Impact of General Systems theory

The impact of general systems theory has been vast and significant. Its supporters believe in its inherent humanistic and ethical qualities. Von Bertalanffy was concerned with the meaning of life and the interconnectedness that exists among various entities, such as the relationship between humanity and the physical environment. As a therapeutic perspective, it guides the practitioner to appreciate the complexities of human behavior and invites the health care provider to *think outside of the box*.

The 1990s offered a new approach to practice that is based on system and holistic theory with distinctive interventions for occupational therapists. The occupational performance models identify and define the inter-relationship of multiple systems, including various elements of the person, the environment, and occupation. These models focus on the central role of occupation in human life and in society, providing support for the fundamental tenets of OT as a profession. The reader will find a thorough explanation of these concepts in Section II.

A recent application of systems theory is clearly evident in the OT Practice Framework (AOTA, 2002). The process diagram of intersecting circles describes the system of OT service delivery in which the client–therapist relationship moves through cyclical phases of evaluation, intervention, and outcome within multiple contexts. In the professional interaction, these elements are never viewed as separate from one another.

The OT Practice Framework demonstrates a constructionist or postmodern philosophy of science, in which reality is "constructed dependent on context and socially based" (Stewart & Law, 2003, p.5). Within the systems that make up the world around us, multiple realities exist, each one emerging from the person's own subjective experience. The shift from objective to subjective realities is a part of the overall paradigm shift that has occurred in a wide range of disciplines including the basic sciences, occupational science, health care, and OT. The client's subjective reality becomes the focus of OT, giving further theoretical support for the value of client-centered practice. More about these aspects of the OT Practice Framework is addressed in other chapters.

A systems perspective is further implied by the OT Framework's stated outcome of OT services, the "engagement in occupation to support participation in context" (AOTA, 2002, p. 611). This suggests that therapists enable clients to engage in occupations that help them to effectively interact within multiple systems. Systems that incorporate specific client roles may be called contexts. The OT Framework defines contexts as "a variety of inter-related conditions within and surrounding the client that influence performance" (AOTA, 2002, p. 623). The seven contexts listed in the OT Framework domain are cultural, physical, social, personal, spiritual, temporal, and virtual.

Contexts as Subjective Systems

The contexts that influence performance are unique for each client. This section will focus on how these contexts may be identified, defined, and evaluated. The categories of

Figure 3-1. Levels of Context according to Spencer. (Adapted from Bronfenbrenner, U. [1993]. Toward an experimental ecology of human development: Research models and fugitive findings. In R. H. Wozniak & K. W. Fischer [Eds.], *Development in context: Acting and thinking in specific environments* [pp. 3–44]. New York, NY: Erlbaum.)

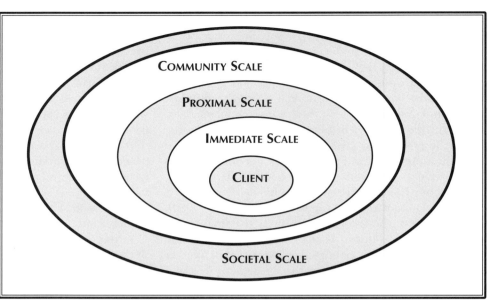

context to be addressed vary with each theorist, although the OT Practice Framework includes the largest number, seven.

According to Spencer (2003), consideration of context represents a systems (as opposed to individual) approach to disability, a view that is shared by the International Classification of Function (ICF) (WHO, 2001).

Four Levels of Context

Spencer defines four scales or levels of context, which might be viewed as concentric circles (Figure 3-1), beginning with the individual at the center:

1. Immediate Contexts

Immediate contexts include the client and his immediate surroundings such as work area, home environments, and caregiver–client relationships. The concept of interacting systems applies to the human open system and the immediate effects of feedback on a client's occupational performance. Evaluating immediate contexts is best accomplished by observing specific task performance within the client's natural environment.

2. Proximal Scale Contexts

Proximal scale contexts are the next concentric circle, which includes frequently encountered behavior settings, such as home, office, classroom, and clinic. Here, the client interacts within the systems of work settings, educational systems, family systems, and health care systems.

3. Community Scale Contexts

Community scale contexts include geographic neighborhoods and communities known to the client. In the community contexts, clients encounter transportation systems,

local social and political systems, religious group systems, and economic systems such as banking and marketing.

4. Societal Scale Contexts

Societal scale contexts include public policies, widely held beliefs and attitudes, and major social institutions. Clients may interact with the Medicare or welfare systems, insurance systems, and national political and legal systems. Thus, each context has multiple levels. As a general postulate, the smaller scale contexts are easier to influence than the larger scale contexts. Each scale implies different strategies for adaptation and change in order to overcome barriers to participation for clients with disabilities (and others). As scale expands, the complexity and number of systems encountered also increases, making the larger scale contexts more difficult to evaluate.

Seven Contexts of the OT Practice Framework

Physical Contexts

Physical contexts are defined in the OT Practice Framework as "nonhuman aspects of contexts, including accessibility to and performance within environments having natural terrain, plants, animals, buildings, furniture, objects, tools, or devices" (AOTA, p. 623). The term *nonhuman* narrows this category, which normally includes environmental factors such as supplies and equipment used when performing a task; properties such as light, temperature, and workspace; and other physical features of the task environment. Many evaluation tools for evaluating home safety, for example, suggest that occupational therapists often consider proximal physical contexts when assessing a client's occupational performance. The emergence of the *universal design* concept represents a public health movement that encourages the design of products and environments that make occupational performance easier for everyone regardless of age, physical fitness, or health status. The concept of universal design represents an intersection of physical context with systems such as building codes and construction guidelines, ergonomics, assistive technology, laws such as those concerning human rights, and public policy such as the independent living movement (Ringaert, 2003). Recent legislation has fueled the independent living concept, which moves persons with disability into communities to enable social participation with nondisabled persons.

Another recent perspective on physical context is the concept of place as a component of self identity. Rowles (2003) alludes to the blending of person, place, and human experience, a holistic view in which client and physical context are inseparable. Rowles differentiates *place* from *space* or objective physical environment based on patterns of use and emotional connections. A place may be individually defined or shared with others, such as a childhood home shared by family members or a high school for members of a graduating class. "The spaces of our life become transformed into places of our life through a variety of physical, cognitive, emotional, and imaginative processes of habituation that imbue existence with meaning and personal significance" (Rowles, 2003, p. 115). Thus, the experiences within specific places become, over time, a part of one's identity. This connection of person, context, and occupation illustrates Schkade and McClung's view of contexts as *occupational environments*, which call for an occupational response (p. 23). The terms context and environment are not interchangeable.

Social Contexts

Systems theory helps us understand the multiple levels of social context. Social context, according to the practice framework, includes "the availability and expectations of significant individuals, such as spouse, friends, and caregivers. [It] also includes larger social groups that are influential in establishing norms, role expectations, and social routines" (AOTA, p. 623).

Many theorists have described the social systems within which our clients perform occupations. Bronfenbrenner defined three dimensions of social systems, which he called "levels of environmental analysis" (Bronfenbrenner, 1993). They are *macrosystems*, a societal level that establishes public policy, *mesosystems*, or local environments that clients frequent in the course of carrying out social activities and fulfilling roles, and *microsystems*, which are the client's immediate living environments where daily social activities are performed with family and friends. Similarly, Spencer (2003) uses the terms immediate, proximal, community, and societal levels to categorize contexts (Table 3-1).

Another way to understand social contexts is through the concept of *social roles*. Social psychologists (e.g., Sullivan and Mead) have defined roles as positions in society having expected responsibilities and privileges. Christiansen

and Baum (1997) define a role as a "set of behaviors that have some socially agreed upon function, and for which there is an expected code of norms" (p. 603). Occupational Therapists often use roles as a way of organizing a client's occupations. For example, the role of "mother" carries with it care-giving tasks such as helping children bathe and dress, fixing meals, and doing laundry. It also implies more subtle expectations such as setting safe limits on the child's behavior and planning educational experiences that encourage both learning and socialization.

A related concept is role competence, meaning that tasks of a given social role are performed according to the expectations of a client's social group. For example, a car salesman is expected to meet a certain quota set by the organization for which he or she works. Tasks within this work role might be finding or attracting customers, persuading them to buy a car, collecting payment, and arranging for product delivery or installation. Roles may also be understood as the things a person must do to contribute to the goal of an entire group. Many work groups represent team efforts, within which each person does what he or she does best. For example, each faculty member of an OT department teaches subjects about which he or she has developed expertise in order to meet the common goal of preparing students for an entire range of practice areas. Benne and Sheats (1948) identified three types of group roles: 1) task roles such as initiator and recorder, which help the group to accomplish its task; 2) group maintenance roles, such as energizer and harmonizer, which help the group to communicate and function as a team; and 3) individual roles, such as aggressor or blocker, which serve the individual member at the expense of the group. Work groups might be considered mesosystems, which flow smoothly in accomplishing goals when each member performs according to his or her expected role. Effective role performance within a group or system is called role reciprocity.

Social support is an important dimension of social context. The OT Practice Framework definition of social context implies several levels of social support. On an immediate level, caregivers and family members provide support for client occupational performance. Caregiver attitude has a profound influence on client occupational performance (Spencer, 2003). Ideally, caregivers enable clients to perform tasks independently and/or to work toward a desired goal. However, if caregiver attitude is critical or judgmental, a social barrier may be created. Within a systems perspective, both client and caregiver may need support, and the therapist can fulfill this need. For example, an occupational therapist can enable a family member to plan needed adaptations to the home environment to increase client safety, security, and function.

Proximal social contexts, according to Spencer (2003), include the social systems of classroom, workplace, and clinic. Each of these mesosystems has its own set of norms (rules), roles (expectations), and standards (goals). Here, the social and cultural contexts overlap in creating environments that can either enable or disable participation for

		Table 3-1		
		Examples of Scales for Context		
Context	**Immediate Scale**	**Proximal Scale**	**Community Scale**	**Societal Scale**
Physical	Wheelchair; adaptive devices; ergonomic chair	Computer workstation; access ramp	Parks, beaches, restaurants, athletic clubs, etc.	Public transportation; handicap parking
Social	Caregivers; spouse; family interactions	Extended family role; work role	Service agency; social support network	Attitudes toward diversity/disability; social stigmas
Cultural	Household culture; style of clothing; choice of foods; mealtimes	Classroom/work routines; appropriate behavior in public	Restaurant dining; dating behaviors; holiday celebrations	Language of personhood; acceptance of diversity; rights of individuals
Personal	Gender roles; place of residence; marital status	Age, income level, financial resources	Educational status, position	Socioeconomic status; class
Spiritual	Sense of well-being; satisfaction	Enacting values, meaning in everyday activities	Religious gatherings, rituals, and traditions	Patriotism; broad belief systems; youth culture
Temporal	Time of day; duration; daily schedule	Age groups; seasons; annual goals	Transitions or marker events (i.e., graduation)	Life stages, separation, and individuation
Virtual	Telephone, cell phone, e-mail, and pagers; use of software and computer games	Virtual home visits, providing information via video, television, or radio; use of the Internet to gather information	Online banking and shopping; computer chat rooms, bulletin boards, mailing lists, and networks	Internet use; posting information on websites; reaching large numbers of people via WWW

Adapted from Spencer, J. C. (2003). Evaluation of performance contexts. In E. Crepeau, E. Cohn, & B. Boyt Schell (Eds.), Willard & Spackman's occupational therapy *(10th ed.). Baltimore, MD: Lippincott, Williams & Wilkins.*

the client. For example, students' stress level may increase with competitiveness in the classroom. The occupational therapist may recommend encouraging cooperation among students to decrease their anxiety, thereby increasing self efficacy and occupational performance.

Community level social contexts include social networks, community organizations, and agencies that provide services for those with special needs. Societal level includes public policies, such as Americans with Disabilities Act, Social Security and Medicare laws, and prevailing social attitudes such as ageism and social stigma.

Cultural Context

What comes to mind when you hear the word culture? Many people associate culture with race or ethnic background. For example, the university where the authors teach sponsors a monthly event called "multicultural Mondays," which features foods, traditions, decorations, and speakers from different parts of the world. This view represents only one small part of cultural context. Wells and Black (2000) define culture as the "sum total of a way of living, including values, beliefs, standards, linguistic expression, patterns of thinking, behavioral norms, and styles of communication that influence behaviors of a group of people and are

transmitted from generation to generation" (p. 279). On an international student experience in Costa Rica, OT students were asked to interview clients and to learn about the cultural differences between their country and ours. However, when students asked clients directly to "tell me about your culture," the clients did not know what to say. The students learned from this a valuable lesson, that most people take their own culture for granted. It consists of the sum total of what they consider to be normal. This is why occupational therapists need to be aware of their own culture and to develop sensitivity for subtle cultural differences in order to avoid making false assumptions about clients. Culture tends to be invisible and elusive, while having a pervasive effect on one's engagement in occupation and participation in life.

Cultural and social contexts have many points of overlap. Every social system or group has a unique culture that all of its members share. The OT Practice Framework defines cultural context as "customs, beliefs, activity patterns, and expectations by the society of which the individual is a member. [It also] includes political aspects such as laws that affect access to resources and affirm personal rights. [It] also includes opportunities for education, employment, and economic support" (AOTA, 2002). This rather broad definition implies several levels of context.

On an individual level, culture may best be observed within a person's lifestyle. As occupational therapists, we make the assumption that our clients choose occupational roles and perform occupations that enact the values and beliefs of their culture. The way they socialize, interact with others, and plan and structure their time, in fact, their entire way of life, all are culturally based. Culture may not be visible, but when we recommend some actions or behaviors that are in conflict with our client's culture, an ethical dilemma may be the result.

Proximal scale cultural contexts, according to Spencer (2003), exist in the work place, classroom, and clinic. One way to discover the culture of the workplace is by doing a worker role interview. Questions focus on the unique tools and techniques, language or jargon, ways of communicating, and daily structure of a particular job. How one defines success or failure in occupational performance is particularly significant in defining cultural context. For example, success in the classroom may be defined by gold stars, letter grades, verbal praise, or the successful completion of specific tasks. Failure may result in poor grades, parent conferences, revoking of privileges, or detention. Cultural context determines what is acceptable or unacceptable behavior within a given social group.

Community scale cultural contexts may be observed while the client performs occupations within community settings. What are some occupations that are typically performed in the community? Things like shopping, banking, eating out, playing golf, and attending church may come to mind. Krefting (1989) studied persons with head injury living in the community and concluded that the culture of the community may not readily include persons with disabilities.

Societal level cultural context includes specific rights and responsibilities. How one defines a "good citizen" will describe the expected norms of American culture. For example, every good citizen should be well informed about local issues, vote for the most qualified candidate, and perform some sort of community service. Prevailing attitudes concerning disability, or in fact, any type of diversity, define societal level social context. Haller (1995) looked at how the media (e.g., movies, television, newspapers, books) represented persons with disability. He defined the following eight models: 1) Medical model—sick, disfigured; 2) Social pathology model—disadvantaged, needing more support; 3) "Superscript" model—performing superhuman feats in spite of disability; 4) Business model—costly to society; 5) Minority civil rights model—members of a disabled group are denied civil rights; 6) Legal model—illegal to treat persons with disability in certain ways; 7) Cultural pluralism model—multifaceted individuals with disabilities do not receive undue attention; and 8) Consumer model—persons with disabilities are an untapped consumer group.

In assisting clients in re-entering society after illness or injury, many unexpected cultural conflicts may arise. Multiple systems with differing rules and standards need to be negotiated if adaptation is to be successful. Both therapist and client need to realize that adaptation is an evolving process requiring patience and a large measure of frustration tolerance as well as new learning and practice. Therapists may find themselves in the role of advocate as clients struggle with the health care system to obtain needed services.

Spiritual Context

The OT Practice Framework's division of contexts into seven categories helps us to grasp the complexity of interactions among many systems. However, some of the divisions seem artificial at times, and there are many points of overlap. Such is the case for spiritual context. For instance, a client's practice of religion has a spiritual component that gives the performance of rituals personal meaning, a social component when the religious rituals are practiced in a group, and a cultural component that derives from shared beliefs and values.

The OT Practice Framework defines spiritual context as "fundamental orientation of a person's life: that which inspires and motivates that individual" (AOTA, 2002, p. 623). This definition goes beyond one's religion. The broader definition for human spirituality has been defined by Urbanowski (1997) as the *experience of meaning*. Persons presumably choose daily occupations that have personal meaning to them, or that move them toward self-actualization. In client-centered practice, occupational therapists ask clients to prioritize their occupational goals and concerns so that our interventions will have meaning for them. Hasselkus (2002) has discussed the meaning of everyday occupations in terms of cultures, social groups, and emotional connectedness. Fidler and Velde (1999) have studied the symbolic meaning in occupation and its effect on lifestyle choice. The Canadian Model of Occupational Performance (CMOP) (Law et al., 1998) puts *spirit* at the center of all the other components of the person, implying that the human spirit is the essence of one's identity. Occupational science gives priority to the form, function, and meaning of occupation, confirming the central role of spirituality.

It is difficult to separate the spiritual aspects of occupation from all of the other contexts. Perhaps this exemplifies the holistic nature of occupation and the importance of understanding how these multiple systems work together. Some aspects of spiritual context that occupational therapists can evaluate are the person's level of motivation (Kielhofner's [2002] Volitional Questionnaire, Rosenfeld's [1997] Evaluation of Rehabilitation Potential), life satisfaction (Neugarten, Havighurst, & Tobin, 1961), and sense of well being.

According to Spencer, the spiritual context is a growing area without much evidence-based research (2003).

Rosenfeld (1997) suggests that motivation naturally flows from the client's perception that the occupations he or she performs give meaning to life. This connection with a person's essence or "nucleus" through therapist–client collaboration and the therapeutic use of self motivates the client's engagement in occupation.

Personal Context

The OT Practice Framework quotes the ICF in defining personal context as, "features of the individual that are not a part of a health condition or health status" (WHO, 2001, p. 17). Some examples are age, gender, and socio-economic status. Researchers have defined socioeconomic status in the United States as a combination of household income level, place of residence, and years of education, which identify one's class or status within a given society. This part of personal context overlaps with social and cultural contexts by categorizing persons according to specific criteria. Who can argue that poor people have limited occupational choices or that people with a college education have a better chance for higher paying jobs? Age and gender also greatly influence the opportunities and barriers our clients encounter within their social groups and society, but they do so because of prevailing beliefs and attitudes. Race, ethnic background, marital status, religious or political affiliation, and sexual orientation may also have a significant impact on occupational choice and/or opportunity. As an example, try answering the following questions:

1. Who is more likely to become an Army General—a gay man, an African American woman, or a White heterosexual man? Why?

2. What jobs are available to a woman of 60 as compared to a man of 20 when both have a high school diploma and neither has any work experience?

3. Why do so many baby boomers strive to look and feel younger? How does this affect their lifestyle?

4. How are occupational choices for leisure pursuits different for a 10-year-old boy, an 18-year-old girl, and a 40-year-old man? Why?

5. How does one's age affect one's choices of an appropriate dating partner?

Temporal Context

What is the influence of time on a person's occupation? Included in temporal context is "location of occupational performance in time, such as stages of life, time of day or year, and duration" (AOTA, 2002, p. 623). For example, the structure of a child's day consists of tasks that are different from those of an adult. Many theorists have attempted to define the stages of development over the life span. Table 3-2 lists some of the best known age and stage theories of development that have guided occupational therapists' thinking about age-appropriate activities. More contemporary developmental theorists have rejected the notion of critical ages and stages and have given greater importance to individual, subjective experience.

Seasons and holidays often define our social and cultural activities and influence our lifestyle in many other ways. What are some typical summer activities for you? What winter activities do you typically participate in? What environmental factors influence these choices?

The duration of activities and the time of day in which they occur depend on how clients structure their day. Many people have problems with managing their time. A traditional OT assessment tool is the activity configuration that requires clients to account for each hour of the 24-hour day.

Table 3-2						
Traditional Age and Stage Theories of Development (Approximate Ages)						
Theorists and Stages	**Birth to 2 years**	**2 to 3 years**	**4 to 5 years**	**5 years to puberty**	**Puberty to 18 years**	**18+ years**
Freud: Psychosexual stages	Oral	Anal	Phallic	Latency	Genital	Maturity
Erikson: Psychosocial stages	Trust versus mistrust	Autonomy versus shame and doubt (2 to 4)	Initiative versus guilt	Industry versus inferiority	Identity versus role confusion	Intimacy versus isolation (23 to 35)
Piaget: Intellectual stages	Sensory Motor (0 to 2)	Preoperational (3 to 7)		Concrete Operations (7 to 13)	Formal Operations (13 to maturity)	
Kohlberg and Wilcox: Moral development	Preconventional: Stage 1: Egocentric Stage 2: Reciprocity		Conventional: Stage 3: All authority is good Stage 4: Law and order		Postconventional: Stage 5: Right and wrong separate from rules Stage 6: Ideal	

Virtual Context

Virtual context is defined in the OT Practice Framework as "environment in which communication occurs by means of airwaves or computers and an absence of physical contact" (AOTA, 2002). As technology evolves, more occupations involve virtual aspects, including not only computers but also communicating via telephones or cell phones and keeping informed or entertained through radio, television, cable, or other video and audio transmissions. Computers in the workplace, unusual 20 years ago, are standard equipment today. Students from elementary school through college need to continue to build computer skills and to keep abreast of the ever-changing technology.

Think about how many things you do on your computer. Computers become even more important for persons with disability who may use them to augment voice communication, compensate for low vision, or regulate lighting and temperature in the home. Emergency call services such as Lifeline provide older adults living alone with an instant electronic source of assistance.

Some home health agencies now provide "virtual" home visits, which involve computer communication with clients and their families at an agreed upon time. Furthermore, the Internet has opened the door to global networks of persons with common disabilities, concerns, or situations, who discuss issues online and help each other to solve problems.

LEARNING ACTIVITIES

Physical Context

Neighborhood exploration. Draw a diagram of a neighborhood where you grew up. Where were the important places for you, such as friend's homes, corner stores, bus stop, basketball hoop, and nearby park or lot where you played.

Specify your age and describe three important physical features of your neighborhood.

Space versus place. Draw a floor plan of your bedroom. It can be the one you currently occupy or one from your past. Write one paragraph describing the day you moved into this room. What was it like the first time you slept there? What changes did you make that contributed to how you feel about being in your room? Would you describe it as a space or a place? Give reasons.

Hospital room design. Most people have spent the night in a hospital room at least once. If not, perhaps you have visited someone in a hospital. Draw the hospital room as you can best remember it, and label this drawing "before." What occupations did you perform in the hospital room? What occupations were performed by others? Identify any problems you encountered with the physical space, furniture, or equipment.

Now imagine you have a health condition that requires hospitalization. Make it real if you can—such as when you broke your leg in two places, or make up a condition, such as you are a mother who has just given birth to twins. What might be the desirable physical features of the hospital room where you will recover?

On a second sheet of paper, draw a floor plan of your ideal hospital room. Consider both your own comfort, occupations, and feelings about the room and the occupations or tasks others need to perform in order to care for you while in the hospital. How could you make this space a place? How might you assist a client in doing so?

Social Context

Work with a partner for this assignment. There are four parts, worth 25% each.

Personal Network Map

Decide who will be the "therapist." The therapist should use the attached worksheet to guide an informal interview with your "client." Write down on the worksheet first names of people in the client's social network (10 to 20). Do not exclude any areas.

Working from the completed personal network map, identify individuals from whom you could elicit social support, and briefly discuss reasons for your answers or give an example of a real situation, if applicable.*

- *Practical Social Support*
  - o Who would you call if you needed to borrow money?
  - o Who could you count on to help you move to a new apartment?
  - o When you get sick, who do you count on to give you personal care?
  - o If you are planning your wedding, who would you ask to be members of your wedding party (choose 3 or 4 individuals)?
  - o If you were arrested while traveling out of state, to whom would you place your one telephone call?
- *Informational Social Support*
  - o Who would you ask to help you choose or shop for an outfit for a special occasion?
  - o If you had questions about a research project for school, from who would you request help and guidance?
  - o If you had an opportunity to plan a trip to Florida for spring break, with whom would you consult in making the specific arrangements?
  - o Who would you call to help you find a summer job in your home town?

Only one partner, "client," will answer the above questions. You will trade roles for question 2. Please state name of "client" for each question when writing your report.

- *Emotional Social Support*
  - o Who do you count on to give you a sense of belonging (can be more than one person)?
  - o When you are upset about a personal issue, who could you call to discuss it?
  - o If someone bullied or harassed you, who could you look to for help and support?
  - o When something wonderful happens to you, who is the first person you'd tell?
  - o If something terrible were to happen to you, which individuals could you turn to?

Kinship Network Analysis

Trade roles for this next question. The "therapist" uses the family tree model (Figure 3-2) to create a chart; identify two generations back in ancestry. Use genogram symbols: triangle for male, circle for female (McGoldrick & Gerson, 1985). Start with "client" and identify parents and siblings using symbols. Write the first name and age under each symbol. Identify both maternal and paternal grandparents. If deceased, mark with an x.

Separately, list each person named on the chart, and identify the following:

- Date and place of birth; date and cause of death (if applicable)
- Educational level and major; language(s) spoken
- Jobs or vocations; special skills or talents
- Nature of relationship with spouse, children, and parents
- Major accomplishments; significant events
- Chronic diseases or medical conditions/operations or surgery—past or present
- Religious beliefs or other significant information

Community Assessment Wheel

Draw a circle and divide into eight sections (like cutting a pizza). Each section represents one category of social support services in the community.

Categories
1. Health services
2. Religious services or groups
3. Physical fitness
4. Parks and recreation (i.e., hiking, golf, bowling)
5. Entertainment and cultural events
6. Volunteer opportunities
7. Places to go out and celebrate
8. Services to keep you safe (i.e., EMS, police, fire)

Windshield Survey

Use your home or college town as an example. Get a map and select a 2-mile radius that incorporates some residential streets where a potential client might live. Drive through your selected area (excluding campus) to do a "windshield survey" to identify three locations from which your needs in each of these categories could be met. Write down names and addresses for these sites.

Phone Book Survey

Follow up with a telephone book or internet informational website. Make a list of the three places under each category you have selected, along with address and telephone number.

Identify Gaps

If there is lack of availability of any of these categories within the 2-mile radius you selected, briefly describe what is missing. Use the telephone book to identify the

---

This is the type of community survey you might do with a potential client who is disabled and moving to a new location. For clients, the categories may vary.

Figure 3-2. Genogram worksheet.

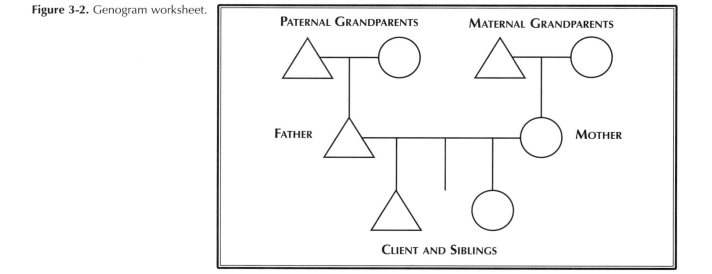

PATERNAL GRANDPARENTS   MATERNAL GRANDPARENTS

FATHER   MOTHER

CLIENT AND SIBLINGS

closest place that would provide the service needed. List addresses and phone numbers.

Societal Level Report

Visit your state capitol and observe a public meeting. Write a short report of the legislative or public hearing you observed. Who led the session, and what was its purpose? What issues were debated or discussed? What did you learn about the political system/process from attending this session?

Cultural Context: Culture and Diversity

This assignment has four parts: exploration of one's own culture (50%), definition of your university's unique culture (10%), magazine picture collage depicting diversity (10%), and analysis of "otherness" interpreting the collage (30%).

Cultural Self-Awareness

Write a minimum of two single-spaced pages answering the following questions:

1. How would you describe yourself in an e-mail to someone you met online?
2. Which physical attributes do you consider your best features?
3. How do you typically greet a close friend or family member?
4. With which ethnic group do you most identify? This includes religion and nationality as well as specific customs, values, and beliefs. Describe.
5. What "customs" (traditions) are connected with your heritage?
6. How does your family typically celebrate a holiday? Give an example.
7. What languages do you speak/understand?
8. Describe your ideal mate, including physical, psychological, and spiritual attributes. Would you marry someone of another culture? Why or why not?
9. How do you think your socioeconomic status affects your view of life and expectations of yourself?
10. People have multiple cultural identities. List and describe three different cultures with which you identify.

Your University's Culture

Write a minimum of one single-spaced page answering the following questions:

1. From your perspective, how diverse is your university? What diverse groups have you seen represented on campus? How welcome do you think students from minority groups feel at your university? Be honest. We are not looking for a "politically correct" opinion but one that is authentically yours. If possible, give some specific examples.
2. What values or standards of behavior are acceptable at your university? What behaviors are unacceptable? Give some examples of each (e.g., Do you call your professors by their title, last name, or first name? What is considered acceptable class participation?).
3. If you were asked to describe the culture on campus to someone unfamiliar with your university, how would you describe it?

Magazine Picture Collage

On a blank sheet of paper, glue six pictures from magazines of persons you would identify as belonging to a culture or having cultural attributes different from your own. Try to select pictures on the basis of appearance only. Sometimes an advertisement will give you some clues, such as if the woman is cooking a traditional Greek dish. Think about the stigmas or stereotypes society sometimes gives people. Label the pictures using identifiers such as race, nationality, religion, class, sexual orientation, gender, and disability status. Give each person pictured a name.

Analysis of Otherness

Using your collage as a guide, answer the following questions about each picture. Choose three pictures to focus on for this section, and identify by using the name you have given him or her (minimum of 2 pages):

- How is this person different from yourself?
- What if he/she were sitting next to you on a train or airplane? How would you feel in this person's presence?
- What would you like to learn about this person? What three questions would you ask in order to learn more about their culture?
- Do you know someone who has similar characteristics? Briefly describe your experiences with the real individual of which this picture reminds you.
- Describe one experience you have had in getting to know someone from a culture different from your own.

Spiritual Context: What Motivates You?

Motivation can be both positive and negative. Persons are motivated to repeat behaviors that they perceive to be effective and meaningful while avoiding those that produce negative feelings or unwanted results. Write a short anecdote about a situation in your own life that evoked strong emotion in you. Explain why you felt the way you did, and describe your own behaviors and attitudes that resulted. What did you learn about yourself? What did this experience motivate you to do? How did the experience affect future behaviors? Choose one positive and one negative emotion from Table 3-3.

Draw two larger circles and divide each into 24 hours. For the next 48 hours, keep track of what you are doing each hour of the day. Create some categories for the tasks or occupations you have charted on your circles. Work, leisure, self care, and socialization might be some typical categories. Name at least 6 different categories, list the activities falling into each category, and tally the number of hours per day you spent within that category. Table 3-4 is an example of average hours per day over 2 days.

Personal Context: What Are My Opportunities and Limitations?

How do your own personal circumstances affect your activity choices? Write one paragraph about how each of the following has affected your life growing up:

- *Age:* Choose two different ages and compare.
- *Gender:* What occupations were encouraged/discouraged by your family?
- *Family income level:* What opportunities/barriers resulted?
- *Place of residence:* How did your home, neighborhood, and community affect your activity choices as a young child and an adolescent?
- *Educational level:* How will your college degree change your life?

As you answer these questions, keep in mind that from a systems perspective, it is expected that all of the contexts have points of overlap, and all act together to influence individual occupational performance.

Temporal Context Learning Activity.

Directions: Use an activity configuration format to keep track of all your activities for 7 days. You may construct a chart with 24 hours per day and seven columns,

one for each day of the week. Exact times are not important, but you should not leave any hour blank.

Next, analyze your activities using the categories in Table 3-4. How well do your activities fit into these categories? What categories would you delete or add?

Finally, consider your life stage. How old are you, and in what developmental stage do you consider yourself to be? Use Erikson's or Levinson's stages as a guide (see Chapter 17 for descriptions of these theories/stages). How does your life stage help to determine your daily activities? How would your activities change if you were in Levinson's Late Life transition? How were they different when you were in Erikson's Industry vs. Inferiority stage?

How do you think the life stage of your clients might affect your approach in occupational therapy?

Virtual Context: Internet Search

Choose a specific health condition such as depression, hearing loss, or multiple sclerosis and complete a computer search. Look for the following:

- Medical information or description
- Remedies or medications
- Resources for self-help

Table 3-3

Spiritual Context Worksheet

Strong Positive Emotions	Strong Negative Emotions
• Excited?	• Angry?
• Overjoyed?	• Ashamed or guilty?
• Cherished?	• Grief stricken?
• Powerful?	• Embarrassed?
• Loved unconditionally?	• Disappointed?

Table 3-4

Example of a 24-Hour Temporal Context Analysis

Self Care	Work	Socialization	Leisure	Rest/Sleep	Errands
Cooking, eating: 2 hours	Driving: 1 hour	Visiting friends: 2 hours	Playing computer games: 1 hour	Sleeping: 6 hours	Grocery shopping: 0.5 hour
Showering, dressing: 1 hour	Computer work: 4 hours	Telephone: 0.5 hour	Workout at gym: 1 hour	Watching television: 1 hour	Bank, post office: 0.5 hour
Cleaning, vacuuming: 1 hour	Writing, taking notes: 1 hour	E-mail: 0.5 hour			Online shopping: 1 hour
Total: 4 hours	**Total: 6 hours**	**Total: 3 hours**	**Total: 2 hours**	**Total: 7 hours**	**Total: 2 hours**

Make sure your list of totals adds up to 24 hours.

- Chat rooms, websites, or bulletin boards
- Books or videos on the topic
- Case examples or personal stories

List the websites for each of these and give references in APA format.

REFERENCES

American Occupational Therapy Association. (2002). Occupational therapy practice framework: Domain and process. *American Journal of Occupational Therapy, 56,* 609–639.

Baum, C. & Christiansen, C. (2005). Person-Environment-Occupation-Performance: A model for planning interventions for individuals and organizations. In C. Christiansen & C. Baum (Eds.), *Occupational therapy: Performance, participation, and well-being* (2nd ed.) (pp. 372–394). Thorofare, NJ: SLACK Incorporated.

Benne, K., & Sheats, P. (1948). Functional roles of group members. *Journal of Social Issues, 2,* 123–135.

Bronfenbrenner, U. (1993). Toward an experimental ecology of human development: Research models and fugitive findings. In R. H. Wozniak & K. W. Fischer (Eds.), *Development in context: Acting and thinking in specific environments* (pp. 3–44). New York, NY: Erlbaum.

Christiansen, C. & Baum, C., (1997). Occupational therapy: Enabling function and well-being. Thorofare, NJ: Slack. Eds.

Dunn, W., Brown, C., & McGuigan, A. (1994). The ecology of human performance: A framework for considering the effect of context. *American Journal of Occupational Therapy, 48,* 595–607.

Hasselkus, B. R. (2002). The meaning of everyday occupation. Thorofare, NJ: Slack.

Haller, B. (1995). Rethinking models of media representation of disability. Disability Studies Quarterly, 15(2), 26-30.

Fidler, G., & Velde, B. (1999). *Activities: Reality and symbol.* Thorofare NJ: SLACK Incorporated.

Kelso, J. A. S., & Tuller, B. (1984). A dynamical basis for action systems. In M. S. Gazzaniga (Ed.), *Self-organizing systems: The emergence of order.* New York, NY: Plenum.

Kielhofner, G. (1978). General systems theory: Implications for theory and action in occupational therapy. *The American Journal of Occupational Therapy, 32,* 637–645.

Kielhofner, G. (1980a). A model of human occupation, part two. Ontogenesis from the Perspective of temporal adaptation. *American Journal of Occupational Therapy, 34,* 657–663.

Kielhofner, G. (1980b). A model of human occupation, part three. Benign and vicious cycles. *American Journal of Occupational Therapy, 34,* 731–737.

Kielhofner, G. (2002). *Model of human occupation* (3rd ed.). Baltimore, MD: Lippincott Williams & Wilkins.

Kielhofner, G., & Burke, J. (1980). A model of human occupation, part one. Conceptual framework and content. *American Journal of Occupational Therapy, 34,* 572–581.

Krefting, L. (1989). Reintegration into the community after head injury: The results of an ethnographic study. *Occupational Therapy Journal of Research, 9,* 67–83.

Law, M., Baptiste, S., Carswell, A., McColl, M. A., Polatajko, H., & Pollock, N. (1998). *Canadian occupational performance measure* (3rd ed.). Ottawa, Canada: Canadian Occupational Therapy Association.

Law, M., Missiuna, C., Pollock, N., & Stewart, D. (2005). Foundations for occupational therapy practice with children. In J. Case-Smith (Ed.), *Occupational therapy for children* (5th ed.). St. Louis, MO: Elsevier Mosby.

Lorenz, E. (1980). Lorenz model. Retrieved September 24, 2006, from http://en.wikipedia.org/wiki/Chaos_theory.

McGoldrick, M., & Gerson, R. (1985). *Genograms in family assessment.* New York, NY: WW Norton & Company.

Neugarten, B. L., Havighurst, R. J., & Tobin, S. S. (1961). The measurement of life satisfaction. *Journal of Gerontology, 16,* 134–143.

Nichols, M. (1984). *Family therapy: Concepts and methods.* Needham Heights, MA: Allyn & Bacon.

Rapaport, A. (1986). *General systems theory: Essential concepts and application.* New York, NY: Cambridge University Press.

Ringaert, L. (2003). Universal design of the built environment to enable occupational performance. In L. Letts, P. Rigby, & D. Stewart (Eds.), *Using environments to enable occupational performance.* Thorofare, NJ: SLACK Incorporated.

Rosenfeld, M. (1997). *Motivational strategies in geriatric rehabilitation.* Bethesda, MD: American Occupatioal Therapy Association Press.

Rowles, G. (2003). The meaning of place as a component of the self. In E. Crepeau, E. Cohn, & B. Boyt Schell (Eds.), *Willard & Spackman's occupational therapy* (10th ed.). Baltimore, MD: Lippincott, Williams & Wilkins.

Royeen, C. B. (2003). The 2003 Eleanor Clarke Slagle lecture: Chaotic occupational therapy: Collective wisdom for a complex profession. *American Journal of Occupational Therapy, 57,* 609–624.

Schkade, J., & Schultz, S. (1992). Occupational adaptation: Toward a holistic approach for contemporary practice, Part 1. *American Journal of Occupational Therapy, 46,* 829–837.

Schultz, S., & Schkade, J. (1992). Occupational adaptation: Toward a holistic approach for contemporary practice, Part 2. *American Journal of Occupational Therapy, 46,* 917–925.

Spencer, J. C. (2003). Evaluation of performance contexts. In E. Crepeau, E. Cohn, & B. Boyt Schell (Eds.), *Willard & Spackman's occupational therapy* (10th ed.). Baltimore, MD: Lippincott, Williams & Wilkins.

Stewart, D., & Law, M. (2003). The environment: Paradigms and practice in health, occupational therapy, and inquiry. In L. Letts, P. Rigby, & D. Stewart (Eds.), *Using environments to enable occupational performance.* Thorofare, NJ: SLACK Incorporated.

Urbanowski, R. (1997). Spirituality in everyday practice. *Occupational Therapy Practice, 2,* 18–23.

VanSant, A. F. (1991). Neurodevelopmental treatment and pediatric physical therapy: A commentary. *Pediatric Physical Therapy, 3,* 137–141.

Von Bertalanffy, L. (1968). *General system theory.* New York, NY: Braziller.

Von Bertalanffy, L. (1969). Chance or law. In A. Koestler & J. R. Smythies (Eds.), *Beyond reductionism.* London: Hutchinson.

Wells, S., & Black, R. (2000). *Cultural competency for health professionals.* Bethesda, MD: American Occupational Therapy Association.

World Health Organization. (2001). *International classification of functioning, disability, and health (ICF).* Geneva: Author.

Chapter 4

ORGANIZATION OF THEORY
IN OCCUPATIONAL THERAPY

"Thoughts without content are empty. Intuitions without concepts are blind."

– KANT

Theory helps us put things we know into categories so that we can more easily remember and retrieve information when we need it. "Disciplines organize knowledge for practical use into theories, models, and frames of reference" (Scaffa, 2001, p. 57). Baum writes, "There is little agreement among writers about how to describe organized knowledge in the field... the terms theory, model, frame of reference, and paradigm have been variously used to describe subsets of the profession's knowledge" (1997, p. 41). Definitions of the terms paradigm, models, and frames of reference in textbooks written in the United States and the United Kingdom were compared by Hagedorn (2001). She writes, "authors all acknowledge that there are no fixed definitions, and on the whole, they appear to have 'agreed to disagree'" (p. 21). Part of the difficulty is that many levels of theory exist in our profession. In this chapter, we will attempt to sort out the terminology and to propose a way for the various levels to be more easily understood. We begin by defining applied theories as those intended to address problems of practical interest in occupational therapy (OT) practice.

WHAT IS THEORY?

Theory helps us describe, explain, and predict behavior and/or the relationship between concepts or events. Each of these purposes requires a different type of research. At first, all theories are hypothetical—our best guess as to why people move, act, or think in certain ways. Theories are built through the systematic gathering of data and through observation. As theories develop, they may be tested through experimentation.

Description

Theories often begin with general descriptions. For example, in observing children, Dr. Gesell (1934), considered

the father of child development in the United States, noticed that children typically begin walking around age one. In his research, he observed thousands of children to determine the typical behaviors of children at different ages. His research resulted in the age-appropriate developmental milestones for children that we take for granted today. Descriptive research often defines a concept, or general idea, of something we wish to better understand.

Explanation

Theories help us understand what we observe. For example, what makes some children clumsy? There are many possible explanations: weak muscles, poor vision, slow reaction time due to fatigue, poor muscle coordination, etc. In research, a possible explanation is called a *hypothesis*. Dr. Ayres hypothesized (after ruling out other explanations) that clumsiness (dyspraxia) results from poor motor planning (1989). She proceeded to study the nature of motor planning in young children by having them try different types of movement tasks, a type of *experimental research*.

Prediction

Much of what we know about different health conditions is based on percentages and *probability*. For example, depression is a common disorder with a lifetime prevalence of about 15% of the United States population, up to 25% in women and up to 50% in older adults (Sadock & Sadock, 2003). This knowledge prepares us to look for signs of depression as possible cause when we encounter clients who lack motivation in OT, especially if those clients are female or over 65. In OT, we might like to be able to predict the extent of recovery our clients can achieve. An episode of depression, if untreated (meaning no antidepressant medication is taken), lasts an average of 6 to 13 months. However, for evidence-based practice, we need to know how

OT interventions can affect the recovery process so that we might help our clients return to healthy functioning faster.

Cause and Effect Relationships

In order to know what strategies really work in OT, we must look at what actually causes therapeutic change. The highest level of theory looks at cause and effect relationships. For example, a group of researchers at the University of Southern California wanted to know what OT interventions *caused* older adults to be able to live independently. Cause and effect relationships are the hardest to prove and require the most rigorous research methods, including a large sample, control groups to eliminate other possible causes, and random selection of subjects. They designed a *randomized controlled trial* in which 361 independent-living adults over 60 years were randomly assigned to control and experimental groups. They conducted an OT program with the experimental group, which included both group and individual OT interventions, and measured the changes in both groups. Their results clearly indicated the positive benefits of the OT interventions in improving both physical and mental health and in quality-of-life measures (Clark, Azen, Zemke, et al., 1997). More cause and effect research is needed to help us understand how OT interventions bring about therapeutic change.

LEVELS OF THEORY

In earlier chapters, we discussed the evolution of theory in OT, leading up to a professional identity crisis in the 1970s and 1980s. This identity problem precipitated a search for theories that would address common threads and unify OT practice. While many diverse frames of reference in the profession had been identified, we now needed to develop a systematic theoretical and scientific basis for occupation itself. Ironically, this is the same goal proposed by our founders (Dunton, 1919; Quiroga, 1995). By the 1990s, scholars had reflected upon the problem of professional identity considerably and had come to understand that the unifying concept for all of the areas of specialization within OT practice was, quite simply, occupation.

While the focus on the broader concepts of occupation seems simple and logical in retrospect, its implications are quite complex. Hooper (2006) explains it as an *epistemological transformation*, or a shift in the way we define knowledge and in the methods by which we acquire knowledge. The mid-century reductionistic approach led occupational therapists to develop and research many specific techniques, such as sensory integration for the treatment of children with learning disability, biomechanical strategies for the treatment of hand injury, and cognitive rehabilitation for the treatment of traumatic brain injury. These applied theories, while useful and valid, represented fragments of

occupation developed in isolation of each other. Broader theories of occupation, such as the model of human occupation (Kielhofner & Burke, 1980), and subsequent occupation-based models, served the purpose of defining the interconnections among the fragments or components of occupation. Furthermore, the application of dynamic systems theories (discussed in Chapter 3) influenced the newer occupation-based models in synthesizing much of the specific knowledge developed earlier within the multiple dimensions of occupation (Hooper, 2006).

However, occupation-based models cannot be expected to replace all of the collected wisdom of OT's more traditional frames of reference. As practitioners, occupational therapists will continue to use specific techniques but will do so within the context of the broader occupation-based models. This requires an understanding and an appreciation of all levels of theory as necessary within our new paradigm of client-centered, holistic, and systems-oriented OT practice.

Understanding the Different Levels of Theory

Mosey (1992) identifies three levels of theory in OT as it had progressed to that point in time—fundamental knowledge, applied knowledge, and practice:

1. *A fundamental body of knowledge* includes philosophical assumptions, an ethical code, a theoretical foundation of both theories and empirical data, a domain of concern, and legitimate tools. In our proposed organization, OT's professional paradigm and the OT Practice Framework fall into the category of fundamental knowledge.

2. *An applied body of knowledge* includes sets of guidelines for practice. Occupation-based models fall into this category in our proposed taxonomy.

3. *Practice* includes action sequences, use of applied knowledge, the clinical reasoning process, and the art of practice. Frames of reference and the assessments and intervention techniques developed from them fall into this category in our taxonomy.

Taking these distinctions into account, we will clarify some different levels of theory as they currently appear to be understood by our scholars and/or defined by the American Occupational Therapy Association (AOTA). Our proposed organization of theory for OT appears in Figure 4-1. It includes three levels: 1) paradigm, 2) occupation-based models, and 3) frames of reference. Each of these terms will be defined in this chapter.

Previously, we said that the *paradigm* in health care has shifted to one that is holistic, client centered, and systems oriented. These broad concepts represent the most general levels of theory. In an attempt to both broaden and unify today's practice, AOTA's Practice Framework has redefined some of the fundamental concepts of OT practice and has incorporated many of the concepts from the International Classification of Functioning (ICF) (WHO, 2001) and several occupation-based models. For example, patients are now called clients or consumers, treatment is redefined as intervention, and disease or illness has been replaced by health condition (AOTA, 2002). These changes in terminology reflect fundamental changes in the way occupational therapists will practice in the 21st century.

The next level includes the occupation-based models which have been called overarching frames of reference (Dunn, 2000), conceptual models (Reed & Sanderson, 1999), or occupation-based frameworks (Baum & Christiansen, 2005). These authors prefer Creek's definition of a model, "a simplified representation of structure and content ... that describes or explains complex relationships between concepts" (1992, in Hagedorn, 2001, p. 23). In OT, occupation-based models help explain the relationships among the person, the environment, and occupational performance, forming the foundation for the profession's focus on occupation. However, according to Reed and Sanderson (1999), conceptual models usually do not provide guidelines for application with specific populations or disabilities.

Theories that explain how therapy works in practice have been called practice models (Reed & Sanderson, 1999; Kielhofner, 2004) or frames of reference (Mosey, 1986, 1992). Frames of reference address specific areas of occupational disability and help practitioners to apply theory with individual clients in specific situations. These represent the most concrete level of theory. Our proposed organization (taxonomy) of the various levels of theory is depicted in Figure 4-1.

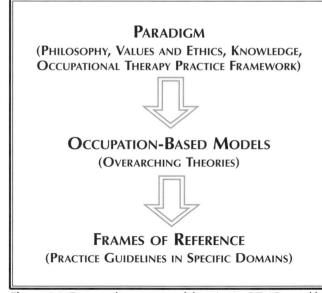

Figure 4-1. Proposed taxonomy of theories in OT. (Created by M. Cole and R. Tufano, 2007.)

PARADIGM

The paradigm for the profession of OT contains the guiding premises and theories behind the profession as a whole. The dictionary definition of paradigm derives from its Greek root, which means model, example, or pattern. In this taxonomy of OT, the term paradigm describes a philosophical viewpoint, whereas the word model is used at a lower level of this theoretical structure to describe a theoretical approach to the human condition.

Kielhofner defines a paradigm as a shared vision encompassing the most fundamental assumptions and beliefs, which serves as the cultural core of the profession (2004). Kuhn (1970) is most frequently cited in defining paradigms in science and the professions. The term *paradigm* was used by Thomas Kuhn to describe the shared vision of a scientific discipline, which includes shared concerns and a common view of the world. A paradigm is a force for unity. It is the most stable element of a discipline, while its models are always changing. Kielhofner (2004) defines the term for OT as the "cultural core of the discipline," which "provides professional identity." He further divides the nature of the paradigm into three content areas: core constructs (concepts), focal viewpoint (world view), and integrating values (values). We will use the term paradigm to incorporate some of what Mosey (1992) called our fundamental body of knowledge—our philosophical base, our values and code of ethics as defined by AOTA, and three concepts most basic to practice in the OT profession: occupation, purposeful activity, and function (AOTA, 2004).

According to Kuhn, scientific disciplines undergo periodic revolutionary shifts in world view, which involve major conceptual restructuring. Kuhn calls these paradigm shifts, such as those described for OT in Chapter 1. In OT, the shared vision incorporates the OT *philosophy*, *core values*, *ethical codes*, and all the collective wisdom of the profession. Paradigms are not always explicit but are implied through professional training and the progression and interpretation of research (Scaffa, 2001). We have identified three general characteristics of the current OT paradigm as holistic, client centered, and systems oriented. These trends are derived from a review of current literature in OT (see Chapter 1) but are also visible in the literature of health care generally (Baum & Christiansen, 2005).

Philosophy

A *philosophy* may be defined as a fundamental belief. Adolph Meyer is credited with the initial articulation of the philosophical base for OT as the valuation of time and work and the role of occupational performance in bringing meaning to life (1921, 1982).

The statement shown in Table 4-1 obviously springs from our humanitarian roots, and the statements closely resemble the humanistic theory described in previous chapters.

Table 4-1
Philosophical Base of Occupational Therapy
"Man is an active being whose development is influenced by the use of purposeful activity. Using their capacity for intrinsic motivation, human beings are able to influence their physical and mental health and their social and physical environment through purposeful activity. Human life includes a process of continuous adaptation. Adaptation is a change in function that promotes survival and self-actualization. Biological, psychological and environmental factors may interrupt the adaptation process at any time throughout the life cycle. Dysfunction may occur when adaptation is impaired. Purposeful activity facilitates the adaptive process. Occupational therapy is based on the belief that purposeful activity (occupation) including its interpersonal and environmental components, may be used to prevent and mediate dysfunction and to elicit maximum adaptation. Activity as used by the occupational therapist includes both an intrinsic and a therapeutic purpose."
Reprinted from American Occupational Therapy Association. (1979). The philosophical base of occupational therapy. American Journal of Occupational Therapy, 33, 785.

In 2004, AOTA reconfirmed its philosophy as the "fundamental concepts of occupational therapy: occupation, purposeful activity, and function" (p. 319). *Occupations* are the ordinary and familiar things people do everyday that fill their time and give their lives meaning (Christiansen, Clark, Kielhofner, & Rogers, 1995). The term occupation forms the basis of AOTA's Practice Framework domain, which includes performance areas (work, leisure, etc.), skills, patterns, contexts, activity demands, and body structures and functions (AOTA, 2002). *Purposeful activity* refers to the goal-directed behaviors or tasks that the individual considers meaningful (Hinojosa, Sabari, & Pedretti, 1993). Purposeful activity is part of the process of OT. This definition implies that engagement in activities may form patterns or clusters associated with occupational roles that make up an individual's lifestyle. *Function* implies the ability to engage in occupations satisfactorily in the eyes of the person and society. Functional outcomes, emphasizing the usefulness of knowledge and skills, often define the value of OT services for individuals (Baum & Edwards, 1995).

Ethics

OT's seven core values are defined in AOTA's official documents as follows: altruism, equality, freedom, justice, dignity, truth, and prudence (2004). Attitudes concerning these basic concepts are ideally shared by all occupational therapists.

1. *Altruism* is the unselfish concern for the welfare of others. Our primary concern should be what is best for the client, not reimbursement or monetary gain, for example.

2. *Equality* recognizes that all persons have the same fundamental rights and opportunities. Nonjudgmental acceptance of all types of diversity should prevail in our practice.

3. *Freedom* implies choice, autonomy, and self-direction. Occupational therapists need to respect a client's choices regarding both autonomy and societal involvement and to consider cultural differences.

4. *Justice* is concerned with what is morally right and what is fair. This refers to legal rights and obligations as well as a sense of fairness in the provision of OT services.

5. *Dignity* may be demonstrated by an attitude of empathy and respect. Occupational therapists interact with clients in ways that nurture their sense of competence and self-worth.

6. *Truth* requires that occupational therapists be faithful to the facts. Practitioners do this by continually updating their knowledge and professional competence.

7. *Prudence* refers to the need for the use of reason in making good judgments. Occupational therapists demonstrate prudence by using caution, vigilance, and moderation in making professional judgments and by carefully reflecting on outcomes.

The principles set forth in AOTA's *Code of Ethics* (2000) form a basis for defining professional behavior, making moral decisions and judgments, and resolving ethical dilemmas. The seven principles are listed in Table 4-2. For further definition, the reader is referred to AOTA's Official Documents (2004).

The *collective knowledge and wisdom of the profession* has also been called OT's fundamental and applied bodies of knowledge (Mosey, 1992) and the OT knowledge base (Reed & Sanderson, 1999). With every new textbook, journal article, research study, and conference presentation, the profession's body of knowledge increases. Learning all of it might seem, at times, an overwhelming task. However, our paradigm helps to organize this vast collection of knowledge by focusing on current perceptions of practice. For example, as we incorporate new scientific research into our knowledge, our understanding of the developmental sequence changes from one of ages and stages to one that portrays the multiple interplay of different systems and varying routes toward maturity. Similarly, our focus on holism leads us to consider components of occupation within the context of their effect on the entire system.

Table 4-2

Occupational Therapy Code of Ethics

Occupational therapy personnel shall:

1. Demonstrate a concern for the safety and well-being of the recipients of their services (BENEFICENCE).
2. Take measures to ensure a recipient's safety and avoid imposing or inflicting harm (NONMALEFICENCE).
3. Respect recipients to assure their rights (AUTONOMY, CONFIDENTIALITY).
4. Achieve and continually maintain high standards of competence (DUTY).
5. Comply with laws and Association policies guiding the profession of occupational therapy (PROCEDURAL JUSTICE).
6. Provide accurate information when representing the profession (VERACITY).
7. Treat colleagues and other professionals with respect, fairness, discretion, and integrity (FIDELITY).

Adapted from American Occupational Therapy Association (2005). Occupational therapy code of ethics (2005). American Journal of Occupational Therapy, 59, 639–642.

Occupational science stands out as the academic and scientific discipline that contributes to our basic knowledge of the form, function, and meaning of occupation. As a discipline, occupational science studies the various aspects of occupation without regard to the usefulness or application of theories and empirical data to address or solve practical problems. Studies within the OT profession are limited to those that can be applied in practice. Therefore, while remaining separate from OT, occupational science continues to contribute valuable research that validates the fundamental concepts of our practice regarding occupations.

Founded in 1989 by Elizabeth Yerxa at the University of Southern California, occupational science was inspired by Mary Reilly's theory of occupational behavior. Some students of *occupational science* are shocked to learn that a basic science has sprung from a profession." Usually it happens the other way around. In 1962, Reilly told the profession, "Occupational therapy can be one of the great ideas of 20th century medicine" (p. 1). Her prophetic statement remains true in the 21st century with one exception: In this current paradigm, many occupational therapists believe that to achieve its rightful position in health care, OT must move out of the shadow of the medical model. Occupational behavior theory recalls the historical roots of OT and conceptualizes human occupation as dynamic and interactive. As such, Reilly's thinking is also the forerunner of many of the occupation-based models, such as the Model of Human Occupation, emerging today. Thus, occupational science and the occupation-based models are linked by a common ancestor. This link helps to clarify the

relationship of occupational science (an academic discipline) with OT (an applied science), even though the two may develop in different directions.

Occupational Therapy Practice Framework

Each level of applied theory helps us to cluster our knowledge in ways that help us apply it. The AOTA OT Practice Framework Document (the Framework) creates a taxonomy, or classification system, for OT knowledge that is consistent with our paradigm.

Domain

The first section of the Framework (2002) outlines what Mosey called OT's domain of concern, defined as "those areas of human experience in which members of a profession have expertise and offer assistance to others" (1992, p. 64). The Framework replaces the third revision of the Uniform Terminology Document, which defined OT's domain of concern as three basic categories: 1) occupational performance areas, 2) contexts, and 3) components of performance. According to Uniform Terminology (AOTA, 1994), OT's domain was limited to three occupational performance areas (activities of daily living [ADL], work, and play/leisure); two occupational performance contexts, including temporal (chronological, developmental, life cycle, disability status) and environmental (physical, social, cultural) aspects; and a much longer list of components of performance (now defined within the Framework categories of client factors, body structures, and functions). The current Framework Domain categories were outlined in Table 2-2. The Framework expands OT's scope to include six different categories (performance areas, skills, patterns, contexts, activity demands, and client factors) within our domain of concern. If each category represented a file drawer and each topic represented a file, we would be able to store much of the content of OT textbooks, journal articles, class notes, and case records in places that could be easily retrieved as needed.

Process

The categories of the Framework Process may be viewed in a similar way: evaluation, intervention, outcome, and context. However, these processes are defined differently within different models and frames of reference. The filing cabinet in Figure 4-2, therefore, contains evaluations, interventions, and outcome measures/research sections for each model/frame of reference. The Process section of the Framework adds guidelines for the practice of OT. The Framework serves practitioners (as Uniform Terminology once did) in giving the profession a common language with which to better articulate and communicate what occupational therapists do. Additionally, it has attempted to unify the profession by defining the fundamental concepts of our

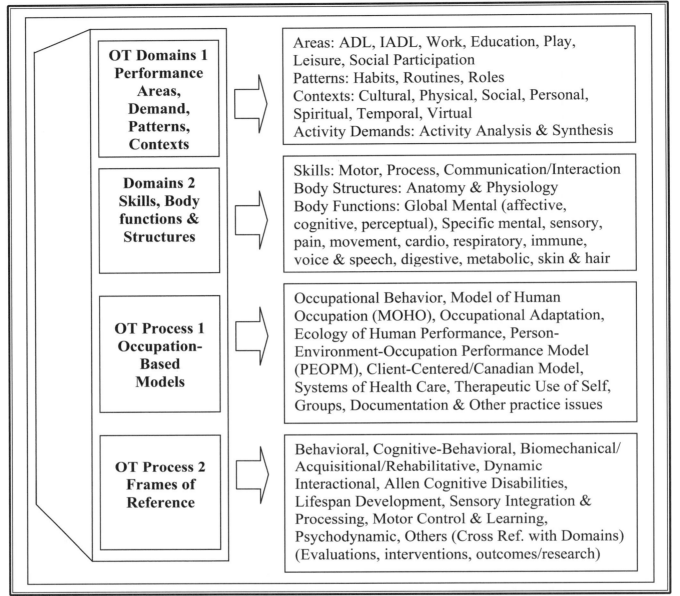

Figure 4-2. Proposed filing cabinet categories based on the OT Practice Framework. (Created by M. Cole.)

practice in ways that apply to a broad continuum of disability, wellness, and prevention.

Proposed Updates to the Framework

As practice and theory in OT evolve, the Framework will periodically need to be revised and updated. Two recent critiques are worthy of review here.

In a recent critique of the Framework domain, Nelson (2006) calls attention to specific "violations" of the rules of scientific inquiry that make the Framework terminology and taxonomy unfit for research. Citing Kerlinger (1986), he applies the following two rules of definition:

- *Precision:* specifies its particulars by listing or applying a set of rules for identifying particulars. For example,

the word adaptation as a *performance skill* differs from the same term adaptation as a *process outcome*.

- *Parsimony:* particulars belonging to one set cannot be assigned to another (cannot overlap). Nelson notes that the terms *occupation*, *activity*, *purposeful activity*, *occupational performance*, *engagement in occupation*, and *participation* seem to "overlap in unexplained ways" (p. 515).

The *rules of classification* applied by Nelson, citing Bailey (1994), further elucidate the Framework's problem with overlapping concepts:

- *Exclusivity:* each subject should have only one place where it fits into the system. Nelson notes 12 examples of terms that are "easily classifiable within (multiple) branches of the classification tree (six domain categories)" (p. 517), among them roles, play, job performance, and functional mobility.

- *Exhaustiveness:* all relevant particulars must be classifiable. When applying this rule to the Framework, all concepts relevant to OT should fit into the classification system. A few that do not are the terms *meaning, purpose,* and *engagement* (p. 519). Nelson had more difficulty in applying this rule because of the Framework's reliance on outside sources for its definitions. An easily understood example is ADL, which is listed as one area of occupation, yet its commonly understood meaning includes some of the other areas that are listed as separate categories, such as play and work.

Another proposed revision concerns the reflection and use of theory within the Framework. Gutman, Mortera, Hinojosa, and Kramer (2007) outline four recommendations. First, they suggest that more emphasis be placed on the importance of theory-based research from both inside and outside the profession (rather than exclusively occupational based) when developing practice guidelines. Second, while acknowledging the benefits of occupation-based theories requiring a "top-down" approach in developing an occupational profile of the client, "the sole reliance on such theories to guide intervention … tends to limit the scope of practice" (p. 120). In this regard, they address the need to acknowledge the reality of clinical care for occupational therapists practicing within the medical model who must select interventions based on 1) medical necessity, 2) the client's health-related goals, and 3) the demands of the practice setting. The third and fourth suggestions also relate to the discrepancy between the medical model and occupation-based practice. Third, they suggest changing some terminology to more accurately reflect the array of clinical problems occupational therapists must identify and treat within the areas of performance skills and client factors. This could take the form of the re-emergence of components of performance within the Framework's domain. Finally, these authors call for the Framework language to more closely resemble that of other professionals, community health care systems, and third-party payers (Gutman et al., 2007). These recommendations, if enacted, would swing the pendulum closer to the center between medical and client-centered (occupation-based) models of health care, making the transition easier for practitioners in medically based settings.

Both the Gutman et al. (2007) and Nelson (2006) critiques acknowledge that the profession's Framework, like the nature of practice itself, is a work in progress. In the meantime, educators and students will need to continue revising and cross referencing the categories of our "filing cabinet" as we update OT's body of knowledge. Further discussion about how models and frames of reference can be integrated with the Framework is discussed in Chapter 21.

OCCUPATION-BASED MODELS

The occupation-based models have also been called overarching theories, umbrella theories, meta-theories, and grand theories. Here we use a broad definition of *model:* an organizing technique designed to assist in categorizing ideas and structuring approaches to thinking about complex problems (Hurff, 1984). These models attempt to incorporate every area of OT practice and to explain the relationship of occupation, person, and environment. Baum and Christiansen (2005) refer to these as occupational performance models. We chose the term "occupation-based" to describe this level of theory because the concept of "performance" implies motor behavior and diminishes the importance of cognitive and affective processes of occupation (Reed & Sanderson, 1999). The Model of Human Occupation (MOHO) was one of the earliest to do this. Originally proposed as a "paradigm" and later described as a frame of reference (both incorrectly in retrospect), MOHO uses systems theory to describe how the human system interacts with various parts of the environment to facilitate or inhibit occupational performance (Kielhofner, 2002). Each occupation-based model has a different focus. Dunn's ecology of human performance model (Dunn, Brown, & McGuigan, 1994), for example, suggests that environments limit the range of tasks that can be performed by a given individual. Schkade & Schultz's occupational adaptation model (Schkade & Schultz, 1992; Schultz & Schkade, 2003) focuses on the internal adaptation process. These models organize and define the broadest concepts of the profession.

The occupation-based models are usually expressed through the use of flow charts, which visually represent the inter-relationship of various components. These systems do not distinguish or focus on any specific disability, age group, or practice area but, rather, apply to all of them. It is expected that OT practitioners will select and apply frames of reference within their structure. An important advantage of practicing within occupation-based models is their ease in generating evaluations and assessment tools that focus primarily on occupation. While the occupational therapist might select other assessments to measure specific components of performance, such as measuring range of motion with a goniometer, the models provide an overarching context of occupation that emphasizes the occupational therapist's unique perspective on a client's ability to engage in activities and participate in life. See Section II for a more in-depth discussion of specific occupation-based models.

FRAMES OF REFERENCE

Current theorists disagree about what to call this concrete level of theory. The Framework uses the term "frames of reference" as the theoretical tool that guides reasoning (AOTA, 2002, p. 616). Kielhofner (2004) uses "conceptual practice models" to address specifics. Dunn (2000) claims that frames of reference provide overarching guidance, while models of practice provide more specific guidance (p. 27). Bruce and Borg (2002) use the terms "frames of reference" and "models" interchangeably (p. 10), while Crepeau and Boyt Schell (2003) acknowledge both terms, but diminish the importance of a distinction (p. 204). In this text, we will follow the Framework's lead in accepting Mosey's perspective that conceptual systems that organize applied knowledge in OT are appropriately referred to as frames of reference (1986, 1992).

Mosey described the purpose of a frame of reference: to structure scientific knowledge so it may be applied in day-to-day situations (1986). We will use Mosey's widely quoted definition (1986, p. 12):

> [A frame of reference is a] *set of interrelated, internally consistent concepts, definitions, and postulates derived from or compatible with empirical data (theory) that provides a systematic description of or prescription for particular designs of the environment for the purpose of facilitating evaluation and effecting change relative to a specified part of the profession's domain of concern.*

Simply put, *a frame of reference is a system of compatible concepts from theory that guide a plan of action for assessment and intervention within specific OT domains.*

While the number of frames of reference has grown significantly since 1986, their structure remains current. The organization Mosey proposes begins by identifying the specific area being addressed within OT's domain of concern. This is followed by a collection of compatible concepts or theoretical base, function–dysfunction continuums, postulates of change, and guidelines for assessment and treatment. If we update Mosey's terminology, we can use this logical breakdown to apply theory in any clinical situation.

Focus

Selected areas of the Framework Domain form the focus of each frame of reference. Since frames of reference have generally been created for use with specific age groups and/or types of disability, this section defines each frame's specific focus. The domain section of the Framework lists and defines all the possibilities, making this a fairly straightforward task. For example, Toglia's multi-contextual approach was developed for persons with brain injury (body structures and functions) and is used to develop cognitive (process) skills. Because the terminology for one or more areas of the Framework Domain are specified for each frame of reference, the authors will update this section title by calling it a *framework focus.*

Theoretical Base: Compatible Concepts

This section collects theoretical concepts from both inside and outside OT's body of knowledge. Theories borrowed from or shared with other disciplines, such as biomechanical theory, are defined and organized in ways that help us to gain insight into the client's problem and what might cause it or contribute to it. Often, different theorists are identified, and their ideas combined or related to one another. For example, concepts from motor learning theory might be combined with task-oriented approach to physical disability (Mathiowetz & Bass Haugen, 1994).

Function and Disability

Function and disability serve the purpose of applying concepts from the theoretical base to individual clients or situations. Mosey originally entitled this step in theory application *function–dysfunction continuums.* Function in a specific area, such as cognition, can be evaluated using the concept of a continuum. A good example is Allen's cognitive disabilities frame of reference (Allen & Blue, 1998). Allen defines six basic levels and 52 modes of cognitive ability, ranging from wellness to semicomatose. This definition of function guides our thinking in setting goals and predicting or evaluating outcomes. These authors prefer the word disability rather than dysfunction because of its more positive view of the client and its congruence with current terminology. Function and disability are both terms used by the International Classification System of Function, Disability, and Health (WHO, 2001), and the Framework (AOTA, 2002).

Change and Motivation

Mosey called this section "postulates of change," which are principles or proposed relationships among variables that explain how therapy works. A *postulate* is a theoretical statement that suggests how two or more concepts are related. Kielhofner called these principles "theoretical arguments," which propose how the basic concepts apply to a specific area of focus (2004). For example, sensory integrative theory suggests that sensory input can influence a client's ability to attend to a task. This postulate (or argument) may or may not have been substantiated with research. However, each frame of reference generates research in areas that support the specific techniques and strategies used for evaluation and intervention. These authors have simplified the terminology for this section title to "change and motivation," which proposes various explanations about how we might assist our clients in making therapeutic change as well as enhancing motivation for engagement in meaningful occupations.

Evaluation and Guidelines for Intervention

Evaluation, from a client-centered perspective, necessitates working in partnership with the client or clients to set occupational goals and priorities. For the occupational therapist, establishing a therapeutic relationship with the

Table 4-3
Structure of a Frame of Reference: Mosey Versus Kielhofner

Mosey	Kielhofner
Frame of reference	Conceptual model of practice
Domain of concern	Focus
Theoretical base	Interdisciplinary base
Function–dysfunction continuum	Theoretical arguments for order and disorder
Postulates of change	Theoretical arguments for therapeutic intervention
Evaluation and intervention	Technology for application
Research	Research

client becomes the initial step in evaluation. Assessment may be less broad, focusing on specific behaviors, skill areas, occupations, tasks, and contexts. Behaviors indicative of function and dysfunction (Mosey, 1992) form the basis for assessment in a client's specific problem areas. In client-centered practice, these may be areas the client has identified as issues or priorities or areas derived from the initial occupational profile. A frame of reference guides the selection of methods used to evaluate the problem based on how disability is defined. The focus may be motor, sensory, psychological, or social functioning or on specific occupational performance areas or contexts. Some frames of reference have produced specific assessment tools designed to measure various aspects of occupational performance.

Intervention, as currently defined, involves doing with the client. Often it involves the analysis and synthesis of activities (Mosey, 1986). Postulates regarding change form the basis for activity analysis and synthesis relative to the change process. For example, Allen postulates that a person with a Level 4 cognitive disability will be confused and distracted by visual clutter, which is defined as objects within the visual field that bear no relevance to the task to be performed. This postulate suggests that the occupational therapist can facilitate task performance (a positive therapeutic change) by modifying the environment in specific ways: 1) by removing unnecessary objects from view and 2) by placing needed supplies within full view of the client. If our assessment tells us that the client has an Allen level 4 cognitive disability, Allen's postulate guides our intervention strategies for setting up a facilitative task environment. According to the OT Practice Framework, during the intervention process, information from the evaluation is "integrated with theory, frames of reference, and evidence" to develop and carry out a plan (AOTA, 2002).

Different Views of Structure for a Frame of Reference

Kielhofner (2004) proposes a slightly different structure for what he calls a conceptual model of practice. Kielhofner discusses the dynamics of a conceptual practice model in terms of concentric circles. The inner circle represents the paradigm of the profession. The next layer, or circle, contains the multiple conceptual practice models, which represent various practical attempts to put the vision of the paradigm into practice. The outer layer or circle represents related knowledge or knowledge generated outside the field of OT. Each practice model draws from this vast array of theories to form its unique interdisciplinary base. Kielhofner's conceptualization is not substantially different from Mosey's but is explained somewhat differently and uses different terminology. A comparison of Mosey's and Kielhofner's terminology is outlined in Table 4-3.

Research: Outcomes

Research, as noted in Table 4-3, is the only component of the structure upon which Mosey and Kielhofner agree. This last step in the structure of a frame of reference represents the evidence that has been gathered by researchers about the validity of the theoretical concepts outlined and the effectiveness of the techniques used by occupational therapists according to its guidelines. The part of the Framework addressed by research is outcomes. In evidence-based practice, the occupational therapist needs to discuss with clients the available evidence that the techniques proposed for intervention actually work or how well they have worked for others with similar problems. Margo Holm (2000) defines evidence-based practice as the "judicious use of current best evidence in making decisions about the care of individual(s)" (2000, p. 576). Gray (1997) put it more simply: "doing things right" and "doing the right things" (p. 17). OT practitioners must develop the habit of reading research studies, attending conferences, or observing videos for practice in the clinic, community, or school, thereby updating their knowledge in order to keep their practice current and evidence-based.

HOW TO EVALUATE MODELS AND FRAMES OF REFERENCE

Crepeau and Boyt Schell (2003) point out that the major theories in OT differ in purpose, scope, complexity, extent of development and validation through research, and usefulness in practice (p. 204). In fact, occupational therapists apply the various levels of theory at different stages of the evaluation, intervention, outcomes continuum. The occupation-based models enter the clinical reasoning process near the beginning of the client–therapist relationship as the occupational therapist develops a perspective about how the client's roles and occupations interact with the outside world (systems, contexts). These theories help to identify the range of possibilities when setting collaborative goals for client engagement in occupations as well as identifying barriers to participation. In addition, occupation-based models help us think about ways in which our clients can find meaningful roles in society. The occupational therapist might select an appropriate occupation-based model by asking the following:

- Which model best explains the way my client wishes to interact with his/her environment?

- Which model offers the best guidelines for identifying the barriers my client has encountered?

- Which model helps me to determine which occupations, roles, and patterns are possible for my client within his or her preferred contexts?

- Which model helps me identify ways to adapt the environment to facilitate engagement in selected occupations?

These questions help occupational therapists determine how well a client, given his or her specific limitations, might fit into a given system, such as a family, a community group, or a work environment.

Frames of reference enter the reasoning process as the occupational therapist thinks about problem areas the client has identified within defined contexts in order to assess occupational skills and guide client choice of appropriate intervention strategies. Occupational therapists need a basic understanding of many different frames of reference in order to select those that best apply in therapeutic situations.

The following are questions we might ask ourselves in order to determine the value and usefulness of a frame of reference for a specific client:

- What frames of reference focus upon the areas my client has identified as priorities?

- What frames of reference help me to understand the problems my client has demonstrated?

- What research has been done to validate the basic concepts of this frame of reference?

- What assessment tools does this frame of reference provide? What is their reliability and validity?

- What concepts guide my thinking when developing intervention strategies?

- What specific techniques have been developed to bring about therapeutic change? What evidence exists in the literature that these techniques are effective?

These questions allow us to share our expertise with clients in ways that focus and clarify specific problem areas. For example, why is a client having problems tolerating wearing certain clothing? The sensory integration frame of reference addresses sensory problems such as tactile defensiveness, an inability to tolerate certain types of tactile stimulation such as the texture of clothing. This frame of reference also provides reliable and valid test instruments for evaluating tactile sensation and perception. A postulate of change is that controlled sensory input can facilitate desensitization and increase tolerance for certain types of tactile input. Tools for doing this, such as brushes, vibrators, and therapeutic activities in which the client encounters graded pressure and texture (finding the pennies in a bucket of sand, rice, or beans), have been researched extensively, and evidence on their effectiveness is readily available. In this example, the sensory integration frame of reference helps to explain the cause of the problem and provides guidelines for evaluation and intervention to address it.

Other frames of reference offer different explanations for difficulty with dressing. If sensory tolerance is not the primary issue, perhaps a lack of motor control (biomechanical, neurodevelopmental), a lack of social awareness (cognitive behavioral, psychodynamic), or a cognitive disability (Allen's cognitive disabilities, Toglia's dynamic interactional) might explain it. Each of these suggests possible frames of reference to consider.

Crepeau and Boyt Schell (2003) suggest that practitioners tend to incorporate theory into their reasoning process in ways that allow them to use it automatically, that is, without conscious awareness. Thus, practicing occupational therapists may not always be able to identify the frame of reference they are using. This does not mean they are not using theory but, rather, that its use has become habitual. However, when students begin to learn clinical reasoning, it is important to consciously think about the choices and to maintain flexibility in using various approaches.

In Section III, we will review some specific frames of reference and demonstrate their application in practice.

Reed's Theory Analysis Method

Concepts form the basis of any theoretical model. Reed and Sanderson (1999) suggest that students define frames of reference that are new or unfamiliar through the use of a Venn diagram (Figure 4-3). A Venn diagram uses three overlapping circles to visualize a practice model (frame of reference) and to compare one model with another. As a starting point in defining a frame of reference, the student needs to identify the most important organizing ideas of the theory being analyzed. The major focus of the model, the central organizing assumption, occupies the center portion of the overlapping circles. Usually, this is the goal or desired outcome of the therapy process. The next step is to identify the three concepts from the same theory that are most likely to produce therapeutic change or to move the client toward the desired outcome. Sometimes, there are many choices, and finding the most useful concepts may take some experimentation. The Venn diagram gives a visual representation of 1) the focus and 2) the basic assumptions of the frame of reference.

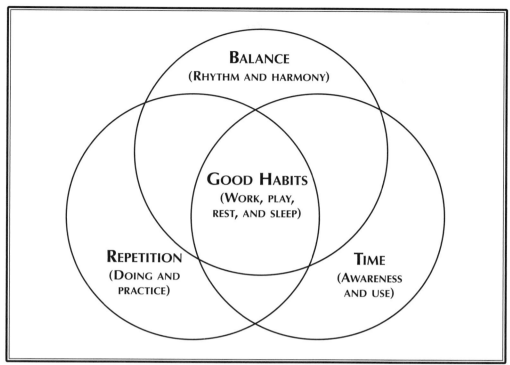

Figure 4-3. Reed's application of a Venn diagram with Slagle's Habit Training Frame of Reference. (Adapted from Reed, K., & Sanderson, S. [1999]. *Concepts of occupational therapy* [4th ed., pp. 239–241]. Baltimore, MD: Lippincott, Williams & Wilkins.)

The remaining steps involve 3) defining function and dysfunction, 4) articulating postulates of change, and outlining strategies for 5) evaluation and 6) intervention. These steps will organize the theoretical ideas in ways that guide occupational therapists' application of the theory to practice. The Venn diagram will be the first step and may not be considered a complete analysis. For a complete understanding of a well-developed theory, many additional concepts will need to be defined. (See Table 4-4 for a list of key terms.)

LEARNING ACTIVITIES

Activities presented here refer to the three levels of theory we propose for the profession: paradigm, occupation-based models, and frames of reference. As an introduction, students may be asked to define each of these levels, to explain how they relate to one another, and/or to give examples of how each might be applied in practice.

Model and Frame of Reference Analysis

Directions: Choose an unfamiliar theory to analyze, and follow these steps:

1. What is the focus or central organizing idea of the theory? This may be thought of as the goal of OT intervention. Write this concept at the center of a Venn diagram like the one in Figure 4-4 (where all three circles intersect).

2. Identify the three most important concepts of the theory that, taken together, will produce the outcome represented at the center. Write these in the three circles of the diagram.

3. Define each concept you have written according to the chosen model or frame (Table 4-5). Explain how these factors produce the outcome represented in the center (intersection).

Additional Learning Strategies

Directions: To help you think about the usefulness of a model or frame of reference, answer the following.

Focus
How broad a focus does this theory have? What areas of the OT practice domain are involved? Does it apply only to one age group? Primarily one type of disability? List the health conditions that might benefit from this approach.

Theorists
Who are the theorists, researchers, or authors who have contributed to this theory? From what disciplines (OT or others) do these concepts originate? To what extent are the concepts compatible, or do they contradict each other?

Function–Disability Continuum
How does this theory apply to individual client functioning? What disabilities might a client have which

Table 4-4

Key Terms

Theory	Describes, explains, and predicts behavior and/or the relationship between concepts or events.
Applied theory	The results of applied research, intended to address problems of practical interest.
Paradigm	A shared vision encompassing fundamental assumptions and beliefs, which serves as the cultural core of the profession (Kielhofner, 2004, p. 19)
Philosophy	A fundamental belief
Model	a simplified representation of structure and content... that describes or explains complex relationships between concepts (Creek, 1992)
Occupational Performance Model	A framework for understanding the individual's dynamic experience in daily occupations within the environment (Baum & Law, 1995)
Occupation-Based Model	Proposed interaction of person, environment, and occupation that guide the organization of occupational therapy practice
Conceptual Models in OT	Graphic or schematic representations of concepts & assumptions that explain why the profession works as it does. (Reed & Sanderson, 1999)
Frame of Reference	System of compatible concepts from theory which guides a plan of action within a specific OT domain of concern. (Adapted from Mosey, 1986.)
Concept	An idea or notion formed by mentally combining characteristics (Reed & Sanderson, 1999)
Construct	An assembly of observable or directly experienced phenomena (Depoy & Gitlin, 2005).
Postulate	A theoretical statement which suggests how two or more concepts are related. (Mosey, 1986)
Assumptions	Broad general statements that are taken for granted for the sake of argument
Epistemology	The dynamics of knowing (Hooper, 2006). How we know what we know.
Taxonomy	System of classification for organizing theory and knowledge in a field.

Figure 4-4. Model and frame of reference analysis worksheet.

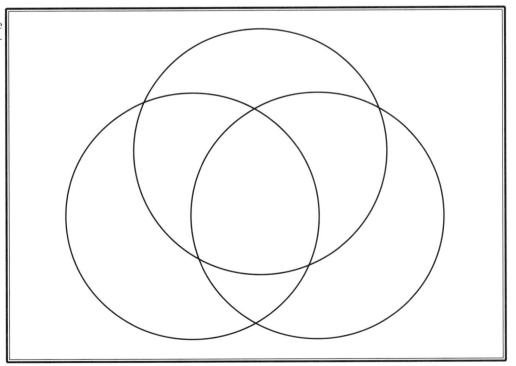

Table 4-5

Template for Analysis Worksheet

Title of Model or Frame of Reference _____

Theoretical Components	Summary
Focus (OT framework domains, practice areas, health conditions, or specific populations)	
Theorists (Whose theories have contributed?)	
Function (How does theory view healthy or optimal functioning?)	
Disability (How is disability defined?)	
Change (How does change occur, according to this theory?)	
Motivation (What motivates a client to change?)	
Evaluation (What formal or informal assessments are offered?)	
Intervention Guidelines (What specific therapeutic techniques or strategies have been developed?)	
Research (To what extent has this theory been validated through research?)	

prevent him or her from achieving the desired outcome? In the example of habit training, disability might be defined as having no habits or routines, and function might be defined as having a daily structure of normal daily activities that include a balance of work, play, rest, and sleep. Create a continuum for the theory you have chosen.

Define the worst possible disability on one end of the continuum and the best possible functioning at the other end.

Change and Motivation

What does this theory tell you about how change occurs for clients? What kinds of things can influence the client's occupational performance in a positive direction? List three strategies that could influence a client's functioning in the focus area defined in the center of your diagram.

Assessment

How could you learn more about a client's functioning in the focus area of this theory? What are some questions you could ask? What might be some ways you could observe occupational performance? What assessment tools are currently available that help occupational therapists evaluate different aspects of human functioning using this theory?

Intervention

What methods or techniques for intervention are defined by this theory? How could you put the postulates of change into action in OT? Give two examples.

Research

What studies provide evidence for this theory? Summarize three studies.

Resolution of an Ethical Dilemma*

1. Gather all relevant information: history, issues, dynamics, and culture.

2. Determine conflicting values and areas of agreement: autonomy, beneficence, and nonmaleficence.

3. Identify relevant actions: seeking alternative courses of action.

4. List possible positive and negative outcomes for everyone.

*Adapted from Reitz, S. (1997). Ethics for students. In K. Sladyk (Ed.), OT student primer: A guide to college success (p. 249). Thorofare, NJ: SLACK Incorporated.

5. Weigh carefully outcomes/consequences (+/–) for each alternative action.

Dilemma: Should Margaret Stop Driving?

Margaret is 83 years old, and has become increasingly forgetful. Her daughter, Lauren, suspects that Margaret might be in the mild stages of Alzheimer's. Greg, Margaret's 90-year-old husband, is legally blind and recovering from a stroke and depends on Margaret to take him to the doctor's office, the bank, to church, and to the diner every day for lunch. One snowy day, Margaret loses her way coming home from the grocery store and drives 10 miles up a country road, finally sliding off the edge in the snow. A policeman offers to move the car to a safe parking spot and drives them home. A week later, Margaret's license is suspended by the state pending a retest and eye exam. Lauren stops in every few days but cannot take time off from work to do all the driving for her parents. A home health agency is contacted, and you, an occupational therapist, are sent to evaluate the situation. You find that Margaret drives extremely slowly, causing traffic jams behind her all the way to the grocery store, about half a mile from her home. She obeys the road signs but gets lost if she drives down an unfamiliar street. She cannot follow directions or read a map. Although blind, Greg is able to help Margaret with judgment in difficult situations, and there is no public transportation in their town. They would be stranded without being able to drive.

Group Learning Strategy

Divide into groups of 4 or 5. Choose a recorder to take notes as you discuss each step in the analysis process. Each member of the group take on one person's role (Greg, Margaret, Lauren, the occupational therapist, and possibly the policeman representing society's perspective) in the above scenario and present the positive and negative consequences for you. Then, as a group, decide on the outcome the occupational therapist should recommend for Margaret. Recorders from each group may present their ethical reasoning process and conclusions to the class.

REFERENCES

Allen, C. K., & Blue, T. (1998). Cognitive disabilities model: How to make clinical judgments. In N. Katz (Ed.), *Cognition and occupation in rehabilitation*. Bethesda, MD: American Occupational Therapy Association.

American Occupational Therapy Association. (2002). Occupational therapy practice framework: Domain and process. *American Journal of Occupational Therapy, 56,* 609–639.

American Occupational Therapy Association (2004). *The reference manual of the official documents of the American Occupational Therapy Association*. Bethesda, MD: Author.

American Occupational Therapy Association (2005). Occupational therapy code of ethics (2005). *American Journal of Occupational Therapy, 59,* 639-642.

Ayres, A. J. (1989). *Sensory integration and the child*. Los Angeles, CA: Western Psychological.

Bailey, K. D. (1994). *Typologies and taxonomies: An introduction to classification techniques*. Thousand Oaks, CA: Sage.

Baum, C., & Christiansen, C. (2005). Person–environment–occupation performance: An occupation-based framework for practice. In C. Christiansen & C. Baum (Eds.), *Occupational therapy: Performance, participation, and well-being* (3rd ed.). Thorofare, NJ: SLACK Incorporated.

Baum, C., & Edwards, B. (1995). Occupational performance: Occupational therapy's definition of function. *American Journal of Occupational Therapy, 49,* 1019–1020.

Baum, C. & Law, M. (1995). Occupational performance: occupational therapy's definition of function. *American Journal of Occupational Therapy, 49,* 1019.

Bruce, M., & Borg, B. (2002). *Psychosocial frames of reference: Core for occupation-based practice*. Thorofare, NJ: SLACK Incorporated.

Christiansen, C., & Baum, C. (1997). *Occupational therapy: Performance, participation, and well-being* (2nd ed.). Thorofare, NJ: SLACK Incorporated.

Christiansen, C., Clark, F., Kielhofner, G., & Rogers, J. (1995). Occupation: A position paper. *American Journal of Occupational Therapy, 49,* 1015–1018.

Clark, C., Azen, S., Zemke, R., Jackson, J., Carlson, M., Mandel, D., et al. (1997). Occupational therapy for independent-living older adults: A randomized controlled trial. *Journal of the American Medical Association, 278,* 1321–1326.

Creek, J. (1992). Models of practice in occupational therapy: Part I defining terms. *British Journal of Occupational Therapy, 56,* 4–6.

Crepeau, E., & Boyt Schell, B. (2003). Theory and practice in occupational therapy. In E. Crepeau, E. Cohn, & B. Boyt Schell (Eds.), *Willard & Spackman's occupational therapy* (10th ed.). Philadelphia, PA: Lippincott, Williams & Wilkins.

Depoy, E., & Gitlin, L. N. (2005). *Introduction to research: Understanding and applying multiple strategies*. St. Louis, MO: Elsevier-Mosby.

Dunn, W. (2000). *Best practice occupational therapy in community service with children and families*. Thorofare, NJ: SLACK Incorporated.

Dunn, W., Brown, C., & McGuigan, A. (1994). The ecology of human performance: A framework for considering the effect of context. *American Journal of Occupational Therapy, 48,* 595–607.

Dunton, W. R. (1919). *Reconstruction therapy*. Philadelphia, PA: W. B. Saunders.

Gesell, A. (1934). Atlas of infant behavior. New Haven, CT: Yale University Press. Retrieved July 5, 2005, from http://info.med.yale.edu/chldstdy/history.html.

Gray, J. A. M. (1997). *Evidence-based healthcare: How to make health policy and management decisions*. New York: Churchill Livingstone.

Gutman, S. A., Mortera, M. H., Hinojosa, J., & Kramer, P. (2007). The issue is: Revision of the occupational therapy practice framework. *American Journal of Occupational Therapy, 61,* 119–126.

Hagedorn, R. (2001). *Foundations for practice in occupational therapy* (3rd ed.). London: Churchill Livingstone.

Hinojosa, J., Sabari, J., & Pedretti, L. (1993). Position paper: Purposeful activities. *American Journal of Occupational Therapy, 47,* 1081–1082.

Holm, M. (2000). Our mandate for the new millennium: Evidence-based practice. *American Journal of Occupational Therapy, 54,* 575–585.

Hooper, B. (2006). Epistemological transformation in occupational therapy: Educational implications and challenges. *Occupational Therapy Journal of Research, 26,* 15–24.

Hurff, J. M. (1984). Visualization: A decision-making tool for assessment and treatment planning. *Occupational Therapy in Health Care, 1*(2), 3–23.

Kerlinger, F. N. (1986). *Foundations of behavioral research* (3rd ed.). New York, NY: Harcourt Brace College.

Kielhofner, G. (2004). *Conceptual foundations of occupational therapy* (3rd ed). Philadelphia: FA Davis.

Kielhofner, G., & Burke, J. (1980). A model of human occupation, Part 1. Conceptual framework and content. *American Journal of Occupational Therapy, 34,* 572–581.

Kuhn, T. (1970). *The structure of scientific revolutions* (2nd ed.). Chicago, IL: University of Chicago Press.

Meyer, A. (1922; 1977). The philosophy of occupational therapy. *American Journal of Occupational Therapy, 31,* 639–642. (Original work published in 1922).

Mosey, A. C. (1986). *Psychosocial components of occupational therapy.* New York, NY: Raven Press.

Mosey, A. C. (1992). *Applied scientific inquiry in the health professions: An epistemological orientation.* Rockville, MD: American Occupational Therapy Association.

Nelson, D. L. (2006). Critiquing the logic of the domain section of the Occupational therapy practice framework: Domain and process. *American Journal of Occupational Therapy, 60,* 511–523.

Quiroga, V. (1995). *Occupational therapy history: the first thirty years 1900–1930.* Bethesda, MD: American Occupational Therapy Association.

Reed, K., & Sanderson, S. (1999). *Concepts of occupational therapy* (4th ed.). Baltimore, MD: Lippincott, Williams & Wilkins.

Reilly, M. (1958). An occupational therapy curriculum for 1965. *American Journal of Occupational Therapy, 12,* 293–299.

Reilly, M. (1962). Occupational therapy can be one of the great ideas of twentieth century medicine. In R. Padilla (Ed.), (2005). *A professional legacy: the Eleanor Clarke Slagle Lectures in occupational therapy, 1955–2004* (2nd ed.). Bethesda, MD: American Occupational Therapy Association Press.

Reitz, S. (1997). Ethics for students. In K. Sladyk (Ed.), *OT student primer: A guide to college success.* Thorofare, NJ: SLACK Incorporated.

Sadock, B., & Sadock, V. (2003). *Synopsis of psychiatry* (9th ed.). Philadelphia, PA: Lippincott, Williams & Wilkins.

Scaffa, M. (2001). *Occupational therapy in community-based practice settings.* Philadelphia, PA: FA Davis.

Schkade, J. K., & Schultz, S. (1992). Occupational adaptation: Toward a holistic approach to contemporary practice, Part 2. *American Journal of Occupational Therapy, 46,* 917–926.

Schultz, S., & Schkade, J. K. (1992). Occupational adaptation: Toward a holistic approach to contemporary practice, Part 1. *American Journal of Occupational Therapy, 46,* 829–837.

Schultz, S., & Schkade, J. K. (2003). Occupational adaptation. In E. B. Crepeau, E. S. Cohn, & B. A. Boyt Schell (Eds.), *Willard & Spackman's occupational therapy* (10th ed.). Philadelphia, PA: Lippincott Williams & Wilkins.

World Health Organization. (2001). *International classification of functioning, disability, and health.* Geneva: Author.

Chapter 5

APPLIED THEORIES OF COMMUNITY HEALTH AND WELL-BEING

"The new millennium will realize the health-enabling, restorative potential of occupation, and the promise of occupational therapy will be fulfilled."

– CHARLES H. CHRISTIANSEN (1999)

The purpose of this chapter is to review current trends of well-being and the impact of occupation in promoting health, particularly from a social community framework. There are multiple reasons why health care trends will continue to evolve from a traditional medical model orientation to a community-based focus. One significant variable to this change process is the management of costs. Medical fees for clients are lessened when conducted in nonmedical settings such as the community. Over the last 20 to 30 years, practitioners have sought and increased employment opportunities in home health agencies, outpatient clinics, private practice, skilled nursing facilities, and school systems. Two major influential resources that help to shape preventive health care, the World Health Organization (WHO) and public health systems, are complementary sectors promoting a more holistic health approach conducive to community practice. Occupational therapy's (OT's) paradigm shift to a more holistic and contextually sensitive practice also supports the promotion of well-being and prevention of illness, a focus that naturally fits a social, community health care model.

There is much to be done to develop the full potential of a national community model for practice. The underlying principles of community-based practice and OT mesh well together, which is evident in similar health objectives and an underlying humanistic, client-centered philosophy. In this new millennium of health care reform and technological development, occupational therapists have a wonderful opportunity to carve a unique role among practitioners in community practice that could restore health and life balance to consumers and promote meaningfulness and distinction of our own profession.

OCCUPATIONAL THERAPY PRACTICE COMES FULL CIRCLE

Carolyn Baum, among other concerned occupational therapists, has written about the changing health system and inclusion of OT services in these times of reform. She supports the idea of a client-centered practice that embraces a social (community) focus (Smith & Eggleston, 1989) as a prototype for future practice:

> [These health system changes] *challenge occupational therapists to extend their interventions beyond the clients' immediate impairments to focus on their long-term health needs by helping them develop behaviors to improve their health and well-being and minimize long-term health care costs associated with dysfunction.* (Baum & Law, 1998; p. 31)

A social model system, as described by Smith and Eggleston, depicts a community-centered focus on wellness. Its approach reflects a collaborative and interdependent relationship between consumer and practitioner that actively engages the client to take personal responsibility and prevent illness. As various countries such as Canada, Australia, Great Britain, and the United States attempt to improve the health of residents, occupational therapists have an opportunity to re-establish their roles and to take action. Within the United States, an example of a governing body that supports a holistic paradigm of care is the Joint Commission on Accreditation of Healthcare Organizations (JCAHO). Its overall objectives are to promote health and to decrease the long-term cost of care associated with chronic conditions (JCAHO, 1995). Occupational therapists can utilize the powerful impact of this governing accrediting agency to justify interventions, match services that fit these objectives, and qualify for reimbursement.

The utilization of a social, community-based practice in health care is a familiar and inbred idea for occupational therapists that has evolved since the origins of the profession. Community-based practice may be defined as the provision of services in community settings where people live and participate in their daily activities (Scaffa, 2001). Current day examples include independent living centers, vocational and residential programs for persons with developmental disabilities, and health and fitness programs.

Originally, George Barton and Eleanor Clark Slagle both designed community-based OT programs in the 1900s. Barton's program, called Consolation House, was located in New York. It was intended to assist veterans to return and re-integrate into healthy and productive living. Slagle's program was called Hull House and was located in Chicago. Its objective was to provide people with physical and mental disabilities a chance to develop work skills to enhance independence. These programs exemplified a treatment approach that constituted the values of morality and humanity coupled with meaningful occupation. It is ironic that the 1999 recipient of the Eleanor Clark Slagle Lecture award, Charles H. Christiansen, is once again reminding OT practitioners that the "... ultimate goal of occupational therapy services is well-being, not health." Christiansen emphasized that "when we build our identities through occupations, we provide ourselves with the contexts necessary for creating meaningful lives, and life meaning helps us to be well (Christiansen, 1999, p. 547)."

Christiansen's (1999) framework, which asserts that occupations serve as the principal means in the formation of one's personal identity, reflects the culminating paradigm shift evident in OT practice over the last 10 years. As previously discussed in earlier chapters of this text, Kielhofner (1997) conceptualized that the purpose of the paradigm shift in OT was an attempt to reclaim our identity and re-focus our intentions back on the nature of occupations. The resulting occupation-based models that emerged in the 1990s were meant to guide practitioners more holistically, with an appreciation toward client capacities and functional ability. A common element among all of these models is the regard for person, occupation, and environment and the inter-relationship of these components. Participation in occupation is viewed as a health determinant and no longer a mere modality to treat patients who are ill. Persons are respected for their inherent qualities, roles, intrinsic and extrinsic pursuits, and free choice and not a culmination of symptoms that needs to be fixed or cured. Practitioners are facilitators; clients are the agents of change. The OT evaluation process includes a balance of scientific knowledge and evidence in conjunction with the phenomenological view of the "problem" as identified by the person. Behaviors are interpreted as an outcome of complex and interacting dynamics (systems theory) and not just a product of one's biological nature (deterministic). Therapeutic intervention is focused on functioning and enabling, not on the disabling causes. Contexts for intervention have been significantly broadened to include physical, social, cultural, personal, spiritual, temporal, and virtual as defined within the OT Practice Framework, a far extension beyond the scope of a medical institution or rehabilitation center. The role of one's environment and its pervasive impact on a client's behavioral outcome is now a heightened focus of OT concern rather than a mere consideration in discharge planning and disposition of the client.

It is a natural fit for occupational therapists to enter partnerships not only with their clients but also with the members of the community where people live and participate in life events. *Community-centered interventions* represent the efforts of multiple coalitions coming together to identify common concerns and to solve community problems (Scaffa & Brownson, 2005). Treatment agencies, who use this model, are now referred to as "systems of care" and consist of multiple and varied services with extended partnerships to other resources in the community. These types of interventions focus on the betterment of a designated population by interfacing with multiple sources for support: consumers, businesses, politicians, law enforcement, religious leaders, and health proponents. This style of intervention is truly a systems theory approach because the identified "patient" is the entire community with its multiple areas of concern. The philosophy that "it takes a village to raise a child" is an example of this system point of view. Other examples of programs include DARE (Drug Abuse Resistance Education), a national program that serves young children in the prevention and education of drug use by law enforcers.

Public health is an example of a field of study that has significant global impact on the direction of health reform in the millennium. Likewise, occupational therapists could have a complementary degree of impact on the study of Public health if they "took a strong educational and political stance aimed at social action for change relating to maximizing the effects of occupation on health and well-being for the wider community as well as individuals with disability" (Wilcock, p. 212, 1998). Public health is slowly gaining more respect as a complement to medical practice. Its national focus areas and leading health indicators, subsequent study of disparities amongst populations, multiple health objectives, and epidemiological research all serve as a guide for both *community practice* and *community-centered interventions* that can be considered by occupational therapists as well as other health practitioners.

OCCUPATION, HEALTH, AND WELL-BEING

Ann Wilcock is an occupational therapist and professor of occupational science and therapy at Deakin University in Victoria, Australia, with a PhD in Public Health. She is recognized as an expert in the role of human occupation as a determinant of health. In her book *An Occupational Perspective of Health* (1998; 2006), now in its second edition, Wilcock prolifically explored the relationship between occupation and health and its importance to public health. Within these texts, Wilcock traces how health promotion and well-being has historically evolved and links the role of OT with these global efforts. Here is a brief highlight of some of her salient points for consideration in current practice.

In 1946, the WHO defined *health* as a state of complete physical, mental, and social well-being not merely the absence of disease or infirmity. While this definition represented a holistic view of health, it was filtered through the lens of people with a medical model point of view. As Wilcock noted for her readers, "health is a concept that many find difficult to define in a positive sense because it is often not thought about seriously until someone experiences a state of illness" (Wilcock, p. 136, 2005).

In 1986, the first WHO Health Promotion Conference was held in Ottawa, Canada. Among the 212 delegates that attended, a document was published called the *Ottawa Charter for Health Promotion*. This document emphasized that health practitioners should fulfill such roles as *advocates*, *enablers*, and *mediators* for their prospective clients and consumers. Wilcock (2005) asserts that as occupational therapists, we should advocate occupation for the development of health and mediation for consumers where occupational injustice has occurred. She defines *occupational justice* as the "... just and equitable distribution of power, resources, and opportunity so that all people are able to meet the needs of their occupational natures and so experience health and well-being" (2005, p. 149). Wilcock proposes that health, as originally defined by WHO, is achievable by participation in occupations, a "fundamental mechanism for realizing aspirations, satisfying needs, and coping with one's environment" (Wilcock, 2005, p. 149).

WHO's definition of health has had far reaching influence since its words hit the page in 1986. For example, WHO and the Ottawa Charter are interlinked in how health is viewed "... as a resource for everyday life that emphasizes social and personal resources as well as physical capabilities (Wilcock, p. 16, 2006). Three further WHO meetings were held in Adelaide (1988), Sundsvall (1991), and Jakarta (1997), and the original Charter initiatives were further broadened and explored. According to Wilcock (2006, p. 17), the three basic strategies proposed in the Charter may be summarized as follows: 1) *advocating* for the political, environmental, economic, social, cultural, biological, and behavioral conditions essential for health; 2) *enabling* people to strive for and reach their health potential; and 3) *mediating* among different sociopolitical interests in the pursuit of health for all people. She also describes how the new public health policy is related conceptually to these initiatives, and this relationship creates a strong bond for world health policy. Wilcock believes that the roles of advocating, enabling, and mediating are complementary to OT practice. "The exploration so far has suggested that public health practitioners and occupational therapists could and should be primary sources of expertise for research and development of population health approaches that take an occupational perspective" (Wilcock, 2006, p. 211).

The concept of *well-being* tends to be more obscure and subjective in its definition as compared to the definition of health. A term that is often associated with happiness and prosperity (Roget's Thesaurus, 1980), well-being may be further defined by physical, mental, and/or social attributes. Physical well-being tends to connote the more objective characteristics related to body structures and physiology. For example, physical well-being may be described in terms of being "strong" or having good body conditioning. Mental well-being includes those characteristics that are often internally experienced and harder to measure objectively. These associations may include feelings, thought processes, and spirituality. Mental well-being is often connoted by "good self esteem" and feeling "self satisfied or complete." Physical and mental capacities are combined under one heading in the OT Practice Framework (AOTA, 2002) and described as "body functions" (a client factor, including physical, cognitive, psychosocial aspects)—"the physiological functions of body systems (including psychological functions)" (WHO, 2001, p. 10). This could be an attempt to integrate rather than separate the functions of the mind, body, and spirit as we become more holistic in practice. Nonetheless, well-being could not be fully understood without including a third component. Social well-being can be defined as having satisfying interpersonal relationships. Social participation is a significant focus area for OT practice as many of our clients seek to "belong" and connect within a social world that is often judgmental and stigmatizing of their disability. In the OT Practice Framework (AOTA, 2002), social participation is defined as an "organized pattern of behaviors that are characteristic and expected of an individual in a given position within a social system" (Mosey, 1996, p. 340). A sense of social well-being reflects social integration and a supportive network. The acquisition and maintenance of social supports, a vital component to recovery, is a primary goal within a social community model. Studies that stress the importance of social participation include one by Nutbeam (1986), who postulated that well-being can be attributed and solely understood within the context of a social model of health, and Doyal and Gough (1991), who concluded that the loss of social participation is like denying one's "humanity" (p. 184).

Wilcock strongly professes that occupational therapists should value and develop a role in community and public health because it is within our scope of practice. From this perspective, she has identified two overarching goals regarding the development of well-being for consumers and OT's role (2005, p. 154):

- To enhance and enrich physical, social, mental, emotional, intellectual, and vocational capacities among clients and consumers

- To utilize wide-ranging, age-appropriate, and balanced occupations for all people

Wilcock also proposes that occupational therapists can have a significant impact in supporting the Ottawa Charter's defined strategies for *health promotion*:

- Assuming the role as "health agents" that enable, advocate, and mediate for consumers
- Creating supportive environments that include safe and satisfying characteristics as defined by inhabitants
- Empowering communities to take ownership and responsible action for their own advancement
- Promoting the personal skills and potential of all consumers in a holistic manner
- Researching the effect of occupation on health and subsequently enlisting and educating the role of occupation among health services

PUBLIC HEALTH AND OCCUPATIONAL THERAPY

Public health may be defined as the "process of mobilizing local, state, national, and international resources to ensure the conditions in which people can be healthy" (Detels & Breslow, 1997, p. 3). It is a culmination of various theories and disciplines including epidemiology, biological and clinical science, biostatistics, nursing, health education, sanitation, industrial hygiene, sociology, psychology, economics, law, and engineering. Its primary source and fundamental science is *epidemiology*, or the study and distribution, frequencies, and determinants of disease, injury, and disability in human populations (MacMahon & Trichopoulos, 1996). Epidemiology offers data on health statistics that can influence health trends, interventions, and ultimately, health policies. Such statistics include reports on *incidence*, which is the number of new cases of disease, injury, or disability within a specified time frame, and *prevalence*, which is the total number of cases of disease, injury, or disability in a community, city, state, or nation existing at one point in time (Pickett and Hanlon, 1990).

Following is an example of how an occupational therapist might incorporate data and the objectives from public health within a community practice setting. An occupational therapist who works in an elementary school completes an assessment on an 8-year-old female named Ariana who shows some difficulty in academic performance and possibly developmental delays. Following an OT assessment, the occupational therapist creates an integrated intervention plan that recommends that Ariana engage in active, physical occupations such as organized sports teams or dance three times per week to promote physical, mental, and social well-being. The therapist recognizes that among various issues of concern, this child has obesity and is starting to develop secondary health concerns related to being overweight with poor nutrition habits. This intervention is an example of a preventive strategy that is meant to diminish the *incidence* of health issues and conditions for this client (obesity, early onset of diabetes, fatigue, physical injuries and strains, poor body image, social withdrawal,

low self esteem, etc.) while also decreasing the overall *prevalence* of children who develop secondary health problems related to obesity in that particular community. In effect, this therapist is also attempting to modify this child's *risk factors*, which may be defined as those variables that increase a person's vulnerability to developing an injury or condition (Scaffa, 1998). Scaffa defines risk factors as physical, behavioral, genetic, social, economic, political, or environmental in nature. In Ariana's case, examples of risk factors for this child may include low tone (physical), sedentary play activities like watching television (behavioral), and a predisposition to weight gain (genetic). Perhaps she lives in a social community where it is unsafe to go outside or her family lives in an apartment complex with no back yard (social). Economically, her family may be on state assistance, and therefore, food selection tends to include lots of carbohydrates with high fat content due to decreased monies. Politically, this child may be "at risk" for developing future health conditions but may not have a specific diagnosis that could warrant OT services at this time according to our current health care codes for reimbursement. Environmentally, this child may not appear "different" from other peers within her culture or among her school mates. It is possible that her habits and routines are typical and reinforced by other children who are "like" her. If this is an impoverished neighborhood (environment), the school may lack resources that could minimize the risk factors described in this child such as organized after school activities, alternative and healthy food options, active play equipment, and alternative learning tools and strategies.

Wilcock (1998) proposes that certain *occupational factors* can lead to ill health, disease, disability, and death. She identifies *occupational risk factors* as 1) occupational imbalance, 2) occupational deprivation, and 3) occupational alienation. In accordance with the Better Health Commission's view of the Social Determinants of Health (1986), Wilcock has postulated that stress is created from experiencing any of these three stated risk factors. With this lack of occupational opportunity, a person does not reach his or her potential. Situations such as overcrowding, loneliness, ecological breakdown, environmental pollutants, imbalance between diet and activity, and substance abuse can all result in *preclinical health disorders*. If these preclinical health disorders are not attended to, they will develop into more serious conditions and possibly lead to death. But what contributes to a person being at risk? According to Wilcock, underlying occupational factors such as economy, policies, governmental priorities, and cultural values are at the base. Note that these factors tend to resemble the risk factors identified by Scaffa. These factors contribute to a social environment and lifestyle that create *occupational institutions and activities*—employment and social opportunities, development of technology, legislation, fiscal management of communities, education, health care systems, etc. When a person's access to the social environment is balanced and one's occupational needs are met, he or she will thrive. If access to the social environment is disrupted

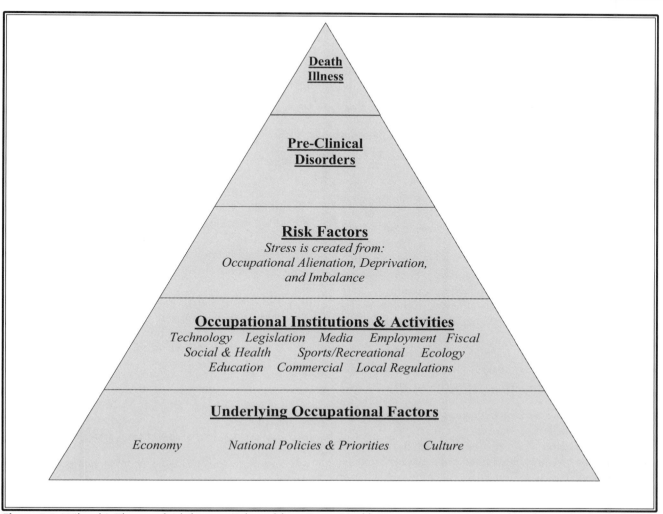

Figure 5-1. Wilcock's Theory of risk factors. (Adapted from Better Health Commission. [1986]. *Looking forward to better health.* [Vols 1–3.]. Canberra, Australia: Australian Government Publishing Service.)

or faulty, he or she will become "at risk" or vulnerable to developing problems. Refer to Figure 5-1 for an overview of these concepts.

Let us further discuss the three risk factors as defined by Wilcock (1998):

1. *Occupational imbalance:* There is an innate tendency within each of us to have our needs met. This hierarchy of needs was defined by Maslow. Persons experience a sense of health and well-being when their physiological, sleep, mental, and social needs are filled. Imbalance is a state that occurs because people's engagement in occupation fails to meet their unique physical, social, mental, or rest needs. There is insufficient time for their own occupational interests and growth and the meeting of expectations of family, social, and community commitments (p. 138). Wilcock asks us to consider how physical, mental, and social capacities; intrinsic and extrinsic factors; activity and food; obligation and choice; excitement and lethargy; the Romantic and the rational;

isolation and togetherness; or boredom and burnout may contribute to a sense of imbalance (2006, p. 170). During an OT assessment, we typically interview and gather an occupational profile that includes a client's occupational balance within the practice domains of activities of daily living (ADL), work/productive activity, leisure, rest, play, and social participation.

2. *Occupational deprivation:* According to Wilcock (2006), deprivation implies dispossession, divestment, confiscation, or taking from and the influence of an external agency or circumstance that keeps a person from acquiring, using, or enjoying something (p. 164). External agencies or circumstances may consist of technology, division of labor, lack of employment, poverty or affluence, cultural values, policies, social consequences of illness and disability, limited social services, and education systems. A typical example of this phenomenon is "failure to thrive" syndrome. When an infant is deprived of needed

sensory stimulation, he may fail to thrive normally and in extreme cases, may die.

3. *Occupational alienation:* This concept suggests that alienation can result when a person's activity is not in natural accordance with our humanity. Possible sources include economic, social, spiritual, and technological activities that create an unnatural shift to human behavior and life patterns. Alienation is a theme that emerged from Marx's philosophy. For example, we are in a turbulent time of information technology and overload. Think about how many forms of communication you use in one day. There is direct and indirect contact such as face to face encounters, voice mail, e-mail, instant messaging, and text messaging. How many PIN numbers and different passwords do you have for identity correspondence? All of this information can create overload and stress as we unnaturally try to multitask, communicate faster, or retrieve and return messages that occurred when we were busy doing something else. There is a marked urge to acquire more and more material wealth as a means to acquire happiness. So, we seek more elaborate cell phones, televisions, and computers with extreme capacities to provide more service options. Some people substitute materialism as a quick means of gratification, often complaining that we are bored if we do not reach our end goal quickly. Think about how technology has taken the place of assembly work that once employed people who are now substituted by machines. Alienation refers to the underutilization or undermining of health by capitalism and technological advancements. While the quest for success and technology is not in itself dangerous, it can create an alienating effect when human occupations are minimized and/or eliminated in the name of progress.

The result of any and all three of these risk factors can lead to stress-related illness. Wilcock suggests that our everyday health and well-being is being challenged by the very entities that were designed to promote an ease in living and prolong life. Her assumption is that the resultant shortage of intervention strategies from public health, social, political or national policies is largely contributing to stress-related disorders (Wilcock, 1998). In like form, Christiansen also directs our concern as occupational therapists to the socially health-related trends of the future. He states that while "biomedicine will experience many great advances in the years ahead, no genetic code, no chemical intervention, and no microsurgical technology will be invented to repair broken identities and the assault on meaning that accompanies them" (Christiansen, 1999, p. 556). He identifies that there are specific areas of concern for this millennium and OT has a rightful place in future treatment and interventions that relate to these practice issues. One well-known area of concern is an aging population and need for expanding geriatric health care. In his 1999 Eleanor Clark Slagle

address, Christiansen cites a study that was completed at Harvard University that sponsored by the WHO and World Bank projected the kinds of health-related problems that this world will encounter in the year 2020 (Murray & Lopez, 1996; Christiansen, 1999). Conclusions from this study show that unipolar major depression will become the second leading threat to life quality in the world with an increase in prevalence in developed countries. Other conditions on the rise include dementia, osteoarthritis, alcohol use, and self-inflicted injuries. On a positive note, infectious diseases in developing countries will show a decrease in incidence and prevalence.

In summary, Christiansen and Wilcock both profess that the health conditions of this millennium are related in part to the imbalance created within social contexts and the inadvertent application of traditional medical model practice for predominantly social conditions. They advocate for the profession of OT to take heed and proactively establish a role in the management of these health concerns. They strongly encourage that we embrace the philosophy of social science and social health models to understand, research, and identify evidence-based interventions that promote health and well-being. The time is now.

Health Promotion and Occupational Therapy

According to the WHO, *health promotion* is the process of enabling people to increase control over and to improve their health (1986, p. iii). It is complementary to client-centered practice in its therapeutic attitude toward consumers. Its foundational premise is to prevent the development of disease and disability in individuals, populations at risk, and communities by providing strategies that are targeted toward risk minimization. Its outcome is to decrease prevalence and incidence of disease. Therefore, health promotion is a therapeutic approach that is suited for social community practice while it also embraces the epidemiological science of recognizing early signs and averting disease from a medical perspective. In the OT Practice Framework, the intervention approach of "creating and promoting" specifically relates to this concept. Occupational therapists can create various occupation-based strategies that can sustain one's well-being and promote health because we are experts in understanding the multi-dimensional benefits of activities. Whenever an occupational therapist encourages recreational and leisure engagement just for "its own sake" (hobbies), he is promoting and encouraging health in that individual.

Prevention may be defined as the "anticipatory action taken to reduce the possibility of an event or condition from occurring or developing or to minimize the damage that may result from the event or condition if it does occur" (Pickett & Hanlon, 1990, p. 81). Within the structure of the public health system, prevention is a distinct strategy to increasing one's quality of life. Prevention attempts to minimize the development and/or occurrence of disease, therefore including the notion of health promotion. Within the OT Practice Framework, prevention is an intervention approach to disability. This intervention (prevention) "addresses clients with or without a disability who are at risk for occupational performance problems ... and is meant to prevent the occurrence or evolution of barriers to performance in context. Interventions (prevention) may be directed at client, context, or activity variables" (AOTA, 2002, p. 618).

There are three types of prevention. *Primary prevention* is directed toward relatively healthy individuals who may have a potential risk of developing a disease or disorder. The sources of these risks could be genetic, socioeconomically driven, age-related, ecologically influenced, politically organized, or occupational factors related to imbalance, deprivation, and alienation. Regardless of the cause, primary prevention acknowledges the potential of a future health problem and provides an intervention to minimize, delay, or avoid its onset. Examples of primary prevention strategies include recommendations like drinking eight glasses of water a day, wearing seat belts in a car, and taking vitamins and nutrients that are specifically targeted to a person's gender and age needs. The use of OT screens, questionnaires, and consumer self-reports rather than assessments are an example of this level of prevention. Recommendations are typically universal for the health patterns that may be noted and can be typically carried out without medical supervision.

Secondary prevention is offered to persons who demonstrate early signs of a disease and/or show preclinical concerns (see Figure 5-1). Strategies are matched to the specific area of health concern and are recommended to maintain positive health status, slow down the development and/or onset of a full-blown outbreak of the disorder, reverse signs and symptoms whenever possible, and prevent complications that are often secondary in nature. An occupational therapist who creates a resting hand splint for a person with arthritis is using a prevention strategy. The splint is designed to treat a specific cause such as arthritis and is individually fitted to a particular client with a diagnosed condition. The splint serves multiple purposes at this time. It will maintain the normal resting position of the person's hand and wrist, it will protect the joints and muscles from overuse and likely slow down the development of swelling and pain that can occur in a full-blown exacerbation, and it will likely prevent the onset of secondary conditions such as further injury to the hand and wrist.

Tertiary prevention is provided when a person is already in a state of ill health and is demonstrating active signs and symptoms. Strategies meant to restore and remediate, maintain, and modify via compensation or adaptation are all OT-based interventions identified within the OT Practice Framework (AOTA, 2002). This mode of intervention most resembles the medical model framework because it specifically is prescribed for the health condition that is now in its active state. For example, for a person with active hallucinations related to chronic schizophrenia, the occupational therapist recommends occupations that can allow for the safe and socially appropriate expression of thoughts and feelings such as drawing pictures, journaling, writing poetry, making up songs, and creative dance. It is unlikely that the symptoms of hallucinations and delusions will ever go away; therefore, the therapist prescribes interventions that can modify the outward expression of perceptual distortions and delusional thinking into adaptive and meaningful occupations. These activities can serve as a means to offer this client a form of self expression with some creative boundaries as a means to substitute for talking about one's hallucinations and delusions in public social contexts where most people will be turned off, judgmental, and stigmatizing ("he's crazy").

Community-based models are conducive for the implementation of primary and secondary interventions with their inherent objectives of promoting health and preventing illness. In reality, all three levels of prevention are needed to sustain health. Managed care companies are slowly beginning to offer reimbursement for primary and secondary intervention such as paying fees toward a fitness membership at a health center or paying for well visits to physicians, dentists, pediatricians, optometrists, etc. We have a long way to go to counter the medical model orientation of waiting for something to go wrong before we attempt to intervene and fix it. It appears that a body of knowledge and research showing the benefits of well-being, life balance, health promotion, prevention, and social impact has existed within the realms of philosophy and the social and behavioral sciences. Attempts to draw attention to these variables has been put forth by multiple systems such as Public Health, WHO, JCAHO, and national health systems that actively attempt to shape an attitude change that is more holistic and less reductionistic. Now, there is a new set of concerns that is emerging within the United States that includes the rising cost of health services and pharmaceuticals, an aging population, the prevalence of chronic conditions coupled with longer life spans, and stress-related conditions. It would seem likely that a social, community-based model for practice is one type of optimal solution.

UNITED STATES HEALTH DELIVERY SYSTEM: A MINI COMPARISON

The United States has a unique health care delivery system among other countries. Some of its unique traits include a lack of a central agency to govern the system, unequal access to health care services due to private health insurance coverage, legal risks, and the existence of subsystems that include multiple payers and third-party insurers who serve as mediators between the patient and insurance company. Health care providers are massive in numbers and there exists a nonstandardized arrangement to financing, insurance, delivery, and payment. Private sectors are attracted by the pursuit of profits, and the system lacks a standard budgetary method of cost control. Therefore, cost containment remains an indefinable goal. The last 20 years have provoked a shift in medical practice with different trends and directions emerging. Promotion of health at lower costs is a basic reason for most of these shifts. Examples of trends in the United States delivery system include the shift from an illness perspective to wellness; focus from the individual patient to community well-being; fragmented care to managed care; and multiple, free-standing institutions to integrated agencies with less duplication of services and a continuum of care (Shi & Singh, 2004).

The unique and controversial issues of service delivery in the United States continue to challenge how occupational therapists will fit in and receive reimbursement for future practice. Occupational therapists are proud of their philosophical beliefs and holistic models for practice but will need to integrate these frameworks into a large system of conflicting and changing health views. It would appear that a viable solution to the problems within United States health delivery is to create a system that merges traditional, medical perspectives with social, community-oriented philosophies. But will this joining really solve our health care needs? Shi & Singh (2004) suggest that this solution is too simplistic and that the "real challenge for the health care delivery system is to incorporate these models within the holistic context of health as defined by the Ottawa Charter for Health Promotion" (p. 64). This new, integrated approach would offer health objectives that include medical care, preventive services, health promotion, and social policy to improve education, lifestyles, employment, and housing (Henry, 1993). This last statement reflects the elements of a biopsychosocial model. Practitioners would need to be diversely trained to influence and change social public policy and actively become part of community partnerships. Let us compare the United States delivery system to other countries that are native to the various cited occupational therapists who are proposing, creating, and practicing (in some cases) a more holistic, client-centered, socially equitable, and community-oriented model to health care.

Canada and most Western European countries have national health care programs that provide universal access. One such structure is called *national health insurance (NHI)*, which consists of governmental financed health care through general taxes with actual service delivery offered by private providers. In Great Britain, a *national health system (NHS)* exists that is similar to NHI except that the government also manages the delivery of medical care. Most health care practitioners in NHS are, therefore, employed by the government in a tightly organized infrastructure. In some European countries, such as Germany and Italy, a *socialized health insurance (SHI)* prevails where health care is financed through government-mandated contributions by employers and employees, and health care

is given by private providers. The government exercises all control. Private "nonprofit" insurance companies collect monies and pay physicians and hospitals. Comparatively, Australia presently has a national program (Medicare) financed by income taxes and a levy. Everyone contributes to the cost of health care according to their capacity to pay with private health insurance representing around 33% of total costs. Public hospitals are funded by the government; private care offers a better choice with Medicare reimbursing all or parts of the entire cost. Australia has a well-organized system of mainly private practitioners who give care mostly on a fee-for-service basis (Shi & Singh, 2004).

Public health has been identified as a social system that can apply the current medical and scientific knowledge about disease and health in ways that will have the most impact on a population (Turnock, 1997, p. 10). Not all Americans agree with this premise, however. Medicine and public health have had a poor history of complementing each other and are often viewed as divergent. The devastating events of "9/11" have brought the services of public health into view. For instance, *environmental health*, a component of public health, is now receiving considerable attention for its role in preventing bioterrorism. Public health embraces the notion of "healthy people" and may be synonymously associated as having similar goals and objectives.

HEALTHY PEOPLE 2010: GOALS AND OBJECTIVES FOR THE UNITED STATES

Healthy People 2010 is a public document that was issued in January 2000. It is a comprehensive set of national health objectives for the decade that is part strategic plan with a summary of public health priorities. Its information can easily be accessed on its Web site (http://www.health.gov/healthypeople), via a toll free number (1-800-367-4725) or read in textbook format. The original concept of *Healthy People* originated from Canada's LaLonde Report (LaLonde, 1974), which described the health status of Canadians. The United States' version of this report was first published by the Department of Health and Human Services (as we now recognize it) in 1979 and emphasized the need for change associated with unhealthy behavioral and lifestyle factors. Since then, there have been several updated documents including *Promoting Health/Preventing Disease Objectives for the Nation* (1980), *Healthy People 2000* (1990), and most recently, *Healthy People 2010* (2000).

There are two overarching goals of *Healthy People 2010*. The first goal is to increase the quality and years of healthy life. This goal is aimed at people of all ages with particular attention given to those populations where there is variation in life expectancy. For example, there are at least 18 countries that have higher life expectancies than the

United States. There is also a disproportionate number of persons who report fair to poor health status with other reports indicating discrepancies in quality of life. The second goal of *Healthy People 2010* is to eliminate health disparities. Another word for disparity is difference. Disparities are studied according to the following categories: gender, race or ethnicity, education or income, disability, living in rural localities, and sexual orientation. Empowering Americans to make informed health care decisions can be accomplished by strategies such as education, increasing participation in community-oriented interventions, promoting safety awareness, and increasing consumer access to health care. Objectives from *Healthy People 2010* (2000) to eliminate the disparity among the rate of asthma within the category of race/ethnicity and within the category of gender and education are shown in Tables 5-1 and 5-2.

Healthy People's two comprehensive goals will be monitored through 467 objectives within 28 national focus areas (Table 5-3). Each focus area is a delineated chapter within the *Healthy People 2010* textbook (2000).

These 467 objectives are diverse in their intentions. Some reflect interventions designed to reduce or eliminate illness, disability, and premature death among individuals and communities. One example is to reduce the proportion of nonsmokers exposed to environmental tobacco smoke currently at a baseline of 65% to 45% by 2010. Other objectives more broadly focus on improving access to quality health care, strengthening public health services, and improving the availability and dissemination of health-related information. A sample objective of this type is to increase the proportion of persons with a usual primary care provider, presently at a baseline of 77%, to 85% by 2010. Among the comprehensive list of 28 focus areas, there are 10 specific leading health indicators (Table 5-4). These 10 areas represent the current and most significant public health concerns within the United States. In likewise

---

Table 5-1

Healthy People 2010 Comparison Rates Among Race/Ethnic Groups

Goal: Reduce asthma deaths (adults aged 35 to 64 years) to 9.0% by 2010

National baseline	17.8%
American Indian or Alaska Native	DSU*
Asian or Pacific Islander	12.8%
Black or African American	52.3%
White	13.3%
Hispanic or Latino	16.4%

DSU = data statistics are unreliable
Adapted from Department of Health and Human Services.
(2000). Healthy People 2010: Understanding and improving health. *2nd ed. Washington, DC: US Government Printing Office.*

Table 5-2

Healthy People 2010 Comparison Rates Among Gender and Education

Goal: Reduce asthma deaths (adults aged 35 to 64 years) to 9.0% by 2010

National baseline	17.8%
Female	22.3%
Male	13.0%
Less than high school education	31.0%
High school graduate	22.9%
At least some college	9.3%

Adapted from Department of Health and Human Services. (2000). Healthy People 2010: Understanding and improving health. *2nd ed. Washington, DC: US Government Printing Office.*

Table 5-3

Healthy People 2010 Focus Areas

1. Access to quality health services
2. Arthritis, osteoporosis, and chronic back conditions
3. Cancer
4. Chronic kidney disease
5. Diabetes
6. Disability and secondary conditions
7. Educational and community-based programs
8. Environmental health
9. Family planning
10. Food safety
11. Health communication
12. Heart disease and stroke
13. HIV
14. Immunization and infectious diseases
15. Injury and violence prevention
16. Maternal, infant, and child health
17. Medical product safety
18. Mental health and mental disorders
19. Nutrition and overweight
20. Occupational safety and health
21. Oral health
22. Physical activity and fitness
23. Public health infrastructure
24. Respiratory diseases
25. Sexually transmitted diseases
26. Substance abuse
27. Tobacco use
28. Vision and hearing

Adapted from Department of Health and Human Services. (2000). Healthy People 2010: Understanding and improving health. *2nd ed. Washington, DC: US Government Printing Office.*

Table 5-4
Leading Health Indicators of *Healthy People 2010*

Ten Major Public Health Issues

1. Physical activity
2. Overweight and obesity
3. Tobacco use
4. Substance abuse
5. Responsible sexual behavior
6. Mental health
7. Injury and violence
8. Environmental quality
9. Immunization
10. Access to health care

Adapted from Department of Health and Human Services. (2000). Healthy People 2010: Understanding and improving health. 2nd ed. Washington, DC: US Government Printing Office.

Table 5-5
Determinants of Health

Biology	Includes genetic factors and acquired problems that render a person at risk. Examples include physical, mental, and familial resources such as aging, diet, physical activity, smoking, stress, alcohol and drug use, injury or violence, infectious or toxic agents. Any of these factors may result in a change in one's biological makeup.
Behaviors	Responses and/or reactions to both internal and external conditions that result in a definable outcome. Examples include both positive and negative behaviors such as exercising, well-being, smoking, and drinking.
Social Environment	Interactions that include family, friends, coworkers, and community members such as social institutions, law enforcement, workplace, places of worship, and school. Other components consist of housing, public transportation, and the absence or presence of violence in the community. Cultural customs, language, and religious and/or spiritual beliefs contribute to the quality of one's social environment.
Physical Environment	Includes those factors that can be identified via our five senses and those intangible elements such as radiation, the ozone, toxic substances, irritants, infectious agents, and physical hazards.
Policies and interventions	Includes health promotion campaigns (smoking cessation), laws (safety belts), prevention services (immunization), clinical services, and agencies (transportation, education, energy, housing, labor, justice, religious, and community).
Access to quality health care	Expanding care will assist with eliminating health disparities and the quality and years of healthy life for persons within the United States.

Adapted from United States Department of Health and Human Services. (2000). Healthy people 2010 (Conference ed.), Washington, DC: United States Department of Healthy and Human Services.

fashion, each leading health indicator has its set of objectives to measure progress. They are meant to augment the already existing 467 objectives identified among the 28 focus areas and can serve as the basic building blocks for community health practice initiatives. *Healthy People 2010* attempts to bridge the importance of a nation's universal set of concerns and objectives (28 focus areas) with a smaller set of health priorities (10 major public health issues).

DETERMINANTS OF HEALTH

Healthy People 2010 represents a systems theory view of health concerns. The factors that influence an individual and/or a community's health are called *determinants of health*. These six determinants act interdependently and ultimately influence one's health status. They include biology, behaviors, social environment, physical environment, policies and interventions, and access to quality health care. Consult Table 5-5 for a brief description of each determinant.

These determinants of health are an important aspect for developing strategies that will improve the health of the United States.

Our understanding of these determinants and how they relate to one another, coupled with our understanding of how individual and community health affects the health of the Nation, is perhaps the most important key to achieving our Healthy People 2010 goals of increasing the quality and years of life and of eliminating the Nation's health disparities. (2000, p. 20)

HEALTH PROMOTION MODELS FOR COMMUNITY-BASED PRACTICE

Occupational therapists can contribute to community and public health in a significant way because the inherent philosophies are very similar. So, what has interfered with this partnership? A strong proponent of the role in OT community practice, Ann Wilcock clearly articulates that occupational therapists should direct some attention and advocate for change within the educational, political, and social venues of our national systems. Wilcock has looked closely at the barriers that interfere with OT's transition to a community practice model. She highlights the historical obstructions of this role from an OT perspective as follows: the OT profession's smallness, gender imbalance, dependence on medicine, its difference, and the difficulty of explaining or understanding its promise without an appreciation of its origins and rich philosophical history (1998, p. 211). She goes on to note that with recent universal social actions (feminist movement) that have changed some traditional values, OT has become more appreciated for its difference. Another significant historical development is the publication of occupation-based theories that continue to be researched for best practice with a diverse application to areas of ability and disability, including public health. It is with this newly established view of occupational performance and evidence-based practice, that occupational therapists can challenge and analyze public health directions and interventions and not succumb to the already existing biases. A distinct link between OT and health promotion needs to be established. A niche market is waiting for the OT profession with its scope of theoretical understanding, evidence-based practice, and moral sensitivity to humanity.

Wilcock's solution for the OT acquisition of a significant role in community practice is to increase action-research that incorporates an alternative approach to health promotion. The following key features reflect her suggested focus areas for research and are directly taken from Wilcock's text, which is so suitably titled *An Occupational Perspective of Health* (1998, pp. 224–225):

- A balance of physical, mental, and social well-being attained through valued occupation

- Enhancement of species' common and individually unique capacities and potential

- Occupational and social support and justice for all people and communities

- Community cohesion through politically supported and socially valued, well-balanced, occupational opportunity

- Research and action aimed at enabling, mediating, and advocating for healthy public policy that is responsive to human needs rather than materialistic wants all within, and as part of, a sustainable ecology

- Health care aimed at the maintenance and enhancement of physical, psychological, spiritual, and social functioning of individuals and communities toward maximum potential and quality in everyday living, in interaction with the natural world that sustains all creatures, and in a way that ensures its healthy survival

Five health promotion models are summarized in Table 5-6 (Wilcock, 1998, p. 230). These approaches specifically represent the factors that influence health promotion from an occupational perspective. The principles of each model represent 8 years of study and offer ways that an occupational therapist can 1) see and understand, 2) organize by setting objectives and deploying resources, and 3) do research, and construct interventions, and programs. Following is some additional information about each model:

1. *Wellness:* considered the closest to traditional, medical practices within OT, offering conventional perspectives. "Wellness is an active process through which individuals become aware of and make choices toward a more successful existence" (Hettler, 1990, p. 1117). Associated as synonymous with health promotion and ill health prevention particularly in the United States where it has been used in industries, business, and corporate works sites. The reader is referred to works of Dossey & Guzzetta (1989), Conrad (1987 & 1992), Walsh, Jennings, Manguine, & Merrigan (1991), and Opatz (1985) for related readings.

2. *Preventive medicine:* considered the closest to public health and defined as "the application of Western medical and social science to prevent disease, prolong life, and promote health in the community through intercepting disease processes" (Wilcock, 1998, p. 233). It has a strong base in epidemiology and is therefore an illness model; it is confused often with health promotion. The reader is referred to works of Last (1987) for further resources.

3. *Social justice:* defined as the "promotion of social and economic change to increase individual, community, and political awareness, resources, and equitable opportunities for health" (Wilcock, 1998, p. 235). Ill health is often an outcome of disparities related to resources and power, economy, national priorities and policies, and cultural values. See Figure 5-1, which highlights these factors as *underlying occupational factors* in the hierarchy of social determinants of health. The reader is referred to the works of Gallagher & Ferrante (1987), Le Grand (1987), and Townsend (1993) for related readings.

4. *Community development:* defined as "community consultation, deliberation, and action to promote individual, family, and community-wide responsibility for self-sustaining development, health, and well-being" (Wilcock, 1998, p. 238). A holistic approach, its therapeutic aim is directed toward the betterment of the entire community through strategies that encourage social and economic development, a community analysis, use of local resources, and self-sustaining programs. In the United States, this ideology became

national policy under Title II of the Economic Opportunity Act of 1964. The *Community Based Rehabilitation model*, defined as a "strategy within community development for the rehabilitation, equalization of opportunity and social integration of all people with disabilities," has a similar focus in that services are offered by persons with needs themselves (WHO, 1994). The reader is encouraged to consult the works of Thomas (1990) for an example of this type of program.

5. *Ecological sustainability:* perhaps the least understood, it is defined as "the promotion of healthy relationships between humans, other living organisms, their environments, habits, and modes of life" (Wilcock, 1998, p. 240). It is based on biological and natural sciences and includes such issues as population growth, restructuring of economic and societal values, reformation of resource policies to reflect community interests, and a merging of economic and biological in ecological decision making. The reader may want to consult the works of MacNeill (1989), Egger et al. (1990), and Corson (1994) for related readings.

In summary, Wilcock continues to explore and research the role of occupation in health promotion as evidenced by the second edition of her textbook (2006). The following five specific issues have been identified by Wilcock as a summary of the second edition, and the reader is encouraged to consult this text for understanding and appreciation of the following topics (Wilcock, 2006, p. 336):

1. Health (natural) and its dependency on occupation to maintain and enhance it

2. The place of occupation in human life, health, and survival

3. Occupation defined as doing, being, and becoming as a positive and negative influence on health

4. The potential contribution of occupation-focused approaches to population health based on current WHO directives

5. Possible occupation-focused action-research for occupational therapists and others to improve ecosustainable community development, occupational justice, health, and well-being worldwide, and to prevent illness, disability and premature death

LEARNING ACTIVITIES

Community Visit: Reflection/Journal

Directions: Attend a community health promotion activity of your choice. You may use your own resources or consult public directories for self-help groups and health promotion programs. Complete the following reflection questions:

1. Briefly describe the community program. How did you learn about it? Include any publicized information you may have read or received about the program.

2. Identify what "Health Promotion Model" (Wilcock, 1998) was exemplified at this program. List any observations to help substantiate your answer.

3. What focus area(s) from *Healthy People 2010* were incorporated?

4. What leading health indicator(s) from public health and *Healthy People 2010* was best represented by this program?

5. What is your overall reaction to this community experience? In your opinion, how does this program reflect the needs of the community?

6. What impact could OT have on this program? How would you organize this program to promote a healthy relationship between occupations and well-being?

Health Promotion Models: Application to Occupational Therapy Practice

Objective: To understand and apply the five health promotion models defined by Wilcock (1998) and relate to OT practice.

1. Review all five health promotion models.

2. Search for examples of each model by using various sources—newspapers, Web sites, phone directories, self help directories, etc.

3. Identify those programs that can be integrated into OT practice by referring to the OT Practice Framework (AOTA, 2001) as the guideline for practice.

Community Health Promotion Program

Objective: To encourage the student to integrate physical, psychosocial, cultural, and public health issues within OT practice.

Description: Students may work in pairs for this assignment. Each pair will develop an original, creative, and innovative Community Based Health Promotion program and complete a written assignment. Students are required to use lectures, assigned texts, reserved library resources, references, and individually researched materials.

Please include the following components and use the following headings for this paper.

• Describe your Community Health Promotion Program by including the following areas (20 points):

o Review the list of 10 leading health indicators in *Healthy People 2010*. Select one, possibly two, area(s) that are pertinent for this project. Describe how your knowledge as an occupational therapist could promote this indicator.

o Research and discuss the community *need* and *rationale* for this program. Discuss the reasons why you think that this program could benefit individuals and the community. Refer to the goals and objectives of your focus areas from *Healthy People 2010* for justification of this program.

o Select the focus areas from *Healthy People 2010* that are related to your leading health indicator—be sure that your indicators and focus areas complement each other.

• Consider systems theory and the six determinants of health as they will influence the outcome of your community project. (35 points)

o Who is your population, the individuals, that you wish to serve? Include identifying data such as typical ages, occupations, gender, race/ethnicity, income and education, geographical location, and sexual orientation. What are some health disparities within your population that relate to your project? What population could specifically benefit from this program based on the research regarding health disparities?

o What behaviors presently exist within this population and how do you wish to impact their present behavioral outcomes to foster a sense of well-being?

o What biological factors/conditions exist within this group? How do you aspire to influence these individuals' physical well being?

o How does this population's physical environment contribute to their present status of health? How will you adapt your program to meet the needs of your population's physical and geographical needs?

o What is your population's social support system? How will you foster a sense of social well-being and integration within this community setting?

o What are the existing policies and interventions that influence your community program? Briefly explain how this population is positively and/or negatively effected. (Also look at trends in health care.)

o What is your population's typical experience with access to health care? How will you influence this factor by offering your community service program?

• Select a "Health Promotion Model" (Wilcock, 1998) for your community program. Describe whether your service will be primary, secondary, or tertiary. Briefly give the reasons why you have selected this particular model and level of intervention for this population. (15 points)

• Identify 6 overall goals for your program. (Your goals should directly relate to all previously stated components including *Healthy People*'s goals, objectives, determinants of health, and health promotion model. (10 points)

• List all staff, supplies, equipment, and resources needed for this program. (10 points)

• What are the roles that you will need to play in this Community Health Promotion Program? How will you positively impact the future direction of the OT profession? (10 points)

REFERENCES

American Occupational Therapy Association. (2002). Occupational therapy practice framework: Domain and process. *American Journal of Occupational Therapy, 56,* 609-639.

Baum, C. M., & Law, M. (1997). Occupational therapy practice: Focusing on occupational performance. *American Journal of Occupational Therapy, 51*(4), 277-288.

Baum, C., & Law, M. (1998). Community health: A responsibility an opportunity, and a fit for occupational therapy. *American Journals of Occupational Therapy, 52*(1), 7–10.

Better Health Commission. (1986). *Looking forward to better health* (Vols 1–3.). Canberra, Australia: Australian Government Publishing Service.

Christiansen, C. H. (1999). Defining lives: Occupation as identity. An essay on competence, coherence, and the creation of meaning. *American Journal of Occupational Therapy, 53,* 547-558.

Conrad, P. (1987). Wellness in the workplace: Potentials and pitfalls of worksite health promotion. *Milbank Quarterly, 65*(2), 255–275.

Conrad, P., & Walsh, D. C. (1992). The new corporate health ethnic: Lifestyle and social control of work. *Journal of Public Health Policy, 22*(1), 89-111.

Corson, W. H. (1994). Changing course: An outline of strategies for a sustainable future. Futures, 26(2), 206–223. Gallagher, E. B., & Ferrante, J. (1987). Medicalisation and social justice. *Social Justice Research, 1*(3), 377–392.

Detels, R., & Breslow, L. (1997). Current scope and concerns in public health. In R. Detels, W. W. Holland, J. McEwen, & G. S. Omenn (Eds.), *Oxford textbook of public health.* New York: Oxford.

Dossey, B. M., & Guzetta, C. E. (1989). Wellness, values clarification and motivation. In B. M. Dossey, L. Keegan, L. G. Kolkmier, & C. E. Guzzetta (Eds.), *Holistic health promotion: A guide for practice.* Rockville, MD: Aspen Publishers.

Doyal, L., & Gough, I. (1991). *A theory of human need.* London: Macmillan.

Egger, G., Spark, R., & Lawson, J. (1990). *Health promotion strategies and methods.* Sydney, Australia: McGraw-Hill.

Gallagher, E. B., & Ferrante, J. (1987). Medication and social justice. *Social Justice Research, 1*(3), 257–274.

Henry, R. C. (1993). Community partnership model for health professions education. *Journal of the American Pediatric Medical Association, 83,* 328–331.

Hettler, W. (1990). Wellness: The lifetime goal of a university experience. In I. D. Matarazzo (Ed.), *Behavioral health. A handbook of health enhancement and disease promotion.* New York, NY: Wiley & Sons.

Joint Commission of the Accreditation of Healthcare Organizations. (1995). *Assessing and improving community health care delivery.* Oakbrooke Terrace, IL: Author.

Kielhofner, G. (1997). *Conceptual foundations of occupational therapy.* Philadelphia: F. A. Davis.

LaLonde, M. (1974). *A new perspective on the health of Canadians: A working document.* Ottawa: Ministry of National Health and Welfare.

Last, J. M. (1987). Public health and preventive medicine. CT: Appleton & Lange. In B. MacMahon & D. Trichopoulos. (1996). *Epidemiology principles and methods.* Boston: Little & Brown.

Le Grande, J. (1987). Equity, health, and health care. *Social Justice Research, 1*(3) 257–274.

MacNeill, J. (1989). Strategies or sustainable development. *Scientific American, 261*(3), 155–165.

Mosey, A. C. (1996). *Psychological components of occupational therapy.* Philadelphia, PA: Lippincott, Williams, and Wilkins.

Murray, C. J., & Lopez, A. D. (1996). *The global burden of disease: A comprehensive assessment of mortality and disability from diseases, injuries, and risk factors in 1990 and projected to 2010.* Cambridge, MA: Harvard University Press.

Nutbeam, D. (1986). Health promotion glossary. *Health Promotion, 1,* 113.

Opatz, J. P. (1985). *A primer of health promotion: Creating healthy organizational cultures.* Washington, DC: Oryn Publications.

Pickett, G., & Hanlon, J. J. (1990). *Public health: Administration and practice.* St. Louis, MO: Times Mirror/Mosby.

Roget's Thesaurus (1980). Boston, MA: Little, Brown & Company.

Scaffa, M. E. (2001). *Occupational therapy in community-based practice settings.* Philadelphia, PA: F.A. Davis.

Scaffa, M. E. (1998). Adolescents and alcohol use. In A. Henderson, S. Champton, & W. Evashwick (Eds.), *Promoting teen health: Linking schools, health organizations & community.* Thousand Oaks, CA: Sage.

Scaffa, M. E., & Brownson, C. (2005). Occupational therapy interventions: Community health approaches. In C. H. Christiansen, C. M. Baum, and J. Bass-Hargen (Eds.), *Occupational therapy: Performance, participation, and well-being* (3rd ed.). Thorofare, NJ: SLACK Incorporated.

Shi, L., & Singh, D. A. (2004). *Delivering health care in America: A systems approach.* Sudbury, MA: Jones & Bartlett Publishers.

Smith, V., & Eggleston, R. (1989). Long-term care. The medical versus the social model. *Public Welfare, Summer, 26*–29.

Thomas, K. (1990). Comments on working in Sudan and Ethiopia. In A. A. Wilcock (Ed.), *Health promotion and occupational therapy.* Melborne, Australia: World Federation of Occupational Therapists Congress.

Townsend, E. (1993). Muriel Driver memorial lecture: Occupational therapy's social vision. *Canadian Journal of Occupational Therapy, 60,* 174–183.

Turnock, B. J. (1997). *Public health: What it is and how it works.* Gaithersburg, MD: Aspen Publishers, Inc.

United States Department of Health and Human Services. (1980). *Promoting health/preventing disease: Objectives for the nation.* Washington, DC: United States Government Printing Office.

United States Department of Health and Human Services. (1990). *Healthy people 2000: National health promotion and disease prevention objectives* (Publication No. 017-001-00474-0). Washington, DC: United States Government Printing Office.

United States Department of Health and Human Services. (2000). *Healthy people 2010:* (Conference ed.), Washington, DC: United States Department of Healthy and Human Services.

United States Department of Health, Education, and Welfare. (1979). *Healthy people: Surgeon General's report on health promotion/disease prevention* (Publication No. 79-55071). Washington, DC: United States Government Printing Office.

Walsh, D. C., Jennings, S. E., Manguine, T., & Merrigan, D. M. (1991). Health promotion versus health protection? Employees perceptions and concerns. *Journal of Public Health Policy, 12*(2), 148–164.

Wilcock, A. A. (1998). *An occupational perspective of health.* Thorofare, NJ: SLACK Incorporated.

Wilcock, A. A. (2005). Relationship of occupations to health and well-being. In C. H. Christiansen, C. M. Baum, and J. Bass-Haugen (Eds.), *Occupational therapy: Performance, participation, and well-being* (3rd ed.). Thorofare, NJ: SLACK Incorporated.

Wilcock, A. A. (2006). *An occupational perspective of health* (2nd ed.). Thorofare, NJ: SLACK Incorporated.

World Health Organization. (1946). Constitution of the World Health Organization. International Health Conference, New York.

World Health Organization. (1986). Constitution of the World Health Organization. International Health Conference, New York.

World Health Organization. (1994). Constitution of the World Health Organization. International Health Conference, New York.

World Health Organization. (2001). *International classification of functioning, disability and health (ICF).* Geneva, Switzerland: Author.

OCCUPATION-BASED MODELS

Section II will summarize the occupation-based models within the practice of occupational therapy (OT). Although each one is distinctive in its own right, there are some common features as well. The most obvious common denominator is that each model is founded by an occupational therapist(s). Each model also describes the process of occupational performance and extrapolates concepts from Mary Reilly's theory on occupational behavior (1966). Also embedded in each of these models are the foundational theories of humanism and holism, systems theory, and developmental and social psychology. The client-centered approach is also emphasized when discussing the evaluation and intervention process, accentuating a collaborative relationship between the person and occupational therapist. Reed (2005), in a review of current literature, derives six assumptions about occupation that support current occupation-based models of practice.

1. Occupation is a basic human need.

2. Occupation is an essential component of human life.

3. Occupation organizes behavior.

4. Occupation gives meaning to life.

5. Occupation enables a healthy lifestyle.

6. Occupation improves an individual's quality of life.

These models are more alike than different, as each focuses on the interdependent relationship among three significant variables: person, environment, and occupation.

At the same time, each model provides a unique integration of theory and concepts that influence the clinical reasoning process of occupational therapists. Some of these models are more developed and further along in the research process than others. There is a distinctive focus and emphasis about each one. The authors of this book believe that it is in a practitioner's best interest to learn about many models rather than to limit one's knowledge to only a few. Effective clinical reasoning involves the practitioner's ability to perform a comprehensive occupational profile and then to choose the models and frames of reference for evaluation and intervention that best suit the needs of the individual client. In order to accomplish this, the practitioner must have a good repertoire of theories from which to select and apply.

In this next section, the reader will find a description of each model according to Chapter 4, adapted from Mosey's organization of theory (1986, 1992). Each model will be described according to the following components: focus within OT's domain of concern, theoretical base and underlying concepts, how function and disability are defined according to the model, explanations of how therapeutic change occurs and how clients are motivated, various evaluation examples, and finally, guidelines for intervention. A research summary and learning activities follow.

At the end of Section II, the reader will find an integrative case example that is meant to compare and contrast the clinical reasoning components of each model.

REFERENCES

Mosey, A. C. (1986). *Psychosocial components of occupational therapy*. New York, NY: Raven Press

Mosey, A. C. (1992). *Applied scientific inquiry in the health professions: An epistemological orientation*. Rockville, MD: The American Occupational Therapy Association.

Reed, K. L. (2005). An annotated history of the concepts used in occupational therapy. In C. Christiansen & C. Baum (Eds.). *Occupational therapy: Performance, participation, and well-being*. Thorofare, NJ: SLACK Incorporated.

Reilly, M. (1966). A psychiatric occupational therapy program as a teaching model. *American Journal of Occupational Therapy, 20*, 61–67.

Chapter 6

OCCUPATIONAL BEHAVIOR

"Man, through the use of his hands as they are energized by his mind and will, can influence the state of his own health"

– MARY REILLY, 1962

Mary Reilly is the founder of the term *occupational behavior*. As evidenced by her early publication in the *American Journal of Occupational Therapy (AJOT)* (1958), Reilly firmly believed in the need for comprehensive theories to guide the practice of occupational therapy (OT). She introduced her own model in 1969 as a means to identify a general theory of OT. Reilly defined occupational behavior as activities that occupy a person's time, involve achievement, and address the economic realities of life (Reilly, 1962, 1966).

Reilly has been credited by many proponents in the OT field as the catalyst for the paradigm shift back to occupation (Kielhofner, 1997). In 1961, Mary Reilly presented the Eleanor Clark Slagle Lecture titled "Occupational Therapy Can Be One of the Great Ideas of the 20th Century Medicine" (Reilly, 1962). Her overall message stated that occupational therapists must look beyond the medical community and redefine their mission and role with a much broader scope. Occupational therapists, as other health professionals, were highly influenced by the medical model and advances of medicine in the 1960s and 1970s. Much of the clinical reasoning among practitioners at that time reflected a reductionistic approach. OT treatment often included modalities and techniques to fix the "problem." As Reilly reminded us, the purpose of occupational therapists as identified by our original forefathers Meyer and Slagle "is to prevent and reduce the incapacities resulting from illness" (Reilly, 1969, p. 300). Hence, she re-directed our attention back to the disruption in function rather than focusing on the medical cause. In our current paradigm, occupational therapists recognize the importance in promoting health through meaningful occupational behavior and intervening when someone experiences a disruption in functioning due to illness or disability.

While Reilly's occupational behavior theory is a challenge to apply directly to practice because of its broad nature, the authors of this text have attempted to summarize this model according to Mosey's organization of theory. Reilly offered futuristic insight about the practice of OT. Her concepts are clearly relevant to practice within this new millennium. As a direct result of her study and publications, Kielhofner and Burke, originally two students of Mary Reilly, incorporated the concepts of occupational behavior into a model of practice called the Model of Human Occupation (MOHO). In 1972, Shannon proposed a "work-play" theory that encouraged occupational therapists to refocus their clinical attention on the behaviors and skills of an individual rather than on illness or injury. He later published an article in the *AJOT* titled "The Derailment of Occupational Therapy" (1977). Like Reilly, he was very concerned with the reductionistic nature of practice. Reilly's concepts also inspired the formulation of "occupational science," a significant research endeavor that led to the creation of an academic discipline by occupational therapists at the University of Southern California.

FOCUS

The occupational behavior model is meant to assist persons of all ages and abilities. Reilly's proposed focus for practice is to prevent and reduce the disruptions and incapacities in occupational behavior that result from injury and illness (Reed & Sanderson, 1999, p. 244). Reilly believed that occupation could best be understood and studied via the behavioral sciences such as psychology, sociology, and anthropology and may be defined as anything that engages one's time, energy, and resources (Reed & Sanderson, 1999, p. 240). While some occupational therapists might associate her theory as directed toward children, perhaps because her book was titled *Play as Exploratory Learning* (1974), she was also concerned with adult development. Reilly believed that an overall emphasis of OT practice should be on work satisfaction. Another way to describe Reilly's theory is to define it as a "work-play" approach to OT practice (Stein &

Cutler, 2002, p. 172). In essence, Reilly's model stressed the significance that childhood play has on the development of work and productive activity throughout adulthood. Therefore, her model could easily be applied to the domains of work and play within our present framework. Reilly suggested that health and well-being were represented by a balance of occupational behavior in self care, work, and play/leisure.

FOUNDATIONS

Theoretical influences to Reilly's model include developmental theory (work-play continuum), achievement theory (exploration and competence), and role theory (occupational role learning and choice) (Reed & Sanderson, 1999, p. 241). Concepts from these theories may be found within the occupational behavior model's assumptions. One significant concept is the notion of *occupational competence*. Developmental theory helps us to understand how early play and occupational experiences will influence our sense of mastery in the future (Case-Smith & Shortridge, 1996). Reilly emphasized that occupational behavior is developed according to a developmental continuum and includes the child's need to 1) explore, 2) achieve, and 3) reach competency. These three levels can all be reached within the realm of play. Following is a further definition of these three main constructs (Reed & Sanderson, 1999; Kielhofner, 1985):

- *Exploration* includes the search for new experiences, for its own sake, that leads to the development of new skills.
- *Competence* is having sufficient or adequate behavior to meet the demands of a situation and involves mastery of skills.
- *Achievement* is an identifiable level of success, attainment, or proficiency.

Occupational behavior is further observed in one's roles. Occupational role systems are defined as gender identification and group membership. The roles of work include being a housewife, student, preschooler, volunteer, or retiree.

THEORETICAL BASE

Following is a list of assumptions or postulates that form the theoretical base Reilly's occupational behavior model. This summary includes her views as well as those of her constituents (Case-Smith, 2005; Florey, 1969; Kielhofner, 1977, Matsutsuyu, 1971; Reilly, 1962, 1966).

- Man has a need to master, alter, and improve his environment.
  - o *Practice application:* clients show the capacity for self-direction and self-actualization. Occupational therapists need to discover what is meaningful and

interesting to the client as a way to motivate and initiate treatment.

- Occupation is intrinsically motivating, and people engage in occupation for its own sake to experience learning, control, and mastery that occurs during performance.
  - o *Practice application:* as clients engage in occupational behavior, the process will become self-reinforcing and self-enriching. The occupational therapist should grade the activities and select tasks to be meaningful for the client so that he or she experiences competency and success.

- Humans have a psychological need for occupation, and when they lack occupation, they suffer. Occupation is the main way that people 1) occupy time, 2) find meaning, and 3) establish the ability to contribute productively to society through life roles. Roles are the primary ways that persons express occupational behavior.
  - o *Practice application:* clients who experience disruption in occupational behavior and role functioning due to illness, disability, environmental barriers, etc. will show signs of distress. Occupational therapists understand that these disruptions in occupational behavior will impact one's psychological profile, psychosocial attitudes, and health conditions and will contribute to stressful events.

- Normal development influences the process of occupational behavior evident in a continuum of play (childhood) to work (adult). In childhood, persons engage in occupations for exploration; this evolves into the desire to learn and gain a sense of competence. Finally, this process culminates in adulthood with the urge to master and achieve in tasks such as work and productive activity.
  - o *Practice application:* occupational therapists can learn a lot about a client's interests, values, desires, etc. in the present by taking a play/leisure history. Patterns of occupational behavior can be understood by reviewing one's past interests and experiences. Persons who experienced disruption in childhood play experiences are likely to show disruptions in adult occupations.

- Society and culture highly influence the specific occupations chosen by a person.
  - o *Practice application:* there is a phenomenological experience to participating in occupations. Clients' occupational behavior is influenced by many components, including one's cultural beliefs and societal norms. Culture and society are part of the contextual features that occupational therapists assess during an occupational profile.

- Occupational behavior involves the daily routine of work, play, and rest within a physical, temporal, and social environment.
  - o *Practice application:* occupations take on many forms in a client's day. Some are necessary for self-maintenance while others are exploratory and performed by choice. The environment both consciously and unconsciously influences the person's choice to engage in occupational behaviors.
- Through participation in occupations, persons learn how to cope and adapt by responding to societal expectations and validating themselves as contributing members of society. As persons are challenged to deal with tasks of everyday life, occupation allows for adaptation to occur.
  - o *Practice application:* occupations are instrumental in providing opportunities for a person's psychological growth and development. The natural challenges of engaging in typical occupations foster one's ability to cope and adapt in productive ways. Occupational participation requires a certain degree of flexibility and adaptation by its own nature.
- Health is realized in the rhythm of activity and rest and includes the need for balance and habits. Balance is achieved by managing the demands of work and play. Habits are the basic structures that give order to daily behavior in time.
  - o *Practice application:* persons with healthy occupational behaviors demonstrate a balance of activities that meet the demands of oneself and society. Habits provide a healthy structure and sense of order to our lives on a daily basis.
- Occupational behavior includes both physical and visible forms as well as a subjective and affective experience for the person.
  - o *Practice application:* occupational therapists use observation as a means to understand the objective nature of occupational performance as well as client interviews/self reports to understand the emotional and phenomenological experiences of the client.
- Learning takes place as a person compares external facts and realities to one's internal, subjective self. A person derives meaning in occupational behavior by exploring one's internal values in relation to the external environment and its demands.
  - o *Practice application:* there is a reciprocal nature to developing one's occupational behavior profile. Clients constantly attempt to integrate feedback from the environment. It is natural to compare and contrast one's internal perceptions with external demands. It is possible to experience

occupational behaviors that are congruent (matching) with one's inner core of values and/or incongruent (mismatching). Clients often assign value to occupations that are also appreciated by society.

FUNCTION AND DISABILITY CONTINUUM

According to Reilly's model, *function* is evident within a person when he or she is capable of seeking, undertaking, and adapting occupations that meet personal needs as well as those of society. *Disability* is evident when a person "suffers" from the lack of occupational fulfillment, competency, and/or achievement. Persons may report or exemplify a lack of self-competence and mastery in occupational behavior. Role functioning is likely to be impaired.

CHANGE AND MOTIVATION

Change is a complex process because it often involves personal dynamics that the occupational therapist cannot measure nor observe. According to this model, change can be encouraged by enlisting a person's intrinsic drive toward mastery, which is assumed to be innate within each one of us. In other words, a person can be *motivated* to alter his occupational behavior if he or she finds something rewarding and meaningful about the process. An appropriate way to motivate a client from this model's perspective is to utilize the person's internal resources by inquiring about one's interest. It is safe to assume that if the client is interested in therapy and can identify the benefits for therapeutic change, he or she is more likely to have a positive therapeutic experience.

EVALUATION PROCESS

Mary Reilly did not identify specific assessments for her model. However, assessments such as those designed by Kielhofner et al. for the MOHO (see Chapter 7), Matsutsuyu's "Interest Check List" (Matsutsuyu, 1969), "Takata's Play History Questionnaire" (Takata, 1974), and Shannon's "Inventory of Occupational Choice Skills" (Shannon, 1974) are relevant choices for the evaluation process.

INTERVENTION PROCESS

OT interventions include the use of occupations to promote adaptation and life satisfaction (Bruce & Borg, 2002). Reilly did not identify specific intervention strategies as part of her model. Remember, she reacted strongly to the trend in the 1960s and 1970s where the use of techniques was a means to "fix" a person's problems. Rather, she described a therapeutic process for enhancing personal life satisfaction. As previously stated, Reilly believed that OT should prevent and reduce the incapacities in occupational behavior that result from illness. The following is a list of therapeutic strategies for your consideration that have been summarized (Bruce & Borg, 2002; Stein & Cutler, 2002; Reed & Sanderson, 1999):

- Enhance a person's strengths to promote competence and individual achievement.

- Incorporate one's interests, and increase occupational exploration for pleasure's sake.

- Enhance a child's development of sensory motor, reality testing, self-concept, and self-expression through the occupations of play.

- Assist adults to explore capacities for occupational behavior, and express feelings through the medium of play and/or leisure.

- Utilize a variety of media to assist a person to identify satisfying occupations, and experiment with appropriate role functioning.

- Develop the ability to adapt one's subjective response and external behavior in order to meet and satisfy role functioning and the demands of an occupation.

- Promote coping skills with the person who experiences difficulties in daily living, work, and leisure.

- Establish a collaborative relationship whereby the person is an active part of the change process.

RESEARCH

Occupational behavior has been criticized by occupational therapists for being difficult to apply to practice, mostly because of its general use of concepts. Case methods have been the primary source of exploring its application to OT practice. Two examples include a study by J. Line (1969) and Reilly herself (1969). As stated at the beginning of this chapter, occupational behavior served as a conceptual inspiration for the development of other occupation-based models. Occupational behavior had farther-reaching results than most other practice models. One can conclude that its most significant impact is the enhancement of the OT profession itself.

SUMMARY

In summary, Mary Reilly instilled a vision about the value of OT that has been appreciated and incorporated into various models and theories of current practice. In keeping with the original mission of occupation therapy, Reilly has served to remind us that occupational behavior is a process through which persons can enhance and promote health. While advances in technology and research will further inspire the development of evidence-based strategies to be used in OT, the principles of her model will remain the constant thread that unifies our profession. Meaningful occupations will continue to provide the means for a person to enhance a sense of well-being and promote healthy role functioning.

LEARNING ACTIVITY

1. Define the following key terms and concepts that are part of the occupational behavior model:
   - Occupation
   - Occupational behavior
   - Habits
   - Roles
   - Occupational competence
   - Occupational achievement
   - Occupational balance
   - Occupational proficiency

2. Construct a Venn diagram that depicts how the occupational behavior model is an outcome of: 1) developmental theory, 2) role theory, and 3) achievement theory.

3. Complete Table 6-1 on the occupational behavior model.

REFERENCES

Bruce, M. G., & Borg, B. A. (2002). *Psychosocial frames of reference* (3rd ed.). Thorofare, NJ: SLACK Incorporated.

Case-Smith, J. (2005). *Occupational therapy for children* (5th ed.). St. Louis, MO: Elsevier Mosby.

Case-Smith, J., & Shortridge, S. D. (1996). The developmental process: Prenatal to adolescence. In J. Case-Smith, A. S. Allen, & P. N. Pratt (Eds.), *Occupational therapy for children* (pp. 46–66). St. Louis, MO: Mosby.

Florey, L. L. (1969). Intrinsic motivation: The dynamics of occupational therapy theory. *American Journal of Occupational Therapy, 23*, 319–322.

Kielhofner, G. (1977). Temporal adaptation: A conceptual framework for occupational therapy. *American Journal of Occupational Therapy, 31*, 235–242.

Kielhofner, G. (1985). Occupational function and dysfunction. In G. Kielhofner (Ed.). *Model of human occupation.* Baltimore, MD: Williams & Wilkins.

Kielhofner, G. (1997). *Conceptual foundations of occupational therapy* (2nd ed.). Baltimore, MD: Williams & Wilkins.

Line, J. (1969). Case method as a scientific form of clinical thinking. *American Journal of Occupational Therapy, 23*, 308–313.

Table 6-1

Template for Analysis Worksheet

Title of Model or Frame of Reference _____

Theoretical Components	Summary
Focus (OT framework domains, practice areas, health conditions, or specific populations)	
Theorists (Whose theories have contributed?)	
Function (How does theory view healthy or optimal functioning?)	
Disability (How is disability defined?)	
Change (How does change occur, according to this theory?)	
Motivation (What motivates a client to change?)	
Evaluation (What formal or informal assessments are offered?)	
Intervention Guidelines (What specific therapeutic techniques or strategies have been developed?)	
Research (To what extent has this theory been validated through research?)	

Matsutsuyu, J. S. (1969). The interest check list. *American Journal of Occupational Therapy, 34,* 368–373.

Matsutsuyu, J. S. (1971). Occupational behavior: A perspective on work and play. *American Journal of Occupational Therapy, 25,* 291–294.

Reed, K. L., & Sanderson, S. N. (1999). *Concepts of occupational therapy* (4th ed.). Philadelphia, PA: Lippincott Williams & Wilkins.

Reilly, M. (1958). An occupational therapy curriculum for 1965. *American Journal of Occupational Therapy, 12,* 293–299.

Reilly, M. (1962). Occupational therapy can be one of the great ideas of 20th century medicine. *American Journal of Occupational Therapy, 16,* 1–9.

Reilly, M. (1966). A psychiatric occupational program as a teaching model. American Journal of Occupational Therapy, 20, 61–67.

Reilly, M. (1969). The educational process. *American Journal of Occupational Therapy, 23,* 299–307.

Shannon, P. (1972). Work-play theory and the occupational therapy process. *American Journal of Occupational Therapy, 26,* 169–172.

Shannon, P. (1974). Occupational choice: Decision making play. In M. Reilly (Ed.), *Play as exploratory learning* (pp. 285–314). Beverly Hills, CA: Sage Publications.

Shannon, P. (1977). The derailment of occupational therapy. *American Journal of Occupational Therapy, 31,* 229–234.

Stein, F., & Cutler, S. (2002). *Psychosocial occupational therapy: A holistic approach* (2nd ed.). Canada: Delmar.

Takata, N. (1974). Play as a prescription. In M. Reilly (Ed.), *Play as exploratory learning* (pp. 209–246). Beverly Hills, CA: Sage Publications.

Chapter 7

MODEL OF HUMAN OCCUPATION

"Occupation is a dynamic process through which we maintain the organization of our bodies and minds."

– GARY KIELHOFNER

The Model of Human Occupation (MOHO) is a conceptual model of practice that evolved from Reilly's occupational behavior model and general systems theory. Gary Kielhofner was a student of Mary Reilly who originally created this model as a Master's thesis in 1975. Within five years, Kielhofner and his colleagues published MOHO (representing initial efforts to study and apply this model to occupational therapy [OT] practice) (Kielhofner, 1980a, 1980b; Kielhofner & Burke, 1980; Kielhofner, Burke, & Heard, 1980). Kielhofner's most recent and third edition of his book *Model of Human Occupation: Theory and Application* was published in 2002. Since its original form in 1975, MOHO has continued to flourish as a practice model for OT. Many of Reilly's assumptions can be found embedded in MOHO although Kielhofner and colleagues have greatly expanded and further researched this model's earlier form. It was intended for use by everyday practitioners and has been exposed to continuous research and revision to reflect current themes in OT practice.

The MOHO is a conceptual practice model defined as "... a set of evolving theoretical arguments that are translated into a specific technology for practice and are refined and tested through research" (Kielhofner, 2002, p. 3). Occupational behavior is an outcome of a dynamic process that helps us to shape and organize ourselves as human beings:

The model of human occupation emphasizes that through therapy, persons are helped to engage in occupational behaviors that maintain, restore, reorganize, or develop their capacities, motives, and lifestyle. Through participation in therapeutic occupations, persons transform themselves into more adaptive and healthy beings. (Kielhofner & Barrett, 1997, pp. 204–205)

FOCUS

MOHO offers a systemic, holistic approach for persons of varying needs and populations across the lifespan. MOHO stresses the importance of the mind/body connection in its depiction of how motivation (internal) and performance of occupations (external) are interconnected. Human occupation is described as the "doing" of work, play, or activities of daily living (ADL) within a temporal, physical, and socio-cultural context. These are the practice domains for human performance that this model highlights. MOHO was the first OT model to conceptualize the interactive and cyclical nature of human interaction with one's environment. Therefore, the major focus for practice according to this model is on the person and how the environment contributes to one's source of motivation, patterns of behavior, and performance.

An important construct for us to define and clarify at this point is how humans or persons are conceptualized according to this model. Kielhofner's theoretical view of the person reflects how motivation, behavior, and performance are integrated. There are three interrelated parts that exist within each person:

- Volition is the motivation for occupation.

- Habituation refers to the process by which occupation is organized into patterns or routines.

- Performance capacity refers to the physical and mental abilities that underlie skilled occupational performance. This subsystem is also called mind–brain–body performance.

Each of these subsystems will be described in further detail as they relate to the open system cycle.

THEORETICAL BASE

Following is a summary list of assumptions that have been gathered among the literature and resources included in the reference section (Kielhofner, 2002; Bruce & Borg, 2002; Kielhofner, Forsyth, & Barrett, 2003):

- Humans are biologically mandated to be active. Spontaneous action is the most fundamental characteristic of all living things (Boulder, 1968; von Bertalanffy, 1968).

- o *Practice application:* Persons have a fundamental and neurologically based need for action and doing. This innate need is the dominant source of motivation for participation in occupation.

- Thinking, feeling, and doing are influenced by a dynamic interaction between one's internal components and the environment. Situations and conditions within the environment will influence a person's motivation.

- o *Practice application:* systems theory helps the practitioner to understand that there are multiple factors within the person and the environment that influence each other. A variation (positive or negative) in any one factor will result in a change in one's motivation, behavior, and/or performance.

- A human is an open system that can change and develop through interaction with the environment. The parts of the open system cycle include input, throughput, output, and feedback.

- o *Practice application:* persons are continuously impacted by input and feedback from the environment. Clients learn about themselves by experimenting with behaviors and receiving feedback about this behavior (output). There are multiple cycles that occur everyday. Some are positive, and some are negative.

- Heterarchy is the principle that parts of any system will interact with each other in ways that depend on the situation. In a heterarchy, each component contributes something to the total dynamic.

- o *Practice application:* all thoughts, emotions, or actions are an outcome of how a person and environment interact together under certain specific conditions. An occupational therapist cannot treat a client's problem in a vacuum. There are multiple and diverse factors that contribute to the client's outcome. It is important to understand how these factors interface with each other.

- Participation in occupations helps to create our occupational identity, which is formed by the person's internal structures defined by volition, habituation, and performance capacity. It is a subjective construct.

- o *Practice application:* clients develop an identity over time. It is believed that this identity begins with self-appraisal and extends toward more challenging dynamics such as accepting responsibility and knowing what one wants in life.

- *Occupational competence* is the degree to which one sustains a pattern of occupational participation that represents one's occupational identity. Competence is the ability to put into action what a person internally regards as meaningful.

- o *Practice application:* a client demonstrates competency when that person can organize his or her life to meet the basic responsibilities to the self and the role obligations of society in satisfying and meaningful ways.

- *Occupational adaptation* is the outcome of a positive occupational identity and achievement of occupational competence. It is dynamic and context dependent. OT can promote change in clients. The parts within the person (throughput) that include motivation, life patterns, and performance lead to behaviors in work, play, and self-care.

- o *Practice application:* the internal parts of the person are responsible for one's occupational performance and adaptation. OT acts as a form of feedback, coming from one's environment and, therefore, capable of impacting how one changes and alters behaviors.

ORDER/DISORDER CONTINUUM: FUNCTION AND DISABILITY

Reilly's assumptions about occupational behavior constitute the basic premise of how practitioners view function and dysfunction. The reader may recognize the similarity in representation among occupational behavior and MOHO.

Kielhofner defined *function* as *order* (a status of health and competent performance of daily living, work, and play). A person displays function when he or she is able to choose, organize, and perform occupations that are personally meaningful. It is a process whereby a person continuously learns how to balance his or her own expectations with those of society. A person demonstrates a sense of competence and role fulfillment. On the other hand, Kielhofner described dysfunction as *disorder* (the inability to perform occupations, an interruption in role performance, and an inability to meet role responsibilities) (Barris, Kielhofner, & Watts, 1983). A person with dysfunctional behavior patterns does not experience a basic quality of life, nor can he meet personal and societal expectations.

Kielhofner et al. expanded Reilly's thinking in many ways, as seen in the design of a function–dysfunction continuum. Three of the constructs to this continuum are identical to Reilly's development of occupational behavior. *Exploration, competence,* and *achievement* (see Chapter 6 for definitions) represent the function levels while *helplessness, incompetence,* and *inefficacy* represent the levels of dysfunction (Kielhofner, 1985). Following are the definitions that represent the dysfunction portion of the continuum:

- *Helplessness* may be defined as having inadequate skills or few to no interests and roles.

- *Incompetence* is demonstrated by the lack of routine, poor skill functioning, and decreased interests and values.

- *Inefficacy* is defined as decreased function and dissatisfaction with one's performance.

Following, we will review the internal and external components that comprise this systemic view of man. See Chapter 3 for a review of systems theory.

THE PROCESS OF HUMAN OCCUPATION

The two main constructs to this model are the *person* and *environment*. Tables 7-1 describes the interactive process of these components.

Man is an open system made up of three interacting subsystems: 1) volition, 2) habituation, and 3) mind–brain–body performance. Each subsystem is comprised of smaller parts that are defined in Table 7-1. These components are internal and, therefore, invisible to the practitioner. These dynamics lead directly to a person's occupational performance, also described as skilled action.

Person constructs (volitional, habituation, and mind–brain–body subsystems) plus one's occupational performance contribute to the development of *occupational identity*, *occupational competence*, and *occupational adaptation*. Occupational performance and skilled actions take place within one's environment and are, therefore, highly influenced by the feedback that is generated from this component.

THE OPEN SYSTEM CYCLE

MOHO's open system cycle shows the interdependence of various factors that influence a person's motivation, behaviors, and performance. Kielhofner has identified four major components within the human system that contribute to successful or disruptive engagement in occupations (Table 7-1).

1. Input

Input may be defined as external information that typically and naturally surrounds a person and is taken in via one's five senses. This input may or may not be meant for the person directly. Input impacts the person who takes in this information. For example, Mary works in an office as a travel agent. Today there is constant construction noise coming from outside her work place. This noise will provide auditory input to Mary. The noise is out of Mary's control and is coming from an external source (outside). It has nothing to do with Mary's job functioning, but it may directly impact her occupational performance for the day.

2. Person

Person is composed of three subsystems: volition, habituation, and mind–brain–body. The person internally processes the information that enters via input within the three subsystems. Once this internal processing is complete, the person then takes some form of skilled action. For example, Mary is trying to work in her office, and yet, she constantly hears construction noise from outside the window (input). She processes that she is highly distracted by the noise. Mary has the following internal thoughts:

- *Motivation:* "I can't seem to get anything done today, but I really want to accomplish a bunch of things."
- *Interests and values:* "I am interested in completing my job tasks, and I value doing a good job."
- *Personal causation:* "I know that I can handle this somehow because I am an adaptive person. There has to be a way that I could figure this whole thing out for myself."
- *Habits:* "My usual ways of doing these job tasks are not working for me today, and my routine is disrupted."
- *Role:* "I am not feeling very good about my worker role and my sense of accomplishment today because I can't get anything done."
- *Mind–brain–body:* "I am feeling hyper-sensitive, jumpy, and overloaded by all this noise."

Based on these internal processes and her perception of the problem, Mary will take some form of action.

3. Skilled Action or Occupational Performance

Skilled action or *occupational performance* is goal-directed action that can be externally witnessed. Skills can take the form of motor, processing, or communication/interaction responses. In the above example, a healthy reaction would show occupational adaptation. In the case of Mary, an adaptive response would be a decision to take her work into another office where it is quieter, or she may decide to wear ear plugs to diminish the outside noise. If Mary had a poor adaptation response, she may become belligerent, go outside and scream at the workers, or walk out of her job in protest. Whichever response the person shows (external skilled action), there will always be some form of feedback (external) from the environment about her performance behavior. Remember, even silence or ignoring someone is a form of feedback.

4. Environment

Environment is composed of both physical and social components. In the above example, an adaptive response would be to approach another coworker about sharing space in his or her office area. Mary will seek and receive feedback from her coworker about the feasibility of sharing office space. On a social level, Mary will likely choose to ask a coworker that she has some rapport with and who is likely to accommodate to her needs. An example of positive feedback that creates an opportunity for Mary would be "Sure, Mary. Come on in and work over here. I will make some room for you. It's a lot quieter in here." A form of negative

Table 7-1

Person

- *Volitional subsystem:* source of motivation that guides individuals to anticipate, choose, experience, and interpret what they do; thoughts and feelings about doing occupations that reflect a sense of mastery, enjoyment, and value judgments. Composed of three smaller parts:
  - o *Personal causation:* one's sense of competence and effectiveness; what a person feels capable of; a person's awareness of his or her abilities; includes feelings of self-efficacy (perception of control over one's own behavior, thoughts, and emotions including a sense of control in achieving desired outcomes). Example: "I am an intelligent person who can succeed in occupational therapy."
  - o *Values:* beliefs about what is right, important, and good to do that influences one's goals; includes personal convictions, principles, and a sense of obligation. Example: "I value helping others, and therefore, my goal is to become an occupational therapist."
  - o *Interests:* what a person finds enjoyable, pleasing, and satisfying. Example: "I enjoy studying the arts and science that underlie occupational therapy as a profession."
- *Habituation subsystem:* made up of the behaviors and roles that help persons to organize their daily lives. Composed of two smaller parts:
  - o *Habits:* automatic and repetitive behaviors that influence how persons perform routine activities, use time, and behave on a daily basis.
  - o *Internalized roles:* a source of identity with inherent obligations and expectations; also called scripts or ideas of what is expected of oneself in a particular situation; these enable individuals to fulfill needs for self and society.
- *Mind–brain–body subsystem:* composed of four constituents that represent one's capacity for occupational performance; one's underlying ability:
  - o *Musculoskeletal:* bones, muscles, and joints comprising one's biomechanical structure
  - o *Neurological:* central and peripheral nervous systems
  - o *Cardiopulmonary:* cardiovascular and pulmonary systems
  - o *Symbolic:* abstract images that guide and give meaning

Skilled Action or Occupational Performance

Goal-directed actions that constitute occupational performance fall into the following categories:

- *Motor skills:* used to move one's self or objects
- *Process skills:* thinking and planning actions used to help one organize and adapt
- *Communication and interaction skills:* observable operations used to verbalize needs and intentions that are part of social behaviors

Environment

Physical and social features in which a person does something that are shaped by culture; provides opportunities and resources (positive) and demands and constraints (negative). A significant source of feedback that can maintain or extinguish one's occupational performance. Constitutes our occupational settings, which are made up of the following components:

- *Physical environment:* composed of spaces (schools, buildings, etc.) and objects (toys, books, etc.)
- *Social environment:* consists of two entities:
  - o Groups of persons that come together for a purpose and have a major impact on the development of role behavior (social context)
  - o Occupational forms or conventionalized ways of doing things like manners, standing in line at the grocery store, etc.

feedback that would impose a barrier or restriction would be "Sorry, Mary. I have too much going on in here. I can't make any room for you. Tough luck."

The cycle appears complete. However, according to systems theory, cycles are dynamic and in constant motion. The feedback from the environment will act as a form of input and another open system cycle will be enacted. For example, if Mary moves into another office where the input is "quiet," she now has the opportunity to process her work in a quiet and modified way. If Mary encounters a barrier from the environment, she will now have to process both the noise from the outside (original input) and the negative feedback response that she just received.

CHANGE AND MOTIVATION

The concept of *change* is reflected in the systemic nature of this model and the principle of heterarchy. Any shift in one part of a person's open system cycle will result in a change in one's overall dynamic. An alteration in one's internal or external structure will create a shift in that person's thoughts, feelings, and behaviors. As a person experiments with novel behaviors and repeats them over time, these behaviors will become more automatic and habitual. Persons create a sense of *occupational competence* when they are capable of engaging in productive and meaningful actions. Therefore, sufficient repetition and environmental feedback is required to assimilate new performance patterns. *Motivation* is influenced by a person's interests, values, and a sense of personal causation, all aspects of the volitional subsystem. Therefore, the volitional subsystem becomes a significant focus area for motivation and change. Kielhofner's assumptions about motivation are strongly rooted in ego psychology and cognitive theory.

EVALUATION PROCESS

The main role of occupational therapists in the evaluation process is to conduct a thorough and client-centered assessment. Kielhofner refers to this process as *data gathering* (Kielhofner, 1995). There are two recommended general steps to this data gathering process:

1. Use the data to find out about a client from the viewpoint of an outsider looking in.

2. Collect and use data to help clients understand how their personal perceptions and subjective views lead to occupational performance actions and patterns.

MOHO assessment instruments are both structured and unstructured. Structured assessments typically include observational measures, self-report questionnaires and checklists, and structured interviews. Unstructured assessments allow the therapist to be more informal and spontaneous in response to a client's needs. Both types of assessments are recommended to attain a more typical picture of the client's performance patterns. There has been an extensive development of MOHO assessment tools over the last 25 years. Kielhofner et al. have created an online reference Web site (http://www.uic.edu/hsc/adad/cahp/OT/MOHOC). Most assessments can also be obtained through the MOHO Clearinghouse at the University of Illinois in Chicago. Examples of typical and juried publications include the following:

- Assessment of Motor and Process Skills (Asher, 1996; Fisher, 1999)
- Volitional Questionnaire (Asher, 1996; del las Heras, 1993)
- Role Checklist (Asher, 1996; Oakley, Kielhofner, & Barris, 1985)
- Occupational Questionnaire (Asher, 1996; Smith, Kielhofner, & Watts, 1986)
- Occupational Case Analysis Interview and Rating Scale (Asher, 1996; Cubie & Kaplan, 1982)
- Occupational Performance History Interview (Kielhofner, Mallison, Crawford, et al., 1997)
- Worker Role Interview (Asher, 1996)

INTERVENTION GUIDELINES

Kielhofner provided general guidelines for intervention in his 1995 text. Underlying principles to intervention include the assumption that OT can help people to change. The aim of intervention is to enhance the open system cycle so that it yields competent and adaptive performance. Practitioners are expected to appreciate the internal processing subsystems of the person (client) and how one's environment provides opportunities and/or barriers for occupational performance. Following is a general summary of Kielhofner's guidelines to intervention (Bruce & Borg, 2002; Kielhofner, 1995):

- Interventions must be client specific and related to the unique life circumstances of the individual. No generic intervention can suit every client's needs. Practitioners are expected to offer alternatives and to experiment with the "right fit."
- Interventions should be focused on changing one's occupational performance (skilled action process). Adaptive solutions should be offered in substitution for maladaptive ones.
- Interventions that impact one aspect of the overall human performance cycle (subsystems) will result in a reorganization of the entire process. Therapists must always consider how change in one part of the cycle will impact the whole.
- Interventions typically occur during periods of chaos or crises for clients. Progress, like life circumstances, is often unbalancing and may create periods of stability followed by instability within the person.

- Interventions may be aimed at modifying or altering one's environment to promote opportunities for change.

- Interventions that are aimed at skilled performance are more efficient than those aimed at a client's underlying personal structure. The overall target of therapy is to alter occupational performance; therefore, practitioners should assist clients to find new and adaptive ways to achieve desired actions and performance.

- Interventions may be aimed at skill development and skill substitution, when lacking.

- Interventions that incorporate a client's typical occupational forms will have more meaningful impact than rote learning or mere repetitious behavior.

- Interventions directed at changing one's habits and roles are challenging due to their basic function of preserving patterns for the person. Therapists may need to provide new opportunities within new environments to develop new patterns of habituation.

- Interventions that take place in one's natural environment are more likely to be assimilated by the client. Therapists should be ready to alter or modify the client's environment to increase occupational performance.

- Interventions that are aimed at habituation will need to be applied swiftly to secure one's occupational identity.

- Interventions aimed at acquiring new role scripts and related habits should be practiced in natural and appropriate environments where feedback is typically generated. Therapists can act as coaches and role models.

- Interventions that relate to one's volitional subsystem provide the most meaning and impact for the client. Occupations must be relevant to the client to be effective.

- Interventions should be aimed at improving one's functional level according to the function/dysfunction continuum. Providing occupations as interventions will innately encourage a client to adapt, change, and to learn about himself as an occupational being.

RESEARCH

Extensive research has been conducted since this model's inception. Since 1980, over 80 studies have been conducted and published. A full reference list may be found on the Internet (http://www.uic.edu/hsc/acad/cahp/OT/MOHOC). Many aspects of this model have been refined over the years in response to the various studies. Clearly, a strength of this approach is the ongoing development and research that has transpired over the years. Its practice range offers assessments for children through later adulthood. Its conceptual framework can be applied in multiple settings, from traditional inpatient to community-based settings. There have been many sources of evidence-based research about MOHO's effectiveness concerning various conditions with some of the most recent studies, including traumatic brain injury (Depoy, 1990; Series, 1992), pediatric health (Adelstein, Barnes, Murray-Jensen, & Skaggs, 1989; Geist & Kielhofner, 1998; Schaaf & Mulrooney, 1989), geriatrics (Levine & Gitlin, 1993), HIV and AIDS (Pizzi, 1990), adolescent psychiatry (Baron, 1987; Lancaster & Mitchell, 1991), and adult psychiatry (de las Heras, Llerena, & Kielhofner, 2003). Studies have also been done on the impact of MOHO in general practice areas (Hagulund & Kjellberg, 1999; Laliberte-Rudman, Yu, Scott, & Pajoukandek, 1999; Neville-Jan, 1994; Rebeiro & Allen, 1998; Suto, 1998).

SUMMARY

The MOHO was the first occupation-based model to incorporate the original concepts of Mary Reilly and systems theory. It is truly holistic and client-centered in nature because it conveys the importance of a person's subjective view on life occupations. MOHO attempts to show the complexities that exist within each person and the role of the environment in shaping one's occupational performance throughout the life span. It guides the practitioner in the art of doing therapy from a systemic perspective. Kielhofner and his constituents have offered major contributions to the field including a wide variety of assessments and extensive research concerning the impact of therapy and the positive outcomes achieved from this therapeutic approach. This model is well respected and practiced within the OT profession.

LEARNING ACTIVITY

Directions: Read the following case thoroughly. Ask a fellow student or person of your choice to act as the client for the purpose of this assignment. Indicate to your partner how you would like him or her to respond in the evaluation process.

1. Review the various MOHO assessments that have been published. Administer any two assessments to your "client" that seem to suit his or her needs. Your partner should attempt to respond as the person described in your case. Include the actual completed assessments with the "client's" responses as part of this assignment. (10 points)

2. Write a report based on your findings. Use Table 7-2 to complete this assignment.

Table 7-2

MOHO Case Assignment Sheet

Student's Name: _____

Case Name: _____

Positive Cycle

Input

Person

Volitional:

Habituation:

Mind–Brain–Body:

Occupational Performance or Skilled Action

Feedback

Negative Cycle

Input

Person

Volitional:

Habituation:

Mind–Brain–Body:

Occupational Performance or Skilled Action

Feedback

(continued)

Table 7-2

MOHO Case Assignment Sheet (continued)

Subsystems of the Person

	Strengths	Weaknesses
Volitional subsystem		
Habituation subsystem		
Mind–brain–body subsystem		

Sources for Motivation Within the Volitional Subsystem

Motivator #1:   Rationale:

Motivator #2:   Rationale:

Motivator #3:   Rationale:

Positive and Negative Influences From the Environment

Positive opportunities and resources: Reasons:

Negative restrictions and barriers: Reasons:

Occupational Therapy Occupations as Interventions

	Goal/Purpose/Meaningfulness
Volitional subsystem occupation	
Habituation subsystem occupation	
Mind–brain–body subsystem occupation	

Guidelines

1. Illustrate one example of an open system cycle that leads to adaptive occupational performance for your client. (5 points)

2. Illustrate one example of an open system cycle that leads to maladaptive occupational performance for you client. (5 points)

3. Identify four strengths and four weaknesses for this client within each of the three subsystems. Use information from your case as well as your assessment findings to complete this section. (25 points)

4. List three sources of motivation for change. State why these choices are motivators based on your case study and assessment findings. (Hint: reinforcers can be social, material, or activities.) (15 points)

5. Give one example of how the client's environment is fostering occupational competence by providing an opportunity or resource. Give one example of how the environment is creating a restriction of barrier. Explain the reasons for your choice (10 points)

6. Identify *one* occupation that could be used as an OT intervention to either maintain or change the functions within each of the three subsystems. Briefly describe the occupation. State the actual goal and meaningfulness of this occupation in relationship to your client. This section requires that you come up with three *different* occupations in total. (30 points)

Case Study: Susan

Susan is a 40-year-old homemaker and mother of a 10-year-old daughter, Veronica. Susan was recently admitted to an inpatient psychiatric unit for suicidal ideation. This is her first hospitalization although Susan has been diagnosed with major depression since she was in college. She has seen various counselors over the years, and her internist has prescribed antidepressants for her. She is presently taking Zoloft, 150 mg.

Approximately 1 year ago, Susan separated from her husband. Since the separation, Susan noticed that she has felt "different." She is slowly doing less and less in the house. She reports difficulty with concentration, diminished interests in leisure and social activities, and overall sadness. She was always a meticulous housekeeper but has had difficulty maintaining her daily responsibilities and routines. Susan feels angry at herself for not "doing what I am supposed to do every day."

She comes to the OT interview dressed in a pair of jeans and t-shirt. She looks older than her actual age. She wears no make-up and her hair is in a pony tail. Susan looks like she is about to cry as you introduce yourself and talk about conducting an OT assessment with her.

During the assessment process, Susan tells her life story. She was in an abusive marriage for 10 years. Her husband repeatedly beat her, especially during his drinking episodes. She also felt very controlled by him. He dictated how he wanted things to be done, and Susan was expected to make him happy. He was very perfectionistic and demanding, particularly around the raising of their daughter and the maintenance of their beautiful home.

The final straw happened when Susan and her daughter went to a movie unexpectedly one evening. John came home to an empty house and became suspicious that Susan left him for another man. When Susan and her daughter returned home around 10:00 p.m., John was waiting at the front door. He immediately dragged Susan into the living room by her hair. He physically slapped and kicked her in front of their daughter who witnessed the whole incident. Susan sustained multiple injuries including a concussion from hitting her head

on the floor. Veronica called 911 and the police arrived. John was arrested, and Susan was taken to the emergency room. She was referred to the psychiatric unit of the hospital because of her reports of suicidal ideation.

Susan is an articulate person although she makes infrequent eye contact and speaks slowly. She graduated from a secretarial school and worked as an executive secretary until age 30. John told her to quit her job and stay at home if she wanted to be a "good wife to him." Susan complied. Veronica was born within their first year of marriage.

Susan and Veronica are very close. They spend lots of time together. Susan is very creative and artistic. She enjoys making crafts of all kinds with her daughter. Susan volunteers at Veronica's school and goes into her classroom 2 to 3 times a week. They love to watch videos together, read books, and sew clothes for Veronica's dolls.

Susan's past interests include reading, making elaborate ceramic pieces, playing tennis, and playing the piano. Susan admits that most of her daily routines revolve around what her husband wants her to get done and what Veronica likes to do. Susan often feels lost without both of them around.

Susan states that she no longer wants to live "this life." She reports that her one joy in life is her daughter. She is a very concerned and conscientious mother. Susan feels very guilty for thinking about dying. She also blames herself for the faulty marriage.

Susan indicated that she has few acquaintances but no real friends. Her parents live nearby and have always been a good source of support. She feels that she has let everyone "down" by getting depressed.

Susan has no real plans of what to do from here. She feels at a loss and wants help from the staff. She is willing to participate in occupational therapy. "I could definitely use some of that," she replies as she hears about the OT program on the unit.

REFERENCES

Adelstein, L. A., Barnes, M. A., Murray-Jensen, F., & Skaggs, C. B. (1989). A broadening frontier: Occupational therapy in mental health programs for children and adolescents. *Mental Health Special Interest Section Newsletter, 12,* 2–4.

Baron, K. (1987). The model of human occupation: A newspaper treatment group for adolescents with a diagnosis of conduct disorder. *Occupational Therapy in Mental Health, 7,* 89–104.

Barris, R., Kielhofner, G., & Watts, J. (1983). *Psychosocial occupational therapy: Practice in a pluralistic arena.* Laurel, MD: RAM Association.

Bruce, M. G., & Borg, B. (2002). *Psychosocial frames of reference: Core for occupation-based practice* (3rd ed.). Thorofare, NJ: SLACK Incorporated.

De las Heras, C., Llerena, V., Kielhofner, G. (2003). Remotivational process: Progressive intervention for individuals with severe volitional challenges. University of Illinois. Model of Human Occupation Clearinghouse.

Depoy, E. (1990). The TBIIM: An intervention for the treatment of individuals with traumatic brain injury. *Occupational Therapy in Health Care, 7,* 55–67.

Geist, R., & Kielhofner, G. (1998). The pediatric volitional questionnaire. Chicago, IL: University of Illinois, Model of Human Occupation Clearinghouse.

Hagulund, L., & Kjellberg, A. (1999). A critical analysis of the model of human occupation. *Canadian Journal of Occupational Therapy, 66,* 102–108.

Kielhofner, G. (1975). The evolution of knowledge in occupational therapy: Understanding adaptation of the chronically disabled. Los Angeles, CA: University of Southern California, Unpublished master's thesis.

Kielhofner, G. (1980a). A model of human occupation, part two. Ontogenesis from the perspective of temporal adaptation. *American Journal of Occupational Therapy, 34,* 657–663.

Kielhofner, G. (1980b). A model of human occupation, part three. Benign and vicious cycles. *American Journal of Occupational Therapy, 34,* 731–737.

Kielhofner, G. (1983). *Health through occupation: Theory and practice in occupational therapy.* Philadelphia, PA: FA Davis.

Kielhofner, G. (1985). *A model of human occupation: Theory and application.* Baltimore, MD: Williams & Wilkins.

Kielhofner, G. (1995). *A model of human occupation: Theory and application* (2nd ed.). Baltimore, MD: Williams & Wilkins.

Kielhofner, G. (2002). *A model of human occupation: Theory and application* (3rd ed.). Baltimore, MD: Williams & Wilkins.

Kielhofner, G., & Barrett, L. (1997). An overview of occupational behavior. In H. Hopkins & H. Smith (Eds.), *Willard & Spackman's occupational therapy.* Philadelphia, PA: JB Lippincott.

Kielhofner, G., & Burke, J. (1980). A model of human occupation, part one. Conceptual framework and content. *American Journal of Occupational Therapy, 34,* 572–581.

Kielhofner, G., Burke, J., & Heard, I. C. (1980). A model of human occupation, part four. Assessment and intervention. *American Journal of Occupational Therapy, 34,* 777–788.

Kielhofner, G., Forsyth, K., & Barrett, L. (2003). The model of human occupation. In E. B. Crepeau, E. S. Cohn, & B. A. Boyt Schell (Eds.), *Willard & Spackman's occupational therapy.* Philadelphia, PA: JB Lippincott.

Kielhofner, G., Mallison, T., Cranford, C., et al. (1997). *A user's guide to Occupational Performance History Intervention-II* (OPHI-II) (Version 2.0). Chicago, IL: Model of Human Occupation Clearinghouse, University of Illinois.

Laliberte-Rudman, D., Yu, B., Scott, E., & Pajoukandek, P. (1999). Exploration of perspectives of persons with schizophrenia regarding quality of life. *American Journal of Occupational Therapy, 54,* 137–145.

Lancaster, J., & Mitchell, M. (1991). Occupational therapy treatment goals, objectives, and activities for improving low self-esteem in adolescents with behavioral disorders. *Occupational Therapy in Mental Health, 11*(2/3), 3–22.

Levine, R. E., & Gitlin, L. N. (1993). A model to promote activity competence in elders. *American Journal of Occupational Therapy, 47,* 147–153.

Neville-Jan, A. (1994). The relationship of volition to adaptive occupational behavior among individuals with varying degrees of depression. *Occupational Therapy in Mental Health, 12,* 1–18.

Pizzi, M. (1990). The model of human occupation and adults with HIV infection and AIDS. *American Journal of Occupational Therapy, 44,* 257–264.

Rebeiro, K. L., & Allen, J. (1998). Volunteerism as occupation. *Canadian Journal of Occupational Therapy, 65,* 279–285.

Schaaf, R. C., & Mulrooney, L. L. (1989). Occupational therapy in early intervention: A family-centered approach. *American Journal of Occupational Therapy, 34,* 745–754.

Series, C. (1992). The long-term needs of people with head injury: A role for the community occupational therapist? *British Journal of Occupational Therapy, 55,* 94–98.

Suto, M. (1998). Leisure in occupational therapy. *Canadian Journal of Occupational Therapy, 65,* 271–278.

Chapter 8

OCCUPATIONAL ADAPTATION

"Mastery is more than the ability to perform a discrete task. It is a reflection of the client's experience as an occupational being."

— JANET SCHKADE & SALLY SCHULTZ

During the 1990s, many experts in occupational therapy (OT) emphasized the importance of the adaptation process in maintaining satisfying and meaningful occupational behaviors. Adaptation had been identified as a significant concept in earlier frames of reference for OT, namely Sensory Integration (Ayres, 1972) and Spatiotemporal Adaptation (Gilfoyle, Grady, & Moore, 1981). Mary Reilly, in her occupational behavior model, believed that as persons are challenged to deal with tasks of everyday life, occupation allows for adaptation to occur. While adaptation was not a new concept to the practice of OT, the models of the 1990s studied and applied these concepts in a different way. More recent study of the adaptation process has not only focused on its importance in childhood development but has also been applied to the adult population. Modern studies about the adaptation process also looked more specifically at the relationship between adaptation and occupation. In keeping with the paradigm shift that reflected OT practice during this decade, these occupation-based models also emphasized how participating in occupations maintains one's well-being and quality of life.

Schkade and Schultz first published their occupational adaptation model in 1992. It was developed out of the need to establish a foundational theory for a new research program (Doctor of Philosophy in OT) at Texas Woman's University. Other significant contributors to this model included Anne Henderson, Lela Llorens, and Kathlyn Reed. *Occupational adaptation* is a comprehensive systems model that is based on core concepts and constructs reflective of OT practice. It can be described as consisting of two components: 1) a framework that describes a normal human phenomenon called adaptation and 2) a framework that allows occupational therapists to plan, guide, and implement interventions (Schkade & McClung, 2001).

FOCUS

The focus or domain of practice is meant to be applied across the developmental lifespan with a holistic application to a variety of populations and therapeutic needs. Occupational adaptation focuses on the interactive process between a person and his or her occupational environment. This model can best be understood by listing some key definitions (Kramer, Hinojosa, & Royeen, 2003, p. 185). The following four constructs guide the reasoning process of a practitioner and bring one's clinical focus to specific areas that represent the theoretical assumptions of this model. It is advised that the reader take the time to fully understand the meaning of these terms since they define the basic models and essential components.

1. Occupations

Occupations include the following three components to qualify: 1) they actively involve the person, 2) they are meaningful to the person, and 3) they include a process and a product that may be tangible or intangible.

2. Adaptive Capacity

Adaptive capacity is a person's ability to recognize the need for change, modification, or refinement (adaptation) in order to achieve relative mastery. It is believed that this dynamic has a cumulative effect over the lifetime of the individual, as experience and adaptive responses become self-reinforcing. It occurs when a person's typical response does not meet the challenges of an occupation and the person now has to modify or adjust his or her behaviors to achieve a competent outcome.

3. Relative Mastery

Relative mastery is a person's self-assessment of his or her occupational response that reviews 1) efficiency of response as defined by use of time, energy, and resources; 2) effectiveness in response as defined by successful achievement of one's goal; and 3) satisfaction in response as defined by one's self-perceptions (internal) and societal norms (external).

4. Occupational Adaptation Process

Occupational adaptation process is a complex series of steps and factors that occur when a person is faced with an occupational challenge, which takes place within one's environment and within one's role capacity. Significant components of this process include the following: 1) the person, 2) the occupational environment, and 3) the interaction or process that takes place between the person and the environment. This process depicts how a person can respond adaptively and masterfully when engaged in occupations.

THEORETICAL BASE

Following is a summary list of assumptions to the occupational adaptation model based on various resources and interpretations, including the authors of this textbook (Kramer, Hinojosa, & Kramer, 2003, pp. 185–186; Schkade & McClung, 2001; Schultz & Schkade, 2003, pp. 220–223; Stein & Cutler, 2002, pp. 166–167):

- Occupations provide a life-long opportunity for adaptation as a person attempts to competently meet the internal and external demands created by one's environment. Whenever a person responds to an occupational challenge, one's internal adaptation process is automatically re-enacted.
    - o *Practice application:* all occupations require some degree of adaptation (internal process). Occupational therapists recognize that when clients are unable to engage competently in occupations, it is due to an internal struggle with adaptation.
- A person's occupational roles and the environment in which they occur naturally create a source of demand for a person. Role expectations and demands are determined both by one's internal perceptions and by external social and cultural norms.
    - o *Practice application:* clients assume roles and associated expectations by incorporating their own perceptions as well as those identified by society (norms). Roles have inherent expectations that are influenced both internally and externally. All role participation automatically requires that clients interact within their environment.

- People have an inherent drive for mastery. A person is believed to be influenced by three systems—sensorimotor, cognitive, and psychosocial—all of which are determined by genetics, the environment, and an experiential learning process that allows a person to integrate feedback from the environment about one's performance. All three systems are enforced in every occupational response.
    - o *Practice application:* an occupational therapist believes that it is natural for clients to engage in occupations with a quest for mastery. When a client shows low motivation for occupational performance, it is good practice to assess the person in all three variables for explanation of cause.
- A person's adaptive capacity can be overwhelmed by impairment, physical or emotional disability, and stressful life transitions at any point in one's life. As demands increase within the person and/or environment, the adaptation process becomes more challenging. As dysfunction increases, so does the demand for change in one's adaptive process.
    - o *Practice application:* health conditions and stress will impact one's adaptive capacity by heightening demands. As the levels of disability and stress increase, it becomes harder to adapt and perform occupations. A client's adaptive capacity is compromised by an increase in dysfunction.
- Occupational performance takes place within different environments that pose various demands for mastery. Occupational environments are influenced by physical, social, and cultural components. Occupational performance occurs in the areas of work, play/leisure, and self-care.
    - o *Practice application:* an occupational therapist will observe a client's performance in self-care, work, and play/leisure while inquiring about the physical, social, and cultural demands of the client's environment. Performance is significantly influenced by externalized judgments (proper etiquette, beauty contests, "machismo," etc.) that can be viewed as positive or negative by a client.
- Success in occupational performance is a direct result of the person's ability to adapt with sufficient mastery to satisfy the self and others. Occupational performance is fixed and defined by occupational roles.
    - o *Practical application:* one way to measure "successful" occupational performance is when a person reports feeling satisfied with himself (relative mastery) and capable of meeting the demands of the outside environment. Balancing these two components efficiently requires an intact adaptive capacity.
- A person's desire for mastery coupled with the environment's demand for competency produce occupational

press. Press may be defined as the set of demands or expectations for behavior that is either objectively or subjectively perceived by an individual (Murray, Barrett, & Hamburger, 1938).

   o *Practice application:* clients feel "pressured" to meet both their internal and external demands. This pressure can lead to stress, which can lead to a reduction in one's adaptive capacity.

- The internal adaptation process allows a person to respond to challenges over a lifetime. Occupational challenges naturally require some aspect of change (modification, alteration, refinement) in a person's response in order to achieve competency and mastery.

   o *Practice application:* it is natural to assume that new adaptive strategies will have to be implemented in the course of one's lifetime since we are constantly challenged (press) to perform toward mastery. Persons who are flexible and adaptive will have healthier outcomes. Occupational therapists can normalize the helping process for their clients by stating that is a natural process to need assistance with change.

- Adaptation energy is limited and finite (Selye, 1956). It is also unique to each person. Stress can deplete one's energy source. Therefore, one's adaptive capacity is compromised during periods of transition and stress.

   o *Practice application:* there is only a certain amount of energy that can be dispensed toward adaptation. Occupational therapists can assist clients to minimize their stress and free up the capacity to have more energy for everyday challenges.

FUNCTION AND DISABILITY

Function is evident when a person is able to engage and perform in occupations within a specific environment and with a sense of mastery and accomplishment. This includes a person's ability to meet role expectations that are self-induced and demanded from the external environment. Therefore, a healthy individual shows adaptive capacity and relative mastery. Disability is evident when a person does not show competent occupational performance due to a disruption in one's adaptive capacity. Dysfunctional behaviors occur because the person's ability to adapt has been challenged to the point that the demands for performance are not satisfactorily met (Schultz & Schkade, 2003, p. 220). One's adaptive response can lead to functional and/or dysfunctional behaviors. Faulty mechanisms may exist within the person subsystem and/or the environment when disability is evident.

Adaptation Process

At this point, let's review the *occupational adaptation process,* the core dynamic to understanding and applying this model. Viewed as a *normative* process, occupational adaptation is an innate capacity in every person. Schkade and Schultz originally described this process in 1992. Throughout the normal developmental stages of life, we are all challenged to adapt. Struggles within the adaptation process do not necessarily constitute a disability but may represent a person who is challenged to alter and change his life roles and functioning. We have all had some difficulties with adapting. The following three main constructs define this process further and illustrate the variables that interface within the adaptation process. These variables include the *person, environment,* and the *interaction between the person and environment.* Figure 8-1 offers further orientation to the various terms and concepts and depiction of their interdependent nature.

According to this model, each person is made up of three parts: *sensorimotor, cognitive,* and *psychosocial*

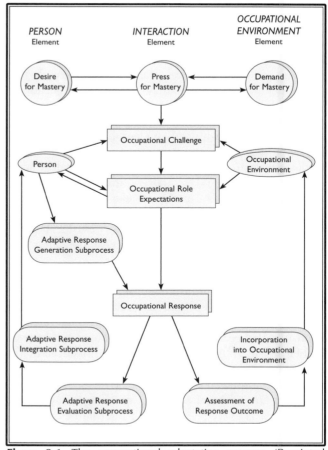

Figure 8-1. The occupational adaptation process. (Reprinted with permission from the American Occupational Therapy Association. Schkade, J. K., & McClung, M. [2001]. *Occupational adaptation in practice: Concepts and cases* [p. 5]. Thorofare, NJ: SLACK Incorporated.)

components. An occupational therapist recognizes that these three components are constructed by physiological, psychological, neurological, cognitive, and intrinsic aspects. It is assumed that every person has an innate propensity to engage in occupations and to aspire toward some form of competency in one's behavioral performance. This phenomenon is called the *desire for mastery*. It is this natural desire to pursue occupational behavior that begins the cycle of the adaptation process. In healthy individuals, the desire for mastery is matched by the person's capacity in sensorimotor, cognitive, and psychosocial functioning. In dysfunctional patterns, the desire may be unrealistic because the person does not have the adaptive capacity to respond competently. Sometimes, one's desire to pursue occupations may be lacking, as evident in persons who are feeling depressed. In accordance with this model, a practitioner can hypothesize that the lack of motivation or desire may be related to the negative responses that the client has received about his past role performance.

The second construct that needs to be analyzed is the *occupational environment*. The environment includes physical, social, and cultural aspects. Persons interact with their environments and engage in occupational performance through work, play/leisure, and self-care/self-maintenance activities. The environment creates its own set of criteria for successful occupational performance. This phenomenon is called the *demand for mastery*. For example, every OT program has to meet certain standards or essentials that are defined by the Accreditation Council for Occupational Therapy Education (ACOTE) in order to meet accreditation status. These standards trickle down to the student as demands for mastery. A student has to demonstrate a specific degree of competency and mastery in order to graduate from an accredited OT program. In healthy adaptive cycles, the demand for mastery from the environment matches the person's capacity to adapt and competently meet those standards of behavior. In dysfunctional patterns, the environmental demands exceed the person's ability to adapt and competently meet those expectations, resulting in inadequate occupational performance.

The third construct to be understood by the practitioner is the *person–environment transaction*. Whenever a person participates in an occupation, he is naturally challenged to meet various expectations of performance. This phenomenon is called *occupational challenge*. Whenever a person participates in an occupation, he is also influenced by the role expectations of that specific environment, which exist to shape one's behaviors and impact one's occupational response. Occupational role functioning is influenced by two factors: 1) every person has an internal perception of how and why one should act a certain way, which contributes to one's personal satisfaction, and 2) every environment also has a set of social and cultural norms that define how one should act in order to fit in. These expected behaviors also impact a person's occupational response. Consider the role of a student. Within each person is an internal set of standards about what constitutes a "good" student. Some

students think that these behaviors include being organized and studying every day to keep up with the content in class. Other students may define what is "good" based on the grades that they get on exams and papers. Coupled with these internal perceptions are the external departmental expectations of being a "good" student. An example of an external competency demand is a departmental policy that states students must achieve a specific GPA (3.0) per each semester. If a student does not meet the minimum GPA criteria, he or she is at risk of being dismissed from that specific OT program. In other words, if the person cannot adapt his or her response and behaviors to meet this occupational challenge (3.0 GPA) and meet this student role expectation (minimal competency to remain in the program), his or her occupational behavior is viewed as incompetent. Occupational challenge, occupational roles, and occupational response all result from the *press for mastery*, which is inherent and originates from the specific environment.

Each day, every person experiences *desire*, *demand*, and *press for mastery* while engaging in his typical occupations. This entire experience is also normative. As originally defined by Maslow, we all have an inherent *desire* to be the best that we can be. *Demands* from the environment are also a given. No one is insulated from having outside expectations and/or rules placed upon him or her. Since the desire and the demand for mastery are typical occurrences in everyday life, we will, in like fashion, experience *press* (a summative outcome of desire and demand put together). This adaptive process is taken for granted when we adapt and competently respond with a successful outcome in occupational performance. It is during those times when a person is unable to meet the internal and external demands of the adaptive process that he or she may come to the attention of an occupational therapist. A problem emerges in occupational performance. The authors have made a significant assumption about occupational performance that is based on these concepts. If a client does not show a desire for mastery, it is incorrect to assume that he is lacking motivation or ambition. Rather, the problem lies within the inability to match the client's occupational role with an occupational goal that will allow this desire to be demonstrated. An occupational therapist must, therefore, collaborate with the client and/or significant others to seek an appropriate choice of an occupation that matches the person's adaptive capacity and environmental demands (Schkade & McClung, 2002). This assumption is critical to the OT intervention process because it minimizes the tendency to blame the client when he or she seems disinterested or unmotivated to change. As occupational therapists, we can offer a different perspective to the reasons why a person may not be showing adequate occupational performance based on a systems view of how the interdependent variables within this model may be misaligned. When a practitioner on the health care team can say that the client is not to blame for poor occupational performance but that there is something faulty about the adaptive process, he or she is using a workable reframe for intervention. The OT needs to analyze the problem within the adaptation process cycle.

The *adaptation process* has also been further decoded for practical application of this model. When facing an occupational challenge, the person calls upon three subprocesses: 1) the adaptive response generation subprocess, 2) the adaptive response evaluation subprocess, and 3) the adaptive response integration subprocess. The function of these three subprocesses is to plan one's occupational response, evaluate it, and promote an adaptive response. Following a breakdown of each subprocess.

Adaptive Response Generation Subprocess

This subprocess is an anticipatory aspect of the adaptation process that consists of two parts. Healthy individuals generate responses with some degree of *relative mastery*.

The components of the adaptive generation subprocess follow:

- *Adaptive response mechanism:* Using the three parts within every person (sensorimotor, cognitive, and psychosocial), this mechanism designs a plan for action for the occupational response.
- *Adaptation gestalt:* Using the three parts within every person (sensorimotor, cognitive, and psychosocial), a holistic plan is executed into action.

Adaptive responses fall into three categories and show the following characteristics:

1. *Primitive:* hyperstable, immobile, appearing "stuck"
2. *Transitional:* hypermobile, highly variable and random, lacking clear direction
3. *Mature:* stable, goal-directed, solution-oriented

Adaptive Response Evaluation Subprocess

In this subprocess, a person assesses his or her relative experience of mastery within three areas. In other words, a person's self-assessment of his or her occupational performance (relative mastery) may be described according to the following criteria.

Areas of relative mastery follow:

- *Efficient* use of time, energy, and personal resources
- *Effective* degree to which one's desired goal was reached
- *Satisfying* expectations of oneself and also those of social and cultural norms

Persons who function well in the adaptation process will often question how masterful was their adaptive response and demonstrate interest and capacity to self-evaluate. The ability to reflect and self-evaluate is a higher order of cognitive reasoning. Persons who show disruption in the adaptation process may neither question nor seek out an explanation about mastery and the reasons why their attempts have failed. They may appear as disinterested, unmotivated, and disheartened to the practitioner. These responses are representative of the discrepancies within the mastery process and may originate in this aspect of the adaptation cycle.

The final subprocess requires that the person be able to synthesize his past experiences and formulate a conclusion about the positive and negative experiences. Once again, synthesis is an executive function of cognitive reasoning, and some persons may not have this capacity. Therefore, it will be important for the OT to assess where the disruption lies within this process.

Adaptive Response Integration Subprocess

Persons demonstrate this subprocess when the following three components are evident. Healthy functioning persons show adaptive capacity, meaning that they can anticipate outcomes of their behavior based on prior experiences of relative mastery. They are also able to self-initiate a new adaptive response when necessary. Figure 8-2 summarizes the cognitive reasoning of a person who shows adequate adaptive responses.

Components of an adaptive response integration subprocess follow:

- The ability to examine the occupational event.
- The ability to determine whether the occupational response was positive or negative.
- The ability to generalize one's adaptive responses for application to new tasks.

Once an *adaptive response* is generated, the environment also has mechanisms for measuring its effectiveness. Feedback is provided to the person about role functioning from a physical, social, and cultural perspective. This information may be positive or negative. When expectations are not met satisfactorily, modifications may be recommended concerning person and/or environment variables. The active role of the environment in evaluating a person's adaptive response is called assessment of response outcome. From the three sources of environmental feedback—physical, social, and cultural—a person is provided with feedback about his or her occupational performance. The last step to the entire adaptation process is the incorporation into one's occupational environment. This last step completes the cycle and allows the person to benefit from feedback that can be used for future occupational involvement.

CHANGE AND MOTIVATION

According to the occupational adaptation model, motivation is impacted by three processes: the desire for mastery, the demand for mastery, and the press for mastery.

Occupational challenges are representative of the interactive nature of these three components. Therefore, a person will be more motivated to change if 1) the occupation itself is personally meaningful and desired by the person, 2) the demands of the occupation can be managed and are within the adaptive nature of the person, and 3) the outside forces or press from the environment equals the person's capacity to adapt and successfully perform. An occupational therapist can recognize that a person has successfully changed or adapted one's occupational behaviors by three indicators: 1) a client's report of improved relative mastery, 2) observation of a client spontaneously generalizing adaptive responses into similar and new situations, and 3) a client's initiation of adaptations not previously seen in the client's repertoire or specifically suggested by an outside source (Schkade & McClung, 2001).

EVALUATION PROCESS

Schultz and Schkade have constructed an assessment questionnaire titled the "Guide to Practice" (1992). These questions focus on three areas: occupational adaptation data gathering, occupational adaptation programming, and evaluation of the occupational adaptation process. These questions guide the occupational therapist to gather information about a client's adaptation process so that a comprehensive view of the client's occupational functioning can be understood. An OT practitioner is also encouraged to consider standardized assessments and observational tools to evaluate the person, analyze the environment, determine role expectations that are both internal and external, and assess the adaptive capacity of an individual. In summary, the evaluation process for a practitioner may include the following points of interest:

1. Determine the strengths and weaknesses that comprise the person in the areas of sensorimotor, cognitive, and psychosocial functioning. These assessments would measure one's physiological, psychological, neurological, cognitive, and intrinsic aspects.

2. Analyze the role expectations and demands within the client's environment as defined by one's physical, social, and cultural contexts.

3. Evaluate a client's capacity to perform activities within the expected role, and identify the strengths that allow for relative mastery and the weaknesses that prevent competency.

4. Utilize standardized OT assessments and tools to determine one's ability for internal adaptation, including ability to generalize learning from one experience to another, self-initiation of new strategies in diverse situations, and an increase in relative mastery.

INTERVENTIONS

Although Schkade and Schultz (1993) have not identified specific techniques for intervention that can be used with this model, they have provided guiding principles that the OT practitioner should consider and integrate within a holistic approach to treatment. "The goal of intervention is to facilitate the client's ability to make his or her own adaptations for engaging in occupational activities that are personally meaningful" (Schultz & Schkade, 2003, p. 222). A collaborative relationship is prescribed; the client is identified as the agent of change while the therapist is a facilitator. An OT practitioner may apply the following strategies during the intervention process:

1. Assist the client to identify a compatible occupational role that is personally meaningful. Encourage the client to tell the therapist about the role expectations according to the client's perceptions. This will help the occupational therapist to understand the client's internal expectations of his role.

2. Facilitate the ability of a client to participate in personally satisfying and appropriate social activities that are permitted by one's sensorimotor, cognitive, and psychosocial capacity. The occupational therapist is interested to learn about how realistic a client's choices may be.

3. Heighten a client's strengths within the three subsystems—sensorimotor, cognitive, and psychosocial—to promote one's adaptive capacity.

4. Facilitate the adaptation process through occupational activities that include active participation of the client, meaningfulness, and result in a tangible or intangible end product.

5. Increase a client's ability to self-evaluate for relative mastery, which includes time, energy, and resource efficiency; overall effectiveness; and satisfaction to oneself and society.

6. Comprise an intervention plan that focuses on 1) occupational readiness—activities that will address deficits in motor, process, and communication/interaction performance skills—and 2) occupational activity—tasks that are related to the occupational role selected by the client.

7. Provide direct feedback about one's occupational performance to enhance the ability to integrate an adaptive response and create a new set of behavioral responses.

8. Assist the client to identify alternative solutions and occupational responses when relative mastery is not achieved.

9. Utilize data from the *Occupational Adaptation Guide to Practice* from Schultz and Schkade (1992) to assist the client to identify his own plan for intervention

and understand patterns of strengths and weaknesses in occupational adaptation.

RESEARCH

Following is a summary list of clinical research that has been conducted on this model by a variety of methods. Outcomes from these studies all show effectiveness and increase in independent functioning related to the use of the occupational adaptation model:

- Impact on independent functioning for persons with cerebral vasular accident (CVA) (Gibson & Schkade, 1997)
- Impact on independence for persons who have had a hip fracture (Jackson & Schkade, 2001)
- Comparison of occupational adaptation interventions versus standard facility protocols for post-hip fracture conditions (Buddenberg & Schkade, 1998)
- Comparison of occupational adaptation interventions versus standard facility protocols for CVA conditions (Dolecheck & Schkade, 1999)
- A case study research for persons with CVA in home care (Johnson & Schkade, 2001)

SUMMARY

In summary, occupational adaptation is a holistic and complex model with various integrated concepts and constructs. It is a client-centered approach that guides the occupational therapist to assess a person's adaptation process from a systems point of view. Its distinctive contribution to OT practice is that it explains how one's adaptive capacity can impact occupational performance successfully or unsuccessfully, drawing a practitioner's attention to faulty processes within this cycle as opposed to faulty people. Persons with disrupted or inadequate occupational performance are assumed to need a change in the adaptation cycle, composed of the various interdependent variables as defined by the authors. The adaptation process is a complex phenomenon that requires a high-level cognitive understanding by the practitioner. It can be used by occupational therapists to fully understand and therapeutically enhance occupational performance for the client, significant others, and health care team members.

LEARNING ACTIVITY

1. Define the following terms and concepts from this model:
   - Occupation adaptive capacity
   - Relative mastery
   - Press for mastery
   - Occupational adaptation process
   - Occupational performance areas
   - Person (components)
   - Demand for mastery
   - Occupational environment
   - Occupational challenge
   - Desire for mastery
   - Person–environment interaction
   - Occupational roles
   - Occupational response
   - Adaptive response generation
   - Adaptive response evaluation
   - Adaptive response integration
   - Adaptive response mechanism
   - Adaptation
   - Three types of adaptation
   - Three areas of relative mastery
   - Occupational readiness
   - Occupational activity
   - Assessment of response outcome
   - Incorporation into occupational environment

2. Construct a Venn diagram that depicts how occupational adaptation is the outcome of 1) the person, 2) the environment, and 3) the transaction of the person–environment.

3. Construct a Venn diagram that depicts how occupational challenge is created by 1) desire for mastery, 2) press for mastery, and 3) demand for mastery.

4. Construct a Venn diagram that depicts how a person creates a response based on 1) the occupational challenge, 2) occupational role functioning, and 3) the occupational environment.

5. Construct a Venn diagram that depicts how adaptive response is the outcome of 1) the generation subprocess, 2) the integration subprocess, and 3) the evaluation subprocess.

6. Complete the worksheet in Table 8-1 on this model.

7. Watch the movie *About Schmidt,* and consider the main character, Warren Schmidt, as your client. Assume that Warren has difficulty in the adaptation process and has been referred to you with the diagnosis of major depression, single episode.
   - Answer the questions included in Table 8-2 based on your observations of Warren.
   - Use your answers to complete a profile about Warren Schmidt.

Table 8-1
Template for Analysis Worksheet

Title of Model or Frame of Reference _____

Theoretical Components	Summary
Focus (OT framework domains, practice areas, health conditions, or specific populations)	
Theorists (Whose theories have contributed?)	
Function (How does theory view healthy or optimal functioning?)	
Disability (How is disability defined?)	
Change (How does change occur, according to this theory?)	
Motivation (What motivates a client to change?)	
Evaluation (What formal or informal assessments are offered?)	
Intervention Guidelines (What specific therapeutic techniques or strategies have been developed?)	
Research (To what extent has this theory been validated through research?)	

REFERENCES

Ayres, A. J. (1972a). *Sensory integration and learning disorders*. Los Angeles, CA: Western Psychological Services.

Buddenberg, L. A., & Schkade, J. K. (1998). A comparison of occupational therapy intervention approaches for older patients after hip fracture. *Topics in Geriatric Rehabilitation, 13,* 52–68.

Dolecheck, J. R., & Schkade, J. K. (1999). Effects on dynamic standing endurance when persons with CVA perform personally meaningful activities rather than non-meaningful tasks. *Occupational Therapy Journal of Research, 19,* 40–53.

Gibson, J., & Schkade, J. K. (1997). Effects of occupational adaptation treatment with CVA. *American Journal of Occupational Therapy, 51,* 523–529.

Gilfoyle, E., Grady, A., & Moore, J. (1981). *Children adapt*. Thorofare, NJ: SLACK Incorporated.

Jackson, J. P., & Schkade, J. K. (2001). Occupational adaptation model vs. biomechanical/rehabilitation models in the treatment of patients with hip fractures. *American Journal of Occupational Therapy, 55,* 531–537.

Johnson, J., & Schkade, J. K. (2001). Effects of occupation-based intervention on mobility problems following a cerebral vascular accident. *Journal of Applied Gerontology, 20,* 91–110.

Kramer, P., Hinojosa, J., & Royeen, C. B. (2003). *Perspectives in human occupation: Participation in life*. Philadelphia, PA: Lippincott Williams & Wilkins.

Murray, H. A., Barrett, W. G., & Hamburger, E. (1938). *Explorations in personality*. New York, NY: Oxford University Press.

Schkade, J. K., & McClung, M. (2001). *Occupational adaptation in practice: Concepts and cases*. Thorofare, NJ: SLACK Incorporated.

Schkade, J. K., & Schultz, S. (1992). Occupational adaptation: Toward a holistic approach to contemporary practice (Part 1). *American Journal of Occupational Therapy, 46,* 829-837.

Schkade, J. K., & Schultz, S. (1992). Occupational adaptation: Toward a holistic approach to contemporary practice (Part 2). *American Journal of Occupational Therapy, 46,* 917-926.

Schkade, J. K., & Schultz, S. (1993). Occupational adaptation: An integrative frame of reference. In H. Hopkins & H. Smith, (Eds). *Willard and Spackman's occupational therapy* (8th ed., pp. 87-91). Philadelphia, PA: Lippinocott.

Schultz, S., & Schkade, J. K. (2003). Occupational adaptation. In E. B. Crepeau, E. S. Cohn, & B. A. Boyt Schell (Eds.), *Willard & Spackman's occupational therapy* (10th ed.). Philadelphia, PA: Lippincott Williams & Wilkins.

Selye, H. (1956). *The stress of life*. New York: McGraw-Hill.

Stein, F., & Cutler, S.K. (2002). *Psychosocial occupational therapy: A holistic approach* (2nd ed.). Albany, NY: Delmar Inc.

Table 8-2

Occupational Adaptation Guide to Practice

Occupational Adaptation Data Gathering/Assessment

What are the patient's *occupational environments* and *roles*?
Which role is of primary concern to patient and family?
What occupational performance is expected in the primary *occupational environment* and *role*?
What are the *physical, social,* and *cultural* features of the primary *occupational environment* and *role*?
What is the patient's *sensorimotor, cognitive,* and *psychosocial* status?
What is the patient's level of *relative mastery* in the primary *occupational environment* and *role*?
What is facilitating or limiting *relative mastery* in the primary *occupational environment* and *role*?

Occupational Adaptation Programming

What combination of occupational readiness and occupational activity is needed to promote the patient's *occupational adaptation process*?
What help will the patient need to assess occupational responses and use the results to affect the *occupational adaptation process*?
What is the best method to engage the patient in the occupational adaptation program?

Evaluation of the Occupational Adaptation Process

How is the program affecting the patient's *occupational adaptation process*?
- Which *energy level* is used most often (*primary* or *secondary*)?
- What *adaptive response mode* is used most often (*pre-existing, modified,* or *new*)?
- What is the most common *adaptive response behavior* (*primitive, transitional,* or *mature*)?

What outcomes does the patient show that reflect change in the *occupational adaptation process*?
- Self-initiated adaptations?
- Enhanced *relative mastery*?
- Generalization to novel activities?

What program changes are needed to provide maximum opportunity for *occupational adaptation* to occur?

Note: The italicized terms are constructs in the occupational adaptation frame of reference.

Reprinted with permission from Schkade, J. K., & Schultz, S. (1992). Occupational adaptation: Toward a holistic approach to contemporary practice (part 2). American Journal of Occupational Therapy, 46, 917-926.

Chapter 9

ECOLOGY OF HUMAN PERFORMANCE

"The experience of being human is imbedded in the sensory events of everyday life"

– WINNIE DUNN

Ecology of Human Performance (Dunn, Brown, & McGuigan, 1994) was designed as a practice framework by Winnie Dunn and her colleagues at the University of Kansas Medical Center. Similarly to Occupational Adaptation, the idea for constructing this model originated with a faculty group. Significant contributors to this model include Catana Brown, Mary Jane Youngstrom, and Linda Haney McClain. The Ecology of Human Performance model serves as the theoretical basis for the OT department at University of Kansas' curriculum, research, and service activities. Unlike the other occupation models, Ecology of Human Performance was designed to be used by various disciplines and not just occupational therapists, including educators and rehabilitation specialists. Its conceptual emphasis is on the role of a person's context and how these features from the environment impact a person and his or her task performance. Many of the concepts, particularly the five intervention strategies proposed by these authors, have been directly integrated into the OT Practice Framework (AOTA, 2002).

Ecology is defined as the transactions between persons and their contexts. Ecology significantly affects human behavior and task performance. Dunn, Brown, and McGuigan, (1994) identified several issues of concern among the current models of practice, which led them to design their model in a different way. They felt that there was not enough attention given to the role of context in OT practice. They also supported the interdisciplinary relationship of OT and educators. Notice the use of the term *task* in place of occupation. The founding authors decided to use *task performance* to describe one of their main constructs because it is a universal notion and, therefore, more likely to be understood by interdisciplinary practitioners in addition to occupational therapists.

The authors designed this model to be applied for a variety of service settings, including community, consumer-based, and wellness programs. Underlying theories that influenced its conceptual base include systems theory

and the social and behavioral sciences, particularly environmental psychology. The OT theorists who influenced the foundational assumptions of this model include Barris (1982)—who discussed the role of the environment in stimulating a client's level of arousal—and Howe and Briggs (1982)—who proposed an ecological systems model that studied the relationship between organisms and their environment and applied it to OT practice.

FOCUS

The focus, or domain, of practice includes persons of varying ages and needs across the life span. The model emphasizes a preventive, health-promotional, and rehabilitative attitude. Its generic focus on task performance allows practitioners of various disciplines to consider activities that fall within the areas of activities of daily living (ADL), work and productive activities, education, leisure/play, and social participation. The focus or targeted area of concern is the role of context in task performance. From an OT perspective, context includes all cultural, physical, and social environments.

There are four main constructs that influence the theoretical assumptions of the Ecology of Human Performance model. Following are some working definitions for the reader to consider and learn (Christiansen & Baum, 1997; Dunn, McClain, Brown, & Youngstrom, 2003; Kramer, Hinojosa, & Royeen, 2003):

1. *Person:* composed of unique and complex skills and abilities that fall within sensorimotor, cognitive, and psychosocial domains. Capable of attaching meaningfulness to tasks within specific environments. As a result of the unique traits of persons, it is often hard to accurately predict someone's level of performance.

2. *Tasks:* objective sets of behaviors necessary to accomplish a goal. There are an unlimited amount of tasks in which a person can engage. Tasks incur demands;

Figure 9-1. Ecology of Human Performance Schemata (Reprinted with permission from the American Occupational Therapy Association, Dunn, W., Brown, C., & McGuigan, A. (1994). The ecology of human performance: A framework for considering the effect of context. *American Journal of Occupational Therapy, 48,* 595–607.)

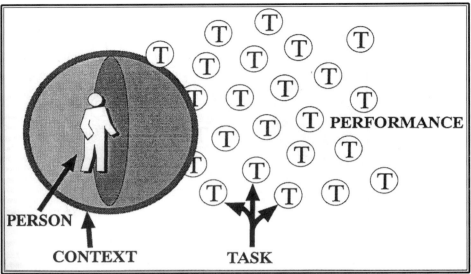

a person's variables determine one's ability to access tasks. Roles shape a person's behavioral expectations while performing tasks. Tasks are the building blocks of occupations and roles. The manner in which a person organizes his or her tasks leads to role performance and occupational performance.

3. *Context:* the interdependent conditions that constitute a person's surroundings and fall into two categories: temporal and environmental.

 o *Temporal aspects:* chronological age; developmental stage or phase; life cycle (career, parenting, educational, etc.); disability status; period or measurable span of time during which a task exists or continues, including the steps, when it takes place, and how long and often it occurs.

 o *Environmental aspects:*

 » *Physical:* nonhuman aspects such as the earth, plants, animals, building, objects, tools, and equipment

 » *Social:* norms, role expectations, and social routines that are part of significant relationships to the person as well as organizations, institutions, political and economic systems, etc.

 » *Cultural:* includes customs, beliefs, activity patterns, and behavioral standards shared by the person's associated group and includes politics, laws, opportunities for education, services, employment, and financial assistance

4. *Personal–context–task transaction:* reflects a process whereby a person engages in a task within his or her context that results in human performance. This transaction is composed of various factors that are interdependent—ecology affects task performance, and task performance, in turn, affects the person, the context, and the person–context relationship.

THEORETICAL BASE

Following is a list of assumptions that form the basis for this model (Christiansen & Baum, 1997; Dunn, Brown, & McGuigan, 1994):

* Ecology is the interaction between persons and their environment. This relationship significantly impacts human behavior and performance.

 o *Practice application:* a client's occupational behavior is viewed as a result of how he or she relates to the environment. A practitioner assesses the reciprocal nature of the person and environment, recognizing that a person isolated from his or her environment may show different behavioral patterns.

* Human behavior or performance can best be understood by examining the relationship of the person, context, and task. Persons are viewed from a systemic and holistic model rather than the sum of their separate parts.

 o *Practice application:* a client's occupational behaviors are meant to be viewed as an interactive and reciprocal process. A change (positive or negative) in any one of the three components will always impact the other two parts and result in a different behavioral outcome. The occupational therapist observes the client performing a task in his natural environment for the best assessment of functioning.

* Performance occurs when a person acts to engage in tasks within a context. Persons use their skills and abilities to "look through" the context and select the preferred tasks. Performance range (number and types of tasks available to the person) is determined by the interaction between the person's variables (skills, abilities, and motivations) and the context variables (supports and barriers).

o *Practice application:* occupational performance represents the client's attempt to complete a task within his or her environment. Performance ranges are high for persons of a healthy status because they are able to successfully match their own personal traits with the demands of the environment. This healthy matching produces appropriate and satisfying occupational performance. Persons with a disability may experience a mismatch of their personal abilities with the contextual demands.

- Each person is an individual with unique skills and abilities within the areas of sensorimotor, cognitive, and psychosocial. Precise predictability about one's performance is unlikely. The meaning a person attaches to task performance as well as contextual influences will highly impact one's overall performance.

  o *Practice application:* since each person is an individual with unique traits, a practitioner must facilitate the client's desire to seek tasks that are of interest to him or her. The assessment process is complex since the practitioner must consider how much value a person associates to the task at hand and how the context or situation is influencing his or her performance on that given day.

- A person's performance range is based on the transaction between the person and context (ecology). Tasks are universally available to everyone. However, it is the summation of a person and the contextual features together that uncover what tasks are available and practical for any one person: 1) The performance range is made up of those tasks that are meaningful and purposeful to the person; 2) the interaction that occurs between the context and person contributes to an individual's sense of meaningfulness; 3) performance range can be narrowed because the person may have limited skills and abilities and, therefore, is unable to utilize the available sources; 4) performance range can be narrowed when the context resources are limited; and 5) persons and contexts transact through engagement in tasks.

  o *Practice application:* even though there may be many options for task performance, clients may not engage in task completion for various reasons. Clients will likely choose tasks that are of interest or meaning to them. Clients may wish to perform certain tasks but may lack the personal traits and abilities that are required. Clients may have the motivation to perform tasks but may encounter limitations within the environment such as money to purchase materials and tools (golf equipment) or the inability to access the specific location in which the occupation takes place (skiing lodge), etc. When clients participate in occupations, they naturally set the person–context relationship in motion.

- A person's variables are continually changing and impacted by past interests and experiences. Skills can be gained and/or lost due to illness or stress.

  o *Practice application:* the practitioner should complete an occupational profile that represents the client's interests and abilities in the present while reviewing the past for patterns of functioning. A therapist can realistically assess the ability of the client to restore and/or relearn skills by standardized and observational evaluations. However, the assessment is a snapshot of the person at that moment in time, and it may be difficult to predict a person's performance in the future.

- Contexts are dynamic. Persons and contexts have a reciprocal impact on each other. The same person acts differently in different contexts. The same context has a unique meaning for different persons. Performance in natural contexts is more accurate as opposed to simulated contexts.

  o *Practice application:* clients can sometimes shape and alter the context to fit their needs (a modified house). Clients show different skills and abilities based on the social expectations and demands of the context (e.g., using an inside-voice tone versus an outside-voice tone). For example, a client may find participating in learning activities to be interesting but may prefer and be more successful at taking an online course versus attending an actual classroom. Clients may show a different level of performance when in a natural context versus a simulated one.

- The transactional relationship among person, task, and context constitutes occupations and roles. Life roles are a constellation of tasks. Tasks may overlap into many roles, and each person has a unique role configuration.

  o *Practice application:* clients have their own interpretation of what tasks are important to them and how they fit into their overall lives as part of role functioning. The practitioner must consider the client's point of view about task preference and participation when designing an intervention plan. For example, a client may view the task of housecleaning as being part of a worker role, a homemaker role, or a leisure role.

- Performance in natural contexts is different from simulated situations. Assessment and intervention best show a person's natural performance when enacted in vivo. Simulated contexts may inhibit or promote performance.

  o *Practice application:* the practitioner should attempt to observe the client performing the same task in different contexts for a complete assessment. The client's natural environment is where the client is likely to show his most typical performance.

- OT includes empowering individuals by enhancing self-determination and including persons with disabilities in all contexts. It is client-centered and includes making changes in systems so that persons with disabilities have full rights and privileges.

  o *Practice application:* an occupational therapist's role includes advocating for the client. When person variables are unlikely to change due to one's health condition, the therapist can seek to alter and modify the environment as a means to promote healthy occupational performance.

- Independence is defined as using contextual supports to meet a person's wants and needs. Adapting and altering the environment are seen as effective means of therapeutic support.

  o *Practice application:* the occupational therapist can reframe the client's problem by seeking to alter and modify the environment. This reframing changes the focus from the client's disability to center on changing the ecology cycle or system. It is not a sign of weakness for persons to rely on assistive and adaptive measures; rather, these measures are enabling occupational performance and supporting healthy role functioning.

Function and Disability

According to this model, persons who show healthy functioning have a high performance range of tasks. This means that they have the capacity to participate in numerous occupations and roles that match their person variables and natural contexts. Persons with adequate human performance 1) show various abilities and interests, 2) can integrate the expectations and supports and manage the barriers of the context, and 3) can fulfill the task requirements that are part of their life roles. Disability is evident when an incongruency emerges within the transaction among the person, the context, and the tasks. This mismatch among the three components results in faulty human performance. There are any number of explanations for inadequate occupational performance. For example, it may be due to *person* variables that may be faulty or due to *contextual* features that are not conducive to human performance. Nonetheless, it is the combination of the person variables and the individual's contextual features that collectively inhibit occupational performance. This unbalanced relationship (ecology) is the cause of faulty *human performance.*

Change and Motivation

According to this model, motivation is enhanced by directly asking the person what he or she wants and needs. Persons are likely to engage in tasks if they have an interest or see its meaningfulness. It is very important to seek the perceptions of the person about his role functioning and

task performance even if the practitioner has a difference of perception or opinion. The person is empowered as the *agent of change*—as having the capacity to be the primary decision-maker. Practitioners within this model will respect the person's opinions and provide an accepting therapeutic environment where the person feels included rather than excluded or "different." Practitioners guide the process as an advocate and a facilitator to enhance independence according to the client's perceptions and needs. From a systems perspective, when further changes in the person (learning new skills) are no longer possible, occupational therapist's can facilitate better task performance by adapting the task or the environment. Unlike people, tasks and environments can be manipulated.

EVALUATION PROCESS

Several checklists have been designed that can be used in the evaluation process. Each checklist is designed to gather data about the four main constructs that comprise this model as well as a reflection of the unique qualities about the client. There is a set of worksheets for each component that make up the person, the context, the tasks, and performance. These include a: 1) person variables worksheet; 2) temporal environment checklist, a physical environment checklist, a cultural environment checklist, and a social environment checklist; 3) task analysis worksheet; and 4) priorities checklist highlighting the various occupational performance areas defined by the client. The reader may consult Dunn, Brown, & Youngstrom's chapter, titled "Ecological Model of Occupation," edited by Kramer, Hinojosa & Royeen, 2003 for a sample of these worksheets. Additional assessments recommended by the authors include *The Sensory Profile Manual* (Dunn, 1997, 1999).

Following is a summary list of guidelines for consideration during the evaluation process (Dunn, Brown, & McGuigan, 1994; Kramer, Hinojosa, & Royeen, 2003, p. 238):

- Identify and prioritize the person's wants and needs. Gather data about task priorities from significant others and the contextual systems in which the client engages on a regular basis.

- Do a task analysis of the designated tasks to understand the skill requirements and demands.

- Observe and evaluate the client's present functional degree of performance while engaged in these tasks. Consider the client's unique interpretation (perception) of how the task should be done, and analyze what contributes to the difficulty in task completion.

- Identify the desired contexts naturally sought by the client. Analyze the context from the client's perspective, and evaluate the external demands that are inherent within the context variables. Look at all variables including physical, social, cultural, and temporal.

- Assess the person variables. Identify strengths and weakness within the areas of sensorimotor, cognitive, and psychosocial functioning.
- Assess the person/task/context match to select reasonable goals and intervention strategies.

INTERVENTIONS

According to this model, there are five specific strategies for intervention. Strategies are targeted to assist the person, the context, the task, or a combination of all three (Dunn, Brown, McClain, & Westman, 1994; Dunn, Brown, & McGuigan, 1994; Dunn, McClain, Brown, & Youngstrom, 2003; Kramer, Hinojosa, & Royeen, 2003). These strategies have also been adopted by the OT Practice Framework (2002).

Establish and Restore

The focus of this strategy is to enhance a person's abilities by teaching skills not previously learned or restoring lost skills due to illness or disability. Practitioners may also educate their clients about tasks such as money management, writing a resume, appropriate ways to discipline children, etc. Person variables fall within sensorimotor, cognitive, and psychosocial areas.

Practice Example

Mary is 21 years old with low self-confidence. She is about to move into her own apartment as a means to enhance her independence. The client identifies cooking as a priority task with which she would like some assistance. The practitioner teaches the client how to cook simple meals that are suited for one person living in an apartment with a small galley kitchen. Some skills will be new and different, while other skills may be restored since the client had some basic knowledge of cooking with her family at home. The practitioner considers how the context (apartment with a small galley kitchen suited for one person) has significant affect on the selection of the menu. Context features will determine such decisions as 1) availability of tools needed to perform task (is there a stove top with multiple burners?, an oven?, a microwave?, a toaster oven?); 2) supports for performance (how much money is allotted for groceries? heat thermometer?, automatic timer with alarm?); and 3) feedback about the performance necessary for the client to learn (cookbooks with step by step directions?, smoke detector to signal if there is smoke and a fire?, person to provide cues and/or assistance as needed?).

Alter

The focus of this strategy is on the context. The practitioner uses his or her assessment of the person's variables in three areas—sensorimotor, cognitive, and psychosocial—to seek the best *match* for one's context. This intervention involves selecting a context that allows the client to perform tasks with his current skills and abilities. Nothing is internally or externally altered or changed about the person, but the context is analyzed by the practitioner to match the person's needs and promote success. In other words, the practitioner seeks the best environment to promote human performance for the individual client.

Practice Example

Mary has intact sensorimotor functioning. She is of average intelligence (cognitive) and learns best by hands-on instruction. She has various psychosocial issues including low self-confidence, overdependency on her family, and a limited social network. She wants to get a new job and meet some new people. The practitioner may suggest that Mary seek a one-bedroom apartment on a central street where she can have easier social and transportation access. Altering the context for Mary may include living on a safe block in a city where she can walk to shops and stores, take public transportation, be close to a gym, and encounter lots of different people in the course of her day rather than living in a quiet, secluded neighborhood with mostly elderly people and no bus transportation.

Adapt/Modify

This strategy focuses on the practitioner's ability to modify the context or task for successful performance. In other words, the practitioner has determined that a way to improve task performance is to adapt/modify the contextual features that best matches one's current level of functioning. Person variables remain as they are, but the task and context are modified to suit the best performance. Modifying approaches include the use of compensatory techniques, which often involve *changing* the physical aspect of one's environment (e.g., assistive devices, ramps, or shower bars). Adapting tasks often includes grading of an activity in the practice of OT. Modification can take place on many levels. For example, social networks (context) can be modified to meet a person's needs by requiring that membership in a support group only includes persons who have a similar condition. Tasks can be modified by substituting ingredients in a recipe that have lesser calories when it is known that the client has high cholesterol and diabetes issues.

Practice Example

Mary gets confused when cooking a meal that has more than three steps. She is also afraid that she will forget food on the stove and cause a fire. The practitioner makes several modifications. First, together, Mary and the practitioner make a list of easy and simple meals that Mary has confidence in cooking. The practitioner modifies the cooking task by simplifying recipes and rewriting each recipe on an index card into three concise steps. Each recipe has been converted to include a microwave set of instructions along with conventional cooking. Second, the practitioner and Mary go shopping together and purchase a simple rotary timer with a bell. Cooking time is highlighted on every recipe card. The practitioner advises Mary to use the rotary timer with a distinctive bell rather than the oven timer that is more cumbersome to understand and sometimes inaccurate. The above modifications modify both the task and the context to suit Mary's unique strengths and weaknesses. Notice that all of these strategies are focused on changing external variables (task and context) rather than internal (person). It is expected that by modifying the task and context, Mary's person variables will also be supported (i.e., her cognitive learning skills will match the level of each task requirement, her self confidence will increase with successful accomplishments, and her level of independence will be heightened overall).

Prevent

The focus of this intervention is to minimize risks and avoid the development of performance problems. Therapeutic strategies can sometimes prevent the occurrence of barriers to performance. This strategy is representative of a health promotional attitude and always takes place before the problem develops. The reader is encouraged to review the definitions of primary, secondary, and tertiary prevention (see Chapter 5).

Practice Application

Mary is encouraged to make a daily planner that will remind her of tasks that need to be done and increase her independent performance in self-care, work, leisure, rest, etc. She is asked to plan one social event every weekend that involves friends rather than family. These strategies are meant to prevent forgetting of necessary daily living tasks, limit dependency on her family, decrease feelings of loneliness and isolation, and ultimately, enhance her independent performance.

Create

This strategy is meant to promote enriching and complex performances in one's context. It supports health promotion and social justice and can be utilized as an adaptable measure to include persons of all abilities in society. The practitioner who advocates for equal rights and fairness of all persons will engage in projects that will enhance the betterment of society in general. This is done in anticipation of a foreseeable problem. Creating contexts that support optimal performance is the goal.

Practice Application

The practitioner suggests roles in the community that will empower Mary and build in inclusive, successful, and enriching experiences. Examples include taking a cooking class at the parks and recreation department for "fun," becoming a "big sister" to a needy child, going to the animal shelter and considering adopting a pet, and joining the gym down the street for women only that offers alternative therapies such as yoga or tai chi.

RESEARCH

Following is a summary list of studies that have been conducted regarding the use of this model in practice. The research team consisted of both occupational therapists and colleagues from other disciplines. Note the application of research study to both health and educational settings such as rehabilitation, adult education, and college.

- Measure of rehabilitation context (Teel, Dunn, Jackson, & Duncan, 1997, 2001)
- Measure of model's effectiveness in adult education and college teaching (Bulgren et al., 1997)
- Effectiveness in teaching grocery shopping to persons with severe mental illness (Brown, Rempfer, & Hamera, 2002)
- Study of model's constructs in the design and validation of the sensory profile measure (Brown, Tolefson, Dunn, et al., 2001)

SUMMARY

The Ecology of Human Performance Model has many unique features in comparison to the other OT models. First, it was created for practitioners of various disciplines, not just OT, and therefore, it supports interdisciplinary collaboration. It emphasizes the importance of one's context or environment and how the interaction between person and context (ecology) influences performance outcomes. The therapeutic approach is client-centered and consumer-centered. It can readily be applied in community-based or social settings. Interventions are suited for health promotion as well as remediation. The authors support a view of social justice—that all people of all abilities deserve to be included in all aspects of society. Practitioners are encouraged to serve as advocates for their clients in supporting this mission. The five intervention strategies are clearly defined and practical in their approach. These strategies have been recognized as model interventions for all OT practice, across all domains and performance areas, as noted by their inclusion in the OT Practice Framework (2002). This model provides an effective alternative from other occupation-based models in that it looks closely at how contexts contribute to faulty human performance. The emphasis is not on the disability of the person but on how to accommodate a person's unique traits and qualities into society by modifying the surrounding conditions. It truly represents a systems point of view—it attempts to change one component of a cycle in a positive way, and recognize that all other components will be affected as well.

Table 9-1	
Template for Analysis Worksheet	

Title of Model or Frame of Reference _____

Theoretical Components	Summary
Focus (OT framework domains, practice areas, health conditions, or specific populations)	
Theorists (Whose theories have contributed?)	
Function (How does theory view healthy or optimal functioning?)	
Disability (How is disability defined?)	
Change (How does change occur, according to this theory?)	
Motivation (What motivates a client to change?)	
Evaluation (What formal or informal assessments are offered?)	
Intervention Guidelines (What specific therapeutic techniques or strategies have been developed?)	
Research (To what extent has this theory been validated through research?)	

LEARNING ACTIVITY

1. Define the following key terms and concepts from this model.
   - Ecology
   - Person (variables)
   - Tasks
   - Context
   - Human performance
   - Performance range
   - Establish/restore skills
   - Alter context
   - Adapt/modify context/task
   - Prevent performance problems
   - Create opportunities
   - Cultural environment
   - Physical environment
   - Temporal environment
   - Social environment

2. Construct a Venn diagram that depicts how human performance is the outcome of 1) person variables, 2) context variables, and 3) task components.

3. Construct a Venn diagram that depicts how context is composed of 1) cultural aspects, 2) physical aspects, and 3) social aspects.

4. Complete Table 9-1 on this model.

REFERENCES

Barris, R. (1982). Environmental interactions: An extension of the model of occupation. *Canadian Journal of Occupational Therapy, 36,* 637–644.

Brown, C., Rempfer, M., & Hamera, E. (2002). Teaching grocery shopping skills to people with schizophrenia. *Occupational Therapy Journal of Research, 22,* Suppl (1), 90s–91s.

Brown, C., Tolefson, N., Dunn, W., Cromwell, R., & Filion, D. (2001). The adult sensory profile: Measuring patterns of sensory processing. *American Journal of Occupaitonal Therapy, 55,* 75–82.

Bulgren, J. A., Gilbert, M. P., Hall, J., Horton, B., Mellard, D., & Parker, K. (1997). *Accommodating adults with disabilities in adult education programs: National field test.* Lawrence, KS: University of Kansas Institute for Adult Studies.

Christiansen, C., & Baum, C. (1997) Theoretical contexts for the practice of occupational therapy. In C. Christiansen & C. Baum (Eds.), *Occupational therapy: Enabling function and well-being* (pp. 74–102). Thorofare, NJ: SLACK Incorporated.

Dunn, W. (1997). The sensory profile: A discriminating measure of sensory processing in daily life. *Sensory Integration Special Interest Section Quaterly, 20*, Bethesda, MD: American Occupational Therapy Association.

Dunn, W. (1999). *The sensory profile manual.* San Antonio, TX: Psychological Corp.

Dunn, W., Brown, C., McClain, L., & Westman, K. (1994). The ecology of human performance: A contextual perspective on human occupation. In C. B. Royeen (Ed.), *AOTA self-study series: The practice of the future: Putting occupation back into therapy* (Module 1), Rockville, MD: American Occupational Therapy Association.

Dunn, W., Brown, C., & McGuigan, A. (1994). The ecology of human performance: A framework for considering the effect of context. *American Journal of Occupational Therapy, 48,* 595–607.

Dunn, W., McClain, L. H., Brown, C., & Youngstrom, M. (2003). In E. B. Crepeau, E. S. Cohn, & B.A. Boyt Schell (Eds.), *Willard & Spackman's occupational therapy* (10th ed.). Philadelphia, PA: Lippincott Williams & Wilkins.

Howe, M. C., & Briggs, A. K. (1982). Ecological systems model for occupational therapy. *American Journal of Occupational Therapy, 36,* 322–327.

Kramer, P., Hinojosa, J., & Royeen, C. B. (2003). *Perspectives in human occupation: Participation in life.* Philadelphia, PA: Lippincott Williams & Wilkins

Reed, K. L., & Sanderson, S. N. (1999). *Concepts of occupational therapy* (4th ed.). Philadelphia, PA: Lippincott Williams & Wilkins

Teel, C., Dunn, W., Jackson, S., & Duncan, P. (2001). Development of the environmental independence interaction scale (EIIS). Unpublished manuscript.

Chapter 10

THE PERSON–ENVIRONMENT–OCCUPATION–PERFORMANCE MODEL

"Occupational therapy practitioners have a unique contribution to bring to health care, to health promotion, to disability prevention, to social problems, and enhancing the quality of life."

– CHARLES CHRISTIANSEN & CAROLYN BAUM

The Person–Environment–Occupation–Performance (PEOP) model was developed in 1985 and published for the first time in 1991 by Charles Christiansen and Carolyn Baum. Since then, it was updated in 1997. Similar to the other occupation-based models presented in this textbook, the three central elements of this model are reflected in its title—person, occupation, and environment. Occupational performance is the outcome of the transaction among people, occupations, and their environments (Law, Cooper, Strong, et al., 1996). It is a client-centered practice approach that can be applied to individuals, organizations, and population groups. The PEOP model can be applied to health promotion programs that are community-oriented as well as rehabilitation centers. The PEOP model highlights the complexity of person–occupation–environment relationships. It defines occupational performance as the outcome of this three-tier transaction in a top-down structure. This model is founded on an extensive body of research that shows the relevance of how a person's behaviors and one's environment are interconnected in a significant way.

The theoretical foundations for this model include general systems theory, environmental theory, neurobehavioral theories, and social and behavioral psychology with particular influence from personality theorists and motivational learning (Maslow). Christiansen and Baum were also influenced by various occupational therapy (OT) theorists who emphasized the role of the environment on occupational behavior. They include Howe and Briggs (1982), Kielhofner and Burke (1980), Reilly (1962), Reed and Sanderson, (1999), and Law (1991).

The PEOP model encompasses concepts and assumptions of several environment–behavior theorists. A critical assumption to PEOP is that occupational performance is influenced by the relationship between person and environment. The theorists and studies that influenced the development of Christiansen and Baum's PEOP model include Bronfenbrenner's ecological systems model (1977),

Lawton and Nahemow's ecological theory of aging (1973), and Csikszentmihalyi's view on adaptation (1988).

The authors were also greatly influenced by the Canadian guidelines for client-centered practice. As described in Chapter 2, the Canadian Association of Occupational Therapists (CAOT) with the Department of Health and Welfare (1983) published the Model of Occupational Performance and Client-Centered Practice, two critical models that have significantly influenced the PEOP model and our current paradigm of OT practice today. These two Canadian therapeutic approaches both emphasized the reciprocal nature of persons and their occupations within social, cultural, and physical environments. The Canadian Occupational Performance Measure (COPM) was published in 1994, offering a well-accepted assessment tool for OT practice (Law, Baptiste, Carswell, et al., 1994). Conceptual constructs from the Canadian authors are not only embedded in Christiansen and Baum's PEOP model but are also inherent in the OT Framework Document (AOTA, 2002). The reader is encouraged to refer to Chapter 2 for a review of the Canadian model of practice.

PEOP also complements the current global health care views as discussed in Chapters 2 and 5 of this text, with particular note to the revised ICF (World Health Organization, 2001), which stresses the importance of health and well-being.

FOCUS

The PEOP model is suited for a variety of individual, group, and institutional needs across the life span. A client-centered and/or consumer-oriented relationship is fostered. The model's focus is on occupations (consisting of valued roles, tasks, and activities) and performance. These occupations, in turn, influence one's life roles. The domain of practice is predominantly selected by the client, who is asked to identify the most important occupational performance issue within the areas of work/productive activities, personal care, home maintenance, sleep, recreation, and leisure. Within the person, the focus areas to be assessed include physiological, psychological, cognitive, neurobehavioral, and spiritual factors. Within the environment, the focus areas to be analyzed consist of one's physical and natural context, cultural and societal norms, social interactions, and social and economic systems.

Christiansen and Baum (2005) have identified four major components to this model. The following four definitions guide the reasoning process of a practitioner and bring one's clinical focus to specific areas that represent the theoretical assumptions of this model. It is advised that the reader keep these definitions in mind when reviewing the basic and essential assumptions of this model:

- *Occupations:* what persons want or need to do in their daily lives
- *Performance:* actual act of doing the occupation
- *Person:* composed of physiological, psychological, neurobehavioral, cognitive, and spiritual factors that are intrinsic in nature
- *Environment:* composed or built of physical, natural, cultural, societal, and social interactive factors and social and economic systems that are extrinsic in nature

Refer to Table 10-1.

THEORETICAL BASE

Following is a summary list of assumptions to the PEOP model based on various resources and interpretations (Christiansen & Baum, 2005; Law et al., 1996) including those of the authors:

- People have an innate drive to explore their environment and demonstrate mastery within it. This process is called *human agency*. Competence is reached when a person is able to perform skills that meet his or her personal needs and utilize the resources (personal, social, material) within one's environment.
  - o *Practice application:* people need adequate emotional maturity and problem-solving ability to set and meet goals that will satisfy their needs over a life-span. Occupational therapists assess a client's competence level as well as personal, social, and material resources within the environment.
- *Adaptation* is defined as a process whereby persons confront the challenges of daily living and are able to use their resources to master these demands.
  - o *Practice application:* occupational therapists realize that environmental demands change and fluctuate over time. A client is viewed as adaptive when he can meet these ongoing challenges and demands over time with an adequate repertoire of resources.

- Persons derive a sense of self-fulfillment from mastery and a sense of self-identity from meaningful participation in occupations.
  - o *Practice application:* Clients accumulate self confidence by experiencing success, and this motivates them to pursue other challenges in their lives. Fulfillment comes from mastering performance as well as accomplishing goals that are meaningful. Persons associate a self-identity based on their accomplishments and roles in life.
- Occupational performance is influenced by many factors. These include the 1) person, 2) unique environment in which one functions, and 3) occupations that consist of one's actions and tasks and ultimately create one's life roles.
  - o *Practice application:* performance is a complex phenomenon that is interconnected among many variables. The occupational therapist understands that a disruption in any one of these components can lead to a negative outcome in performance. Assessments are used to uncover difficulties in all variables.
- The PEOP model represents a transactional relationship that is interdependent among its parts. It studies the health conditions that support or impede performance, environments that allow and/or restrict performance, and an individual's personal profile that includes needs, preferences, and goals. It is client-centered in nature.
  - o *Practice application:* an occupational therapist will inquire about the needs of the client and respect his or her uniqueness. A client is viewed as someone whose performance is influenced by his or her health condition and environmental demands. The focus is always on the person first, rather than on the disability.
- Occupational performance describes the actions that are meaningful to the individual as he or she self-manages, cares for others, works, plays, and participates fully in home and community life. This can be separated into two components: occupations and performance.
  - o *Practice application:* occupational performance is a complex phenomenon that represents more than "doing" or participating in one's environment. Occupational therapists understand the components of occupational performance to include a person's abilities, actions, tasks, occupations, and roles that are performed for a purpose and as a means to express uniqueness.

Here, we review how the process of occupational performance occurs according to this model. The four major components of this model are defined in further detail from earlier descriptions. Each of these four variables has both

Table 10-1

The Four Major Constructs to the PEOP Model

Construct #1. The person is made up of a series of intrinsic factors that make up one's set of skills and abilities.

- *Neurobehavioral factors:* sensory and motor systems that facilitate adaptive and/or compensatory responses

- *Physiological factors:* physical health and fitness, including abilities such as endurance, flexibility, movement, and strength

- *Cognitive factors:* the mechanisms of language comprehension and production, pattern recognition, task organization, reasoning, attention, and memory (Duchek, 1991) that allow the ability to learn, communicate, move, and observe

- *Psychological factors:* personality traits, motivational influences, and internal processes used by an individual to impact what they do, how these events are interpreted, and how they contribute to a sense of self

- *Spiritual factors:* signs and symbols that influence everyday life and provide meanings that contribute to a greater sense of personal understanding about self and one's place in the world

Construct #2. Participation is always impacted by the extrinsic characteristics of the environment in which it occurs.

- *Built environment:* physical properties such as design, use of tools and appliances, and assistive technology devices

- *Natural environment:* geographical features such as terrain, hours of sunlight, climate, and air quality

- *Cultural environment:* values, beliefs, customs, and behaviors that are passed from one generation to the next with influence on social role expectations

- *Societal factors:* social acceptance as a universal need, and interpersonal relationships that influence one's personal development

- *Social interaction:* the experience of social support that enables a person to do what he or she wants or needs (social support)

- *Social and economic systems:* access to health care, policies and procedures, monetary resources, etc.

Construct #3. Occupations are the activities and tasks done in managing a person's daily life. They are a set of tasks that are grouped in some meaningful way so that the person can perform life roles. They are goal-directed pursuits, have temporal meaning, are recognizable by others, have meaning to the person, and involve multiple tasks. Examples include grooming, housekeeping, sports, and studying OT. Christiansen and Baum (2005) have described a hierarchy of occupation-related behaviors. The following sequential pattern depicts the levels of complexity that comprise occupations. The practitioner views occupations as consisting of these basic properties:

- *Abilities:* general traits and characteristics that can lead to occupational performance, including the above-mentioned intrinsic factors. These abilities allow a person to take action (e.g., above-average intelligence will allow for competent pursuit of scholarly occupations).

- *Actions:* observable behaviors. Abilities are applied into action that a person finds personally meaningful. The same action can be used to complete many different tasks (e.g., typing on a word processor to write a paper, answer an e-mail, or complete an online application).

- *Tasks:* the combination of actions for a common purpose that is defined and recognized by the doer. Task analysis involves the practitioner's ability to break down the actions into steps (e.g., practicing the piano, taking a test on OT theory, and driving to the store to buy personal items).

- *Occupations:* tasks become occupations when they have a distinct purpose, are performed with different outcomes in mind, include a social dimension such as fulfilling role obligations, and have a temporal nature (e.g., studying to be an occupational therapist, working as a truck driver, or performing a musical audition).

- *Social and occupational roles:* recognizable positions that define one's status in society. These include specific expectations for behavior and are dynamic. Roles typically involve the performance of many occupations. (e.g., a competent student, a classical pianist, or a "good enough" parent).

Construct #4. Occupational performance and participation is the culmination of doing occupations. It is the interaction of a person's intrinsic factors, the environment (extrinsic factors), and one's chosen activity (occupations) that all lead to occupational performance and participation. It is a complex phenomenon. It describes the actions that are meaningful to a person as he or she cares for him- or herself and for others, works, plays, and participates in home and community life. It is the successful outcome of the transactions among the person, environment, and occupations that the person seeks.

indirect and direct impact on one's occupational performance (Table 10-1).

FUNCTION AND DISABILITY

According to the conceptual notions of this model, a person shows adequate function when he or she expresses a level of competency in his or her ability to perform and master occupations. A healthy individual demonstrates occupational performance in meaningful activities and meets a balance of personal and environmental demands. He or she is, therefore, enabled. This person can self manage, care for others, work, play, and participate fully in home and community life. He or she shows adaptation in occupational performance as he or she naturally meets the challenges in life. This person has established healthy role patterns that fulfill personal and societal expectations.

Dysfunction is observed when a person's occupational performance is limited and restricted. Therefore, occupational competence is not achieved. Persons may demonstrate a lack of goal attainment and participation in activities. The person experiences "occupational performance dysfunction" (Rogers, 1983), which is most evident in role responsibilities. Dysfunction patterns are noticeable when a person cannot perform roles to a level of personal or social satisfaction (competency) because of the following: 1) deficits in abilities and skills due to a health condition (disability), 2) restrictive barriers, or 3) a lack of resources within the environment. The conflicting demands of having multiple roles to negotiate in life (role conflict) and lack of clarity in role expectations from one's culture can have significant impact on poor occupational performance.

CHANGE AND MOTIVATION

According to this model, the person's innate desire to explore his or her environment and demonstrate mastery within it (*human agency*) needs to be activated to enhance motivation. Persons derive a sense of self fulfillment from mastery and a sense of self identity from meaningful participation in occupations. The intrinsic factors within a person are significant to one's occupational performance outcome. Therefore, clients are more likely to persist through change in the clinical process and remain motivated if they perceive their occupational performance as competent and meaningful. Christiansen and Baum have referred to this model as a top-down, client-centered approach. They suggest starting with the client's view of the most important occupational performance "problem" and integrating this perception into an intervention plan. It is critical that the practitioner be sensitive to the inclusion of the client's perception when discussing strategies for change and priorities for treatment. It is also important that the client experience success during interventions since he or she is more likely to

engage and participate in activities that provide a feeling of competency. Successful application of this model involves a practitioner appropriately matching the client's intrinsic factors, also referred to as performance enablers, with the activity or intervention demands. Experiencing a sense of accomplishment will create a reinforcing positive cycle for the client who will experience intrinsic (internal) satisfaction and extrinsic (external) rewards as well.

ASSESSMENTS

This top-down approach begins with the practitioner assessing the client's perception of problems within occupational performance. Examples of assessments include interviews such as the Canadian Occupational Performance Measure (COPM) (Law, Baptiste, Carswell, et al., 1994), Occupational Self Assessment (Baron et al., 2001), Activity Card Sort (Baum & Edwards, 2001), Interest Checklist (Matsutsuyu, 1969), Role Checklist (Oakley, Kielhofner, Barris, & Richler, 1986), Occupational Performance History Interview II (Kielhofner, Mallison, Crawford, Nowak, Rigby, Henry, & Walens, 1997), and Occupational Self Assessment (Baron et al., 2001). The priority goal in the evaluation process is to analyze the client's strengths and issues/problems in occupational performance. Standardized and observational screenings can also be used to assess the person's abilities, intrinsic factors, and environmental (extrinsic) conditions. A task analysis will assist the occupational therapist to assess the performance components of an activity that are not congruent with the client's performance ability at that time.

INTERVENTION PROCESS

"Occupational performance becomes a complex concept affected and changed by individual skills, occupation demands, and environmental supports and barriers" (Reed & Sanderson, 1999, p. 269). In general, intervention strategies should aim to increase occupational performance competency, develop life-long skills, and increase one's sense of health and well-being. The following specific intervention guidelines have been summarized from Baum and Christiansen's (2005) most recent publication on the PEOP model.

- Appreciate the restorative benefits of occupational performance as a means to enhance the person's ability to 1) control movement, modulate sensory input, to coordinate and integrate sensory information, compensate for sensorimotor deficits, and modify neural structures through behavior; 2) maintain physical health and fitness; 3) maintain cognitive skills; 4) increase motivation, develop personal identity, and enhance well-being and self-efficacy; 5) enhance personal meanings and collective or shared meanings. Person factors include the following list:

o Neurobehavioral factors: sensory systems (olfactory, gustatory, visual, auditory, somatosensory, proprioceptive, and vestibular) and motor systems (somatic, cerebellum, basal ganglia network, and thalamic integration)

o Physiological factors: endurance, flexibility, movement, and strength

o Cognitive factors: mechanisms of language comprehension and production, pattern recognition, task organization, reasoning, attention, and memory

o Psychological and emotional factors: personality traits, motivational influences, and internal processes used by persons to influence what they do, how events are interpreted, and how they contribute to one's sense of self

o Spiritual factors: signs and symbols that contribute to a greater sense of personal understanding about the self and one's place in the world

• Recognize the role of the environment as it affects a person's health condition and participation in meaningful activities, tasks, and life roles by the following:

o Employing occupation-enabling resources that include assistive technology devices (built environment) that can modify one's physical environment

o Learning about and adapting to one's natural environment such as air quality, daylight hours, and terrain

o Respecting and accommodating to cultural preferences and norms for occupation participation and views on illness and disability

o Incorporating societal acceptance, one's sense of belonging, and resolving attitudinal barriers within local, state, and national organizations

o Fostering healthy interpersonal skills and social support networks

o Promoting availability of economic supports, access to health care, and client rights

• Enhance occupational performance by structuring occupations for meaningful participation and competent mastery. Adapt and/or modify the actions, tasks, and ultimately, one's occupations to match the abilities of the client (intrinsic factors). Teach compensatory techniques when appropriate. Foster temporal adaptation (process of adjusting to changing temporal requirements in daily life or throughout the lifespan) (Kielhofner, 1977).

• Enhance role functioning by increasing and modeling skill development, managing multiple role participation, and clarifying role expectations from an internal and external perspective

RESEARCH

Various studies have been conducted since 1990 to show the effectiveness of this model. Following is a summary list for review:

• Study of the relationship between older persons and the physical environment (Cooper & Stewart, 1997)

• Persons with mental health problems and the work environment (Strong, 1998)

• Successful work re-entry for persons with disabilities (Westmorland, Williams, & Strong, 2000)

• Environmental factors influencing children's participation in occupations (Law, Milroy, Willms, Stewart, & Rosenbaum, 1999)

• Temporal nature of occupational performance for young people with disabilities in transition to adulthood (Stewart, Law, Rosenbaum, & Williams, 2001)

• Cultural sensitivity of the PEOP model (McKye, Shin, & Letts, 1998)

• Environmental sensitivity on occupational performance (Peachy-Hill & Law, 2000)

• Meaning of occupation as a quality of life factor for older persons in a nursing home (Green & Cooper, 2000)

SUMMARY

The PEOP model is a comprehensive yet user-friendly model that looks at occupational performance as the targeted area of concern. It bears much similarity to the "Person-Environment-Occupation Model: A Transactive Approach to Occupational Performance" designed by Law et al. (1996), and it is somewhat hard to distinguish the two models in earlier OT textbooks. Christiansen and Baum (2005) have recently developed their model to be more expansive and have modified some of its constructs since 1991. One of the model's unique components is that it represents a top-down approach—the client's view of the problem is of primary concern. The client's perceptions of occupational performance issues become the cornerstones for clinical intervention. It is a flexible model that allows occupational therapists to expand on various assessments and strategies to suit the practice setting. It complements and is applicable for the current global concerns of health care—well-being, health prevention and promotion, quality of life, and social inclusion.

LEARNING ACTIVITY

1. Define the key terms and concepts from this model:
   - Occupations
   - Occupational performance
   - Person
   - Environment
   - Human agency
   - Transactional relationship
   - Intrinsic factors of the person
   - Extrinsic factors of the environment
   - Basic properties of an occupation (hierarchy)
     - o Abilities
     - o Actions
     - o Tasks
     - o Occupations
     - o Social and occupation roles

2. Construct a Venn diagram depicting the following:
   - How occupational performance and participation is the outcome of 1) person factors, 2) occupations, and 3) environmental factors
   - How occupations are composed of 1) abilities, 2) actions, and 3) tasks
3. Complete Table 10-2 based on this model.

REFERENCES

American Occupational Therapy Association. (2002). The occupational therapy association practice framework: Domain and process. *American Journal of Occupational Therapy, 56*, 609–639.

Baron, K., Kielhofner, G., Iyenger, A., Goldhammer, V., & Wolenski, J. (2001). *The occupational self-assessment (OSA)* (Version 1.2). Chicago, IL: Model of Human Occupation Clearinghouse.

Baron, K., Kielhofner, G., Iyenger, A., et al. (2002). *The occupational self-assessment (OSA)* (Version 2.0). Chicago, IL: Model of Human Occupation Clearinghouse.

Baum, C. M, & Edwards, D. (2001). *Activity card sort*. St. Louis, MO: Washington University.

Table 10-2
Template for Analysis Worksheet

Title of Model or Frame of Reference _____

Theoretical Components	Summary
Focus (OT framework domains, practice areas, health conditions, or specific populations)	
Theorists (Whose theories have contributed?)	
Function (How does theory view healthy or optimal functioning?)	
Disability (How is disability defined?)	
Change (How does change occur, according to this theory?)	
Motivation (What motivates a client to change?)	
Evaluation (What formal or informal assessments are offered?)	
Intervention Guidelines (What specific therapeutic techniques or strategies have been developed?)	
Research (To what extent has this theory been validated through research?)	

Baum, C. M., & Christiansen, C. H. (2005). Person-environment-occupation-performance: An occupation based framework for practice. In C. H. Christiansen, C. M. Baum, & J. Bass-Haugen (Eds.), *Occupational therapy: Performance, participation, and well-being* (3rd ed.). Thorofare, NJ: SLACK Incorporated.

Bronfenbrenner, U. (1977). Toward an experimental ecology of human development. *American Psychologist, 32,* 513–530.

Christiansen, C., & Baum, C. M. (1991). *Occupational therapy: Overcoming human performance deficits.* Thorofare, NJ: SLACK Incorporated.

Christiansen, C., & Baum, C. M. (1997). *Occupational therapy: Enabling function and well-being (2nd ed.).* Thorofare, NJ: SLACK Incorporated.

Christiansen, C., & Baum, C. M. (2005). *Occupational therapy: Enabling function and well-being (3rd ed.).* Thorofare, NJ: SLACK Incorporated.

Cooper, B., & Stewart, D. (1997). The effect of a transfer device in the homes of elderly women. *Physical and Occupational Therapy in Geriatrics, 15,* 61–77.

Csikszentmihalyi, M., & Csikszentmihalyi, I. S. (1988). *Optimal experience: Psychological studies in flow in consciousness.* Cambridge, UK: Cambridge University Press.

Green, S., & Cooper, B. A. (2000). Occupation as a quality of life constituent: A nursing home perspective. *British Journal of Occupational Therapy, 63,* 17–24.

Howe, M. C., & Briggs, A. K. (1982). Ecological systems model for occupational therapy. *American Journal of Occupational Therapy, 36,* 322–327.

Kielhofner, G. (1977). Temporal adaptation: A conceptual framework for occupational therapy. *American Journal of Occupational Therapy, 31*(4), 235–242.

Kielhofner, G., & Burke, J. (1980). A model of human occupation, part 1: Conceptual framework and content. *American Journal of Occupational Therapy, 34,* 572–581.

Kielhofner, G., Mallinson, T., Crawford, C., Nowak, M., Rigby, M., Henry, A., & Walens, D. (1997). *A user's guide to the occupational performance history interview-II (OPHI II)* (Version 2.0). Chicago, IL: Model of Human Occupation Clearinghouse.

Law, M. (1991). The environment: A focus for occupational therapy. *Canadian Journal of Occupational Therapy, 58,* 171–179.

Law, M., Baptiste, S., Carswell, A., McColl, M. A., Polatajko, H., & Pollock, N. (1994). *Canadian occupational performance measure manual* (2nd ed.). Toronto, Canada: CAOT Publications, ACE.

Law, M., Cooper, B., Strong, S., Steward, D., Rigby, R., & Letts, L. (1996). The person-environment-occupational model: A transactive approach to occupational performance. *Canadian Journal of Occupational Therapy, 63,* 9–23.

Law, M., Haight, M., Milroy, B., Willms, D., Stewart, D., & Rosenbaum, P. (1999). Environmental factors affecting the occupations of children with physical disabilities. *Journal of Occupational Science, 6,* 102–110.

Lawton, M. P., & Nahemow, L. (1973). Toward an ecological theory of adaptation and aging. In W. Preiser (Ed.), *Environmental design research* (pp. 24–32). Stroudsburg, PA: Dowden, Hutchison & Ross.

Matsutsuyu, J. S. (1969). The interest check list. *American Journal of Occupational Therapy, 23*(4), 323–328.

McKye, A., Shin, J., & Letts, L. (1998). *Cultural sensitivity of the person-environment-occupation (PEO) model.* Abstract summaries. Number A142. Montreal, CA: World Federation of Occupational Therapists Congress.

Oakley, F., Kielhofner, G., Barris, R., & Richler, R. K. (1986). The role checklist: Development and empirical assessment of reliability. *Occupational Therapy Journal of Research, 6,* 157–169.

Peachy-Hill, C., & Law, M. (2000). Impact of environmental sensitivity on occupational performance. *Canadian Journal of Occupational Therapy, 67,* 304–313.

Reed, K. H., & Sanderson, S. N. (1999). *Concepts of occupational therapy* (4th ed.). Philadelphia, PA: Lippincott, Williams, and Wilkins.

Reilly, M. (1962). Occupational therapy can be one of the great ideas of 20th century medicine. *American Journal of Occupational Therapy, 16,* 1–9.

Rogers, J. C. (1983). Clinical reasoning: The ethics, science, and art. *American Journal of Occupational Therapy, 37*(9), 601–616.

Stewart, D., Law, M., Rosenbaum, P., & Williams, D. (2001). A qualitative study of the transition to adulthood for youth with physical disabilities. *Physical and Occupational Therapy in Pediatrics, 21,* 3–21.

Strong, S. (1998). Meaningful work in supportive environments: Experiences with the recovery process. *American Journal of Occupational Therapy, 52,* 31–38.

Westmorland, M., Williams, R., & Strong, S. (2000). *Workplace perspectives: Successful work (re)entry for persons with disabilities* (Research report). Hamilton, ON: McMaster University.

World Health Organization. (2001). *International classification of functioning, disability, and health (ICF).* Geneva, Switzerland. Author.

Chapter 11

MODEL INTEGRATION

The purpose of this chapter is to promote the reader's ability to appraise the five occupation-based models that were described in Section II. While each of the models focuses on the role of occupations in enhancing well-being, each model also views the process of promoting occupational performance in a slightly different way. These differences are most apparent within the assumptions of each model. These *assumptions* are the compatible concepts from theory that ultimately guide a practitioner to make the most of related intervention strategies. The learning activities included at the end of each chapter in Section II are guided attempts to increase the practitioner's knowledge, understanding, and application of each model. Ultimately, practitioners must decide what model to clinically apply based on this level of knowledge. The decision-making process of selecting a specific model or theory for practice is complex. In essence, practitioners are being asked to judge the relevancy of a particular model as it pertains to the needs of the client based on one's know-how and best practice evidence.

Each model was created as a practical guideline to support occupation-based concerns; however, each model is not able to solve every problem presented by our clients within our present health care environment. Mary Reilly initiated our profession's attempt to reclaim our role as occupation experts via the occupational behavior model. This inspired others such as Kielhofner, Dunne, Schkade and Schultz, and Christiansen and Baum, along with their colleagues, to synthesize and create new models of their own. Every theorist believes that his or her own model is inclusive enough to be appreciated and applied by all occupational therapy (OT) practitioners within all domains of practice. The authors of this text have refrained from qualifying the work of these theorists because we do not want to bias or limit the individual practitioner's clinical reasoning process. Identified as the *paradigm effect*, Barker described how models and theories both guide our beliefs and values as well as restrict our ability to see beyond their

structure (Barker, 1992). Data that are not in keeping with a paradigm's (or in this instance, a model's) concepts or set of theoretical assumptions tend to be discarded, omitted, or filtered out. Barker concluded that this filtering process results in the omission of new ideas in favor of what is familiar. So, in keeping, the authors of this text support the idea of clinical choice and use of multiple models and/or frames of reference as a means to comprehensibly address the complex needs of our clients.

The principles of holism and client-centered practice that are at the core of OT practice also endorse the idea that the selection of a model for therapeutic application should match the clinical needs and wants of the client rather than based on the comfort level of the therapist. We support the application of multiple models and frames of reference for working within a health care environment that still vacillates among curing illnesses, prevention strategies, and the promotion of health and well-being. Choosing an appropriate theory for OT practice requires the ability to compare and contrast various models and/or frames of reference, assess the relevancy of these models to a specific client, and make reasonable clinical choices based on evidence (Bloom, 1956).

The following learning activity is meant to take the reader through a series of steps that will mimic the clinical reasoning process common in everyday practice. It begins with the introduction of a case and follows with specific questions that help the reader to develop the ability to discriminate and evaluate what model is best suited for this particular client. The objectives of this learning activity can best be identified by referring to Bloom's taxonomy, namely to 1) acquire knowledge; 2) comprehend the information; 3) apply the concepts; 4) analyze for patterns; 5) generalize and synthesize facts; and finally, 6) evaluate, discriminate, and assess the value of the theory presented (Bloom, 1956). Model integration focuses on Bloom's final step, evaluating the usefulness of each model for application in specific client circumstances and clinical situations.

Table 11-1

Template for Analysis Worksheet

Title of Model or Frame of Reference _____

Theoretical Components	Summary
Focus: What are the specific occupational performance domains that Paul, his mother, and the therapist would identify if completing an occupational profile?	
Theoretical Base: According to the basic assumptions of this model, write 2 to 3 paragraphs that explain how a practitioner would "view" this client. Consider this section to be a "clinical dialogue" of how you would organize your clinical reasoning about Paul.	
Function: How does this model view healthy or optimal functioning? What strengths does Paul (as the person) demonstrate that can enhance healthy functioning?	
Disability: How is dysfunctional behavior defined according to this model? What weaknesses does Paul demonstrate that can disrupt his occupational functioning?	
Change and motivation: How does change occur, according to this theory? What specific motivators will you use for Paul that are based on his personal history?	
Evaluation Process: What formal or informal assessments are suitable from this model's perspective? What assessment(s) would you specifically select for Paul and why? How will you go about administering the assessment? Complete the assessment as if you were Paul or ask someone to role play and answer the questions for you.	
Intervention Guidelines What specific therapeutic techniques or strategies are suggested by this model? Based on the completed assessment (simulated), identify 5 OT strategies that are consistent with the client's needs and consistent with the recommendations of this model.	

LEARNING ACTIVITY

Directions: Answer the following questions based on the case of Paul (see p. 137):

After reading and gaining knowledge about Paul, complete the case analysis template according to each of the five occupation-based models (Table 11-1). *Note:* If using this exercise as a group or class activity, assign one group of students to each model. Upon completion of the template, have each student group verbally present their findings to the entire class so that students can 1) understand information and grasp the meaning each model and 2) apply the case of Paul within each model's unique organization. Consider the following steps to assist in the completion of step 1.

1. Imagine that Paul is your client. Ask a fellow student or colleague to role play Paul for you so that you can use your observation skills as well. This may allow for a more realistic impression of a person. Use the adapted template to guide your therapeutic process. Feel free to use all facts from the case as well as logical deductions from the role play. Consult the OT Practice Framework (AOTA, 2002) as a reference and a guide.

2. Complete Table 11-1 based on your knowledge and comprehension of both Paul and each practice model. Be sure to use all *correct* and relevant terminology as identified by each theorist.

After you have thoroughly reviewed the case of Paul and applied each of the five models directly, answer the following questions:

1. In your best clinical analysis, what models (among the five) are a suitable match in meeting the needs of Paul? Explain your rationale.

2. In your best clinical analysis, what models (among the five) are the least suitable match in meeting the needs of Paul? Explain your rationale.

3. Formulate some clinical concerns that were *not* addressed by any of the models. Brainstorm alternative ways to assist Paul with these concerns.

4. Using your best clinical evaluation skills, what OT practice model would you say is the most valuable to Paul? Base your choice on reasonable arguments and conclusions.

Case Study: Paul

General Background

Paul is a 45-year-old, single male of Italian and Irish heritage who lives with his mother in their family home. He is about 5 feet 3 inches tall and weighs 180 lbs. He is of Christian faith and goes to church periodically with his mother. He was diagnosed as having mild mental retardation (IQ level = 75) during early childhood. He was educationally mainstreamed and needed lots of teaching assistance, which his mother was able to provide because she was a public high school teacher. He did complete high school although it took him 5.5 years. He had very few friends growing up and tended to be ridiculed by peers for his different "look." Paul wears glasses for distance, and he has bilateral nerve deafness for which he wears double hearing aids. He tends to waddle when he walks, appears clumsy at times, and trips often. Eye contact is poor, and he tends to walk with his head down. He has mild apraxia. He has also been diagnosed with major depression, a seizure disorder, and dependent personality.

Paul's father died approximately 1 year ago. Since his father's death, Paul has become more dependent on his mother for self-care and social activity. He often appears sad, lonely, and lethargic.

Chief Complaint

Paul's mother reports an increase in aggressive and hostile outbursts at home over the last 6 months. She is questioning whether she can continue to care for Paul at home or whether he should be placed in a group home that includes staff supervision. She has contacted his case worker to request an assessment of his overall functioning.

Present History

Paul works at a dining hall at a nearby community college for 30 hours per week. His work routine consists of stacking the dishwasher, drying dishes, emptying trash cans, and washing floors. His driver's license has been suspended due to his seizure activity. His mother drives him to and from work. Paul has only utilized vocational services via his treatment agency for developmental disabilities, even though multiple levels of service are offered, including residential options and social activities.

His mother officially retired since Paul's father died. She presently enjoys working as a part-time tutor at the local high school and loves her volunteer job as a literacy counselor. About 6 months ago, she noticed Paul appearing more irritable and "edgy." She complains that his anger and impulsivity are getting worse. She is having difficulty setting limits on Paul's behavior. She has tried to punish him for "being bad" by taking his privileges away. This action only makes him more upset and angry. The two of them get into multiple screaming matches every week. Paul's mother is also becoming more symptomatic, reporting high blood pressure and migraine headaches. She is 76 years of age and very worried about who will take care of her son when she dies.

Paul's seizure activity has increased and seems to be related to the increase in his stress level. During a recent angry episode, Paul took a broom and smashed it on the kitchen table, breaking several dishes. He has also punched holes in the walls of his bedroom, where he tends to spend most of his time. His mother is at her wit's end. She threatens Paul with telling him that she is going to place him in a group home if he does not stop misbehaving.

Past History

Paul's parents have provided structure for him all of his life. His mother taught him how to dress himself, make simple sandwiches, wash dishes, and use the telephone. Paul's father was instrumental in setting limits in a firm yet gentle way. He worked as a carpenter and had a workshop in the garage. He and Paul would make different wooden projects together, and Paul loved to do wood burning design. Many of these wood projects would be given to their church for craft sales and fund raising. Paul has always had difficulty initiating routines, and he has no social contacts outside of his work environment. He works well with one-on-one attention and seems to prefer males to females. Paul's mother is concerned about his safety in the home and, therefore, forbids him to use the stove or the washing machine. Paul has difficulty with money management; therefore, his mother keeps track of all his money and gives him a minimal allowance every week. He likes to buy candy and videos. His favorite shows are *Everybody Loves Raymond* and *Star Trek*.

Referral Request

Provide an overall assessment of Paul's functioning with recommendations for self-care and self-management.

REFERENCES

American Occupational Therapy Association. (2002). Occupational therapy practice framework: Domain and process. *American Journal of Occupational Therapy, 56,* 609–639.

Barker, J. (1992). *Future edge: Discovering the new paradigms of success.* New York: NY. William, Morrow, & Company.

Bloom, B., & Krathwohl, D. (1956). *Taxonomy of educational objectives: The classification of educational goals. Handbook I: Cognitive domain.* New York: NY. Longmans & Green.

FRAMES OF REFERENCE

Frames of reference, unlike the models in **Section II**, are not occupation-based. Most have been developed to address specific disability areas, and as such, they are best used as guidelines for addressing the impairments that create barriers to occupational performance. **Section III** reviews and applies some of the frames of reference most commonly used in occupational therapy practice today. It is not intended to be exhaustive, and there are many useful and legitimate frames of reference that have been left out.

Each frame of reference will be structured according to the criteria described in **Chapter 4** using the following outline:

- *Focus*
- *Theoretical Base*
- *Function and Disability*
- *Change and Motivation*
- *Evaluation*
- *Guidelines for Intervention*
- *Research*

Using this format, students and therapists can easily compare one frame of reference with another as part of the clinical reasoning process. **Chapter 21** provides a format for comparison, a guide to the OT Practice Framework (AOTA, 2002), and some case studies and learning activities.

The concepts covered form the basis for learning experiences at both ends of the wellness–disability continuum. The wellness experiences help students to use the theory to increase self-awareness, self-understanding, and regulation/self-improvement. The disability applications require the student to use the theory appropriately with case examples.

REFERENCES

American Occupational Therapy Association. (2002). *Occupational therapy practice framework: Domain and process.* American Journal of Occupational Therapy, 56, 609–639.

Chapter 12

APPLIED BEHAVIORAL FRAMES

"Learning cannot occur in the absence of some kind of reinforcement."

– B. F. SKINNER (1953)

Behavioral theories might be understood as a continuum, beginning with behavior modification and ending with cognitive behavioral therapy. Behavior modification has been used by occupational therapists since the 1940s, applying concepts from Skinner (1953), Pavlov (1927), and Bandura (1977). This frame of reference applies the scientific method to human behavior, focusing on only the external features of human functioning that can be observed and measured. In later decades, therapists objected to the term "behavior modification" because of its implication that the therapist is exerting control over the client (Corey, 1991). Currently, behavioral principles are commonly applied through self-management or self-regulation strategies, which are more compatible with a client-centered approach. Mosey (1970, 1988) adapted behavioral principles for occupational therapy (OT) in defining the acquisitional frame of reference. Therefore, the acquisitional frame of reference will also be described. Cognitive behavioral approaches, which have developed more recently, are described in Chapter 13.

Mosey first applied this frame of reference as acquisitional, or "action-consequence," illustrating its use in the treatment of psychosocial dysfunction based on the principles of operant conditioning (1970, p. 84). Traditional views of the acquisitional frame of reference incorporate concepts from learning theory—such as repetition, practice, and reinforcement—applied by occupational therapists within the context of everyday tasks.

Royeen and Duncan (1999) note that there has been a recent resurgence in applied behavioral therapy based on acquisitional theory. They describe the acquisitional frame of reference as using behavioral principles to facilitate motor and cognitive skill development. As defined by Mosey (1988), acquisitional frames of reference promote the learning of skills for occupational performance without regard to sequence or stage of development.

This distinguishes the acquisitional frame from more developmental approaches. Behavioral principles have also been applied in the motor learning approach described in Chapter 19.

FOCUS

Application of behavior modification in today's OT practice is a useful approach to working with persons with developmental disabilities, mental retardation, or other mental health conditions such as obsessive compulsive disorders or phobias. Occupational therapists facilitate desired behaviors through defining goals and working toward them using skill instruction, modeling, coaching, and behavioral reinforcement (Christiansen & Matuska, 2004). Additionally, behavioral principles are generally used whenever occupational therapists need to create behavioral goals and objectives or to teach clients new occupational skills through grading the steps of a task.

THEORETICAL BASE

Classical Conditioning

Pavlov's (1927) classical conditioning may best be remembered in connection with his experiments with dogs. Pavlov noticed that when dogs were presented with food, they would begin to drool in anticipation. Drooling is an observable behavior, which Pavlov sought to connect with the ringing of a bell. At each mealtime over several weeks, the bell would ring just prior to feeding. After a period of repetition, food was no longer needed as a stimulus. The dogs would drool whenever they heard the bell ring. This experiment demonstrates the most basic level of conditioned learning (*associational learning*), the association of a stimulus (bell) with a response (drooling), motivated by external reinforcement (food). Human behavior may be learned in much the same way. For example, an infant cries

Table 12-1		
Types of Reinforcement and Examples of Their Use		
Continuous reinforcement	Giving rewards every time a desired behavior is seen	Best used when shaping new behaviors, such as using table manners during meals
Fixed-ratio reinforcement	Giving rewards after a specific number of attempts or successful use of skills	Given at later stages of skill learning. Offer praise every fifth time child raises hand to speak instead of interrupting
Fixed-interval reinforcement	Giving rewards at specific time intervals	Giving feedback at the end of each therapy session; allowing one diet-free meal after each whole week of staying on a weight loss diet
Intermittent reinforcement	Giving rewards at random or unpredictable times	Best way to maintain desired behaviors; also explains why children may misbehave (random attention—negative reinforcement), and why adults may have gambling addictions (random wins)
Negative reinforcement	Withdrawal of attention or other expected outcome	Giving child a "time out" during which no attention from others occurs; ceasing to "enable" addictive behaviors by making excuses for consequences (aggressiveness, lateness, etc.)
Token economies	System in which a "token" is given for desired behaviors. Tokens are saved like money and may be cashed in for a choice of rewards	Used in some mental health settings for extinguishing unwanted behaviors and encouraging socially appropriate behaviors
Self-reinforcement	Internalized good feelings that result from successfully reaching a desired goal	Used in self-management programs such as stress reduction or the use of other of self-control strategies

when hungry but soon learns that crying also brings attention from mother. Both mother and child form conditioned responses that can be quite complicated. For the infant, being held and cuddled becomes associated with feeding time, while mother associates her child's crying with more than just hunger. This demonstrates the principle of *response generalization,* where different responses may be associated with the same stimulus.

Operant Conditioning

Operant conditioning, as identified by B. F. Skinner (1953), refers to learned behaviors that occur in one's natural environment as a result of reinforcement. Skinner noted that behaviors that are reinforced tend to be repeated (learning) while behaviors that are not reinforced tend to disappear (extinction). A *reinforcer* is defined as anything that increases the likelihood that a behavior will be repeated. For example, a teacher gives a gold star to the child who completes an assignment correctly. Children quickly learn to recognize other signs of approval, such as smiles, attention, and praise. As occupational therapists, we may use these social reinforcers with clients automatically each time they demonstrate therapeutic strategies correctly. Continuous reinforcement refers to rewarding a desired

behavior each time it occurs. However, reinforcement becomes more effective when given selectively. *Schedules of reinforcement* may be fixed interval (e.g., every 10 minutes), fixed ratio (e.g., after every five correct responses), or intermittent (occasionally and unsystematically). Intermittent reinforcement ultimately produces the most stable learned behavior and is most difficult to extinguish (unlearn). Reinforcement is a double-edged sword. It can be used intentionally to shape positive behaviors but may also occur randomly in the environments in which our clients live, surreptitiously reinforcing negative behaviors. Table 12-1 shows examples of how different types of reinforcement are best used or understood.

In OT, we frequently encounter clients with maladaptive behaviors, those which interfere with engagement in desired occupations and create barriers to social participation. For example, a child may have a temper tantrum when faced with frustration in school. An older adult who has had a stroke may continually neglect the right side of the body or field of vision. As therapists, we need to look at the contexts within which clients demonstrate these maladaptive behaviors, in order to determine what aspects of clients' natural environments might be reinforcing unwanted behaviors. Attention of others, even negative attention such as criticism or punishment, may actually be reinforcing for the client, and this can only change through collaboration with families or other members of the client's social group. Operant conditioning can help occupational therapists understand why clients behave in ways that are self-destructive or otherwise nontherapeutic, even when our treatment approach comes primarily from another frame of reference.

Shaping and Chaining

Shaping and chaining, an outgrowth of operant conditioning, can guide the learning of occupational skills. Skinner demonstrated these principles by teaching a pigeon to turn around. Each time the bird turned in the desired direction, it was given a morsel of food (shaping). Eventually, the bird turned all the way around (chaining), and learned that repeating this behavior brought continued reinforcement. In OT, we often modify tasks to make them less difficult for our clients. As our clients improve, we increase the difficulty and complexity of the task so that continued progress can occur. For difficult tasks, we may reinforce each step until the whole sequence is learned. For example, a person with brain injury, typically having problems with short-term memory, might need to rebuild healthy routines and habits through intentionally repeating sequences until they become automatic. A bedtime checklist may include locking the door, changing into pajamas, brushing one's teeth, and turning off the television. As each sequence is mastered, other routines may be added.

Social Learning Theory

Bandura (1977) added social learning theory, providing additional understanding of how human behaviors are learned. Bandura sees reinforcement as a hierarchy beginning with external reinforcement (such as edible treats, monetary rewards, and public recognition) and becoming increasingly internalized. Internal, or self-reinforcement, includes the satisfaction of having mastered a skill, achieved a goal, or behaved in culturally and morally acceptable ways regardless of the external consequence.

FUNCTION AND DISABILITY

The behavioral term for dysfunction is *maladaptive behavior*. In this frame of reference, every health condition, regardless of its internal properties, is viewed only with respect to its external observable and measurable consequences. Occupational performance deficits fall into this category, making this frame of reference a good fit for OT. Additionally, contextual influences become a focal point in considering barriers to and facilitators of engagement in occupation. Function involves the acquisition of adaptive behaviors that are defined by others, are desirable, or those specific skills that the client wishes to master. Function in the behavioral frame of reference is narrowly defined by setting *behavioral goals and objectives*.

Behavioral Goals

Behavioral goals refer to specific accomplishments that can be observed and measured. For example, a student might choose graduation from college as a goal. This goal is behavioral because it involves meeting specific criteria for completion (taking courses, earning credits) and involves external recognition, such as wearing a cap and gown and being awarded a degree on graduation day. Behavioral goals may be long-term but their accomplishment is easily recognized. For example, you might set a goal to own a home by age 30 or to become a millionaire by age 50. Many professions use behavioral goals in their work, including OT. For practice, try writing some behavioral goals (see Behavioral Goals and Objectives section, p. 146).

Behavioral Objectives

Behavioral objectives are shorter-term steps toward a longer-term goal. Many course syllabi in college list behavioral objectives, which are specific tasks or learning to be accomplished in order to receive credit. Behavioral objectives serve to narrowly define behavior for the purpose of learning or mastering it. Some examples might be writing a term paper on a specified topic or demonstrating one's understanding of the subject by achieving a passing grade on a test. Behavioral objectives often include a time frame, such as a due date for the term paper and specific dates for midterm and final exams. When writing behavioral objectives for clients, occupational therapists often include outcome criteria by which to measure or affirm the accomplishment of the objective. It is important for the occupational therapist to communicate with the client to ensure the objectives are clearly defined and the criteria for their accomplishment is easily recognized. Checklists for recording the completion of each step can be helpful to both client and therapist. For practice, try writing some behavioral objectives for hypothetical clients and situations (see Behavioral Goals and Objectives section, p. 146).

CHANGE AND MOTIVATION

Reinforcement

Both change and motivation are attributed simply to *reinforcement*. Once a desired behavior is defined, cues (or reminders) are given by the therapist, parent, or teacher to help shape the behavior to be learned. When the client demonstrates the desired behavior, reinforcement is provided. To work correctly, the therapist needs to fully understand what is reinforcing to the client. Praise and approval may have a positive effect on some clients and no effect on others. Occupational therapists using this approach need to take the time to find out what things act as motivators for each individual. For clients who lack self-control, external rewards such as food, money, or something of value such as a free movie or other desired activity have a greater effect.

Clients with greater maturity respond better to internalized rewards, such as those described by Bandura (1977). In a study of time management, female subjects with multiple roles were asked what motivated them to keep juggling so many different tasks. Surprisingly, the answer for most had nothing to do with praise or approval of others, nor did it involve achieving an external goal. These busy women kept going like the energizer bunny because of their perceptions of how terrible they would feel about themselves if they did not (Cole, 1998). Bandura (1977) calls this type of reinforcement *self-produced consequences*. Meeting one's own internalized self-imposed standards represents the most effective type of reinforcement.

Critics of behaviorism interpret the use of external rewards as giving too much control to the reinforcer (therapist) in what should be, in client-centered practice, an equal therapist–client partnership. In OT, we need to strive to provide successful occupational experiences for clients that enable them to shift from dependence on external rewards to internal reinforcement based on competence and self-efficacy. Bandura's hierarchy of reinforcement (1977) bridges the gap between behavior modification and the cognitive behavioral approach discussed in Chapter 13. Dunn (2003) suggests that for children, gradually moving from continual to intermittent reinforcement helps the child to internalize expectations and standards for effective occupational performance.

Extinguishing Unwanted Behaviors

Behavior modification is perhaps best known as a method for altering unwanted behaviors, such as compulsive rituals, irrational fears, self-destructive behaviors, and bad habits. *Extinguishing* undesirable behavior involves withdrawal of reinforcement. This is a simple concept that is very difficult to put into practice. When changing problem behaviors are a priority for clients and families, occupational therapists need to pay close attention to the environmental contexts within which the behaviors occur. Removing the cues that trigger the behavior as well as the consequences that may be reinforcing it are necessary for the behavior to change.

For example, suppose you are a smoker and would like to stop smoking. Think about what might be reinforcing about smoking, such as feeling relaxed or reducing stress. How could you remove these reinforcements? Substituting other ways to relax and cope with stress might be needed. Then, you would need to remove the cues that trigger the urge to smoke. Getting all smoking materials, ash trays, and matches out of sight might be an initial step. However, other cues can be more subtle, such as drinking coffee in the morning or watching the tonight show on television, as activities associated with smoking. The process requires a great deal of attention to detail as well as motivation on the part of the client. Try the writing exercise at the end of the chapter to help you think about cues and reinforcers.

EVALUATION

Behavioral assessments always involve the identification and definition of targeted behaviors. Observational assessments that narrowly define problem behaviors or presence and/or absence of skills fit best with this frame of reference. Checklists that assist clients with identifying areas of dysfunction and task or role preferences can help to define the focus of OT intervention. Positive reinforcers also need to be defined during the assessment process. These are external things (treats) or interactions (praise, recognition) that the client finds rewarding and/or meaningful. Stein's (2003) Stress Management Questionnaire is one example of an OT assessment tool that uses a behavioral approach to define specific feeling, behaviors, and circumstances related to client stress. This assessment exists in online and print versions and offers computer scoring.

GUIDELINES FOR INTERVENTION

Intervention tends to be specific to the target behavior, either developing new skills or coping strategies or systematically eliminating unwanted behaviors. Stress management is a common area for intervention. For example, biofeedback technology is utilized in cases where internal state is targeted for change/control (e.g., control of muscle tension in relieving stress).

Teaching Skills

Teaching skills applies early learning theory. New behaviors may be learned through chaining steps of a task and shaping the new behavior through reinforcement. The environment is controlled so that only the target behavior is reinforced. An example of a new behavior that can be learned in this way is assertiveness training.

Behavior Contracts

Behavior contracts have been suggested by Bruce and Borg (2002). This is a written agreement defining what both client and therapist will do with regard to working on specific, defined goals. Behavior contracts are especially helpful when working with mental health clients because they specify the consequences for meeting or not meeting certain expectations, making them more objective (as opposed to emotion based).

Relaxation Training

Relaxation training is a common therapeutic approach for coping with anxiety. Some contemporary methods include deep breathing, progressive muscle relaxation, self-hypnosis (meditation, mantra), and autogenic training (body awareness). These techniques can be used to treat insomnia, pain management, anger management, attention deficit disorders, and impulse control problems. Table 12-2

Table 12-2

Relaxation Technique Example

- Begin by sitting or lying down in a relaxed position with back and head supported.
- Breathe in through mouth, breathe out through nose.
- While breathing out, count slowly to 10.
- Use a tense and relax method for each segment.
- Progress through muscle groups one at a time.
- Separate each muscle group from rest of body.
- Focus your mind on each muscle group in turn.
- It is important to feel the tension while inhaling.
- Practice tensing muscles in foot and ankle.
- Hold 10 seconds, then release (relax).
- Make a cue card, practice sequence consistently.
- Do this twice a day until learned.
- Relax the following muscle groups, beginning with the dominant side.
    - o Foot
    - o Lower leg
    - o Entire leg
    - o Hand
    - o Forearm
    - o Entire arm
    - o Repeat, nondominant side
    - o Abdomen
    - o Chest
    - o Neck and shoulders
    - o Face

shows an example of progressive muscle relaxation. As a learning activity, try searching the Internet for instructions in making your own relaxation audiotape (http://www.guidetopsychology.com/pmr.htm or others).

Systematic Desensitization

The OT Practice Framework (AOTA, 2002) defines dominating habits as "so demanding they interfere with daily life" (p. 623). Occupational therapists may use behavioral strategies to extinguish negative behaviors in children (e.g., tantrums) or adults (e.g., overeating). One method of extinction that has been applied in the treatment of phobias is a technique of systematic desensitization (Sadock & Sadock, 2003). Developed by Joseph Wolpe (1958) in Johannasberg, South Africa in the 1960s, this treatment always begins by inducing a state of relaxation, through slow breathing, progressive muscle relaxation, or hypnosis. Wolpe (1958) considered relaxation to be incompatible with a state of anxiety (such as a phobia). Then, the therapist introduces images of approaching the feared situation through visualization. In the example of fear of flying, the client is asked to identify each step in the process of

taking a trip on an airplane. Perhaps this begins with making a reservation, packing one's bags, driving to the airport, checking in, and continuing toward to most feared steps, such as entering the plane, fastening one's seatbelt, and taking off. Visualizing each step in the sequence that the client identifies as the least to the most anxiety-producing event for him or her is called *successive approximation*, or gradually approaching and facing one's greatest fear (phobia).

The systematic desensitization approach uses both behavior modification and cognitive behavioral concepts, therefore bridging the gap between traditional and current approaches. Current self-help Web sites teach many of these techniques in the context of weight loss, fitness, relaxation, stress reduction, child rearing, and self-management of problem behaviors such as smoking and substance abuse. It is interesting to investigate some of these topics on the Internet. Systematic desensitization is covered in more detail as a self-regulation strategy in Chapter 13.

RESEARCH

Stein (1982) reviewed a large body of behavioral research including that by Pavlov, Skinner, Bandura, and other early behaviorists, continuing through the early 1980s. He interprets these concepts as a frame of reference for OT using social-skills training and stress management as examples. Occupational therapists' use of Stein's Stress Management Questionnaire (2003), a computerized assessment tool, and subsequent techniques for group intervention continues to the present. It measures the effectiveness of behavior modification programs with special populations such as persons with mental retardation and autism (Christiansen & Matuska, 2004), pediatric feeding disorders (O'Brien, Repp, Williams, & Christophersen, 1991), somatoform pain disorders (Palermo & Scher, 2001), thoracic outlet syndrome (Novak, 2003), pancreatic islet transplantation (Barshes, Vanatta, Mote, et al., 2005), and intragastric balloon postsurgical adjustment as a treatment for obesity (Herve, Wahlen, Schacken, et al., 2005). Some of these studies point to the need for behavior modification programs to assist clients in developing new habits as a follow-up to surgical procedures, a possible opportunity for occupational therapists. Behavioral medicine, combining biopsychosocial, holistic health, and behavioral approaches, has led to new areas for practice and research using behavioral concepts and strategies (Stein & Cutler, 2002).

LEARNING ACTIVITIES

Extinguishing Unwanted Behavior

Directions: Choose one of the following "bad habits" that need to be modified. Identify five specific actions you would take to get rid of the problem behavior,

Table 12-3

Example of Forming a Habit of Daily Exercise

Date	30-Minute Workout	Actual Performance Notes/Journal	Reinforcement for Daily Achievement
10/10	Yes	Ran for 20 minutes, and worked abs for 10 minutes.	New sneakers
10/11	No	Too tired.	No candy
10/12	Yes	Ran for 20 minutes, and worked abs for 10 minutes. Exceeded goal by lifting for 20 minutes.	Went out at night
10/13	No	First day of midterms. The night before, I did not get much sleep. After midterms, I worked until 4:00 p.m. and opted to study for the rest of the night because I was too tired to do anything else.	No pizza
10/14	No	Studying for midterms was more important than my previously set reward.	No nonschool-related activities
10/15	No	Still studying.	No television watching
10/16	No	Still studying; very tired.	Did not read a novel
10/17	No	Still studying; very tired. Opted not to go out in the rain.	Stayed dry!
10/18	Yes	Ran in the morning for 20 minutes, and worked abs for 10 minutes. Exceeded my normal running distance.	Got to read my novel
10/19	Yes	Ran in the morning for 20 minutes, and worked abs for 10 minutes. Exceeded my normal running distance.	Watched "Grey's Anatomy" on television
10/20	No	Felt under the weather; did not do anything.	Did not go to hockey game
10/21	Yes	Felt much better. Ran for 20 minutes, and exceeded my running distance. I seem to run better in the morning.	Went out to bar for a few drinks
10/22	No	Woke up late and had too much work to do. When I finished, I was too tired, and it was already dark.	Did not watch a movie
10/23	No	Was not able to sleep well (slept for 4 hours). Went to class from 8:00 a.m. to 12:00 p.m.; worked from 1:00 p.m. to 4:00 p.m.; came home to study in bed and fell asleep.	

(Created with Deana Forlenza, MOT student at Quinnipiac University)

keeping in mind both cues and reinforcers as well as the motivation of the client.

- 5-year-old sucking his thumb
- 16-year-old biting her nails
- 12-year-old boy slapping girls on the behind in lines
- 25-year-old obese woman binging on cake and ice cream late at night
- 3-year-old having temper tantrums when told "no"
- 30-year-old man driving too fast and not wearing seat belt

Behavioral Goals and Objectives

Part 1 Directions: Write three behavioral goals you could set for yourself. Make sure they are truly meaningful to you and that there is an objective way to measure or affirm their accomplishment.

Part 2 Directions: Choose one of the following behavioral goals, and write five behavioral objectives that would help you reach that goal. Use words that convey objectivity, such as "demonstrate" rather than "understand," and include a specific time frame and a measurable outcome for each. (circle your choice)

- Learn to ride a horse.
- Learn to play the guitar like (name favorite guitarist).
- Make exercise a regular part of your weekly routine.
- Save enough money to go to Cancun for spring break next year.

Repeat this exercise using one of your own personal goals. You may do this as a journal writing exercise or get together with a partner and coach each other.

Case Study: Deana

Use Table 12-3 to answer the following questions:
1. If you were Deana's occupational therapist, how would you tally the results?
2. In this 2-week trial, what were the barriers to forming a new habit of daily exercise?
3. How successful were Deana's planned "reinforcements" for meeting her daily goal?
4. What might be some changes you would make to this plan so that Deana might have a better chance of reaching her occupational goal?

Case Study: Anna

Anna, age 4, has entered an early intervention program for attention deficit hyperactivity disorder (ADHD). She has achieved potty training in day care but not at home. While few problems with behavior occur at preschool, mother reports that Anna behaves uncontrollably at home, refusing to sit at the dinner table to eat, leaving play activities unfinished all over the house, and frequently responding to parental demands with temper tantrums. You are the occupational therapist assigned to work with Anna and her family.

On interviewing, you learn that both parents work and the limited time spent at home has little structure and no rules or consequences for bad behavior. Using play activities to evaluate Anna, you discover that she concentrates longer when playing interactive board games and responds positively to requests that the rules be followed in that context. She enjoys creative pretend games like dress up and using finger puppets. A finicky eater, Anna cannot be tempted with food rewards. Anna has a strong will and wants to do more for herself than her parents usually allow.

Theory Application

1. Write three behavioral goals for Anna and three behavioral objectives. Be sure to consider parental priorities, such as preserving family dinner time and getting Anna to bed without creating turmoil.
2. Recommend three things that Anna's parents could use for positive reinforcement.
3. Write a paragraph describing how you would explain the process of behavior modification to Anna's parents.
4. Assuming that you have four weekly sessions with Anna's family, how would you sequence and proceed to implement the goals and objectives during each of the 4 weeks?

REFERENCES

American Occupational Therapy Association. (2002). The occupational therapy practice framework: Domain and process. *American Journal of Occupational Therapy, 56,* 609–639.

Bandura, A. (1977). *Social learning theory.* Englewood Cliffs, NJ: Prentice Hall.

Barshes, N. R., Vanatta, J. M., Mote, A., Lee, T. C., Schock, A. P., Balkrishnan, R., et al. (2005). Health-related quality of life after pancreatic islet transplantation: A longitudinal study. *Transplantation, 79,* 1727–1730.

Bruce, M., & Borg, B. (2002). *Psychosocial frames of reference: Core for occupation-based practice.* Thorofare, NJ: SLACK Incorporated.

Christiansen, C., & Matuska, K. (2004). *Ways of living: Adaptive strategies for special needs* (3rd ed.). Bethesda, MD: American Association of Occupational Therapy.

Cole, M. (1998). Time mastery in business and occupational therapy. *Work, 10,* 119–127.

Corey, G. (1991). *Theory and practice of counseling and psychotherapy* (4th ed.). Pacific Grove, CA: Brooks Cole.

Dunn, W. (2003). *Best practice occupational therapy with children and families.* Thorofare, NJ: SLACK Incorporated.

Herve, J., Wahlen, C. H., Schacken, A., Dallenmagne, B., Dewandre, J. M., Markiewicz, S., et al. (2005). What becomes of patients one year after the intragastric balloon has been removed? *Obesity Surgery, 15,* 864–870.

Mosey, A. (1970). *Three frames of reference for mental health.* Thorofare, NJ: SLACK Incorporated.

Mosey, A. (1988). Role acquisition frame of reference. In S. Robertson (Ed.), *Mental health focus.* Rockville, MD: American Occupational Therapy Association.

Novak, C. B. (2003). Thoracic outlet syndrome. *Clinical Plastic Surgery, 30,* 175–188.

O'Brien, S., Repp, A. C., Williams, G. E., & Christophersen, E. R. (1991). Pediatric feeding disorders. *Behavior Modification, 15,* 394–418.

Palermo, T. M., & Scher, M. S. (2001). Treatment of functional impairment in severe somatoform pain disorder: a case example. *Journal of Pediatric Psychology, 26,* 429–434.

Pavlov, I. (1927). *Conditioned reflexes.* New York, NY: Dover.

Royeen, C., & Duncan, M., (1999). Acquisitional frame of reference. In P. Kramer & J. Hinojosa (Eds.), *Frames of reference for pediatric occupational therapy* (2nd ed., pp. 377–400). Philadelphia, PA: Lippincott, Williams & Wilkins.

Sadock, B. & Sadock, V. (2003). *Synopsis of psychiatry: Behavioral sciences/clinical psychiatry.* Philadelphia, PA: Lippincott, Williams & Wilkins.

Skinner, B. F. (1953). *Science and human behavior.* New York, NY: Macmillan.

Stein, F. (1982). A current review of the behavioral frame of reference and its application to occupational therapy. *Occupational Therapy in Mental Health, 2,* 35–62.

Stein, F. (2003). *Stress management questionnaire: An instrument for self-regulating stress* (CD, individual version). Clifton Park, NY: Delmar Learning.

Stein, F., & Cutler, S. (2002). *Psychosocial occupational therapy: A holistic approach* (2nd ed.). Canada: Delmar

Wolpe, J. (1958). *Psychotherapy by reciprocal inhibition.* Stanford, CA: Stanford University Press.

Chapter 13

COGNITIVE BEHAVIORAL FRAMES

"Cognitive behavioral therapy ... is defined as the application of self-regulation methods and strategies to change thinking and behavior"

– MEICHENBAUM (1977)

This frame of reference builds upon earlier behavioral theory with the addition of thoughts (cognition) as "behaviors" that can be modified. Cognitive behavioral psychologists conceptualized thinking as an intervening factor influencing behavior. This solved the problem of too much control being in the hands of the therapist by essentially putting the client back in the driver's seat. As children mature, they become more capable of thinking about the situations they face in life. Behavior and the process of adaptation involves not only a stimulus and a response that is reinforced. Human behavior is also shaped by internal thought processes that involve beliefs, intentions, emotions, attitudes, cultural expectations, and perceptions based on past experience. For occupational therapy (OT), the cognitive behavioral frame moves beyond the correction of distorted thinking to include teaching-learning and self-management that combine cognitive and behavioral strategies.

This frame of reference has been changed and applied in OT over many years. The theoretical works of social psychologists Bandura (1985), Beck (1970, 1976), and Ellis (1985) have been adapted for OT by Linda Duncombe (2005), Stein and Cutler (2002), and others as an effective model for psychosocial intervention. Specific OT approaches include the following:

1. The psychoeducational group approach (Cole, 2005; Crist, 1986)

2. Self-regulation model (Stein, 1987; Stein & Cutler, 2002; Stein & Smith, 1989)

3. Social and Life Skills training model (Salo-Chydenius, 1996)

4. Coping model (Williamson & Szczpanski, 1999)

In pediatric OT practice, five cognitive approaches have been identified as occupation-based (Law, Missiuna, Pollock, & Stewart, 2005):

1. Cognitive behavior modification (Kendall, 1993; Meichenbaum, 1977)

2. Cognitive strategy training (McCormick, Miller, & Pressley, 1989)

3. Verbal self-guidance (Martini & Polatajko, 1998)

4. Cognitive orientation to daily occupation (CO OP) (Polatajko & Mandich, 2005)

5. Passport to learning (Leew, 2001)

FOCUS

Occupational therapists should consider this frame of reference whenever psychological barriers to activity engagement are encountered. Emotions interfere with participation in occupations across the lifespan: a child's feelings of peer rejection, a brain-injured adult's denial of functional limitations, an older adult's self-imposed isolation due to fear of falling. This frame of reference has been identified as the one most often used in behavioral health settings because it is especially effective in dealing with issues of motivation and emotion. However, physical and mental health cannot be separated when using a client-centered approach. In OT, cognition is the focus of evaluation and intervention as it pertains to all of the occupational performance areas mentioned in the OT practice framework (AOTA, 2002). Additionally, under the domain of occupational performance patterns, the framework discusses dominating habits as "so demanding that they interfere with daily life." Examples given are self-stimulation in autism, use of chemical substances resulting in addiction, and obsessive neatness (p. 623). The cognitive behavioral frame of reference offers useful techniques for self-management that occupational therapists can use in addressing these barriers to occupational performance.

THEORETICAL BASE

First, we will review the basic principles of Albert Bandura, Aaron Beck, and Albert Ellis as they apply to therapy. The application of cognitive behavioral theory fits easily with occupation-based approaches because activities have traditionally played an important role in the empirical process of changing thoughts and behaviors. Subsequently, we will discuss the various OT approaches that have emerged from these concepts.

Bandura's Social Learning Theory

In Chapter 12, we said that Bandura's work (1985) provides a bridge from behavior modification to cognitive behaviorism. Unlike other theories that have diverged from common roots, cognitive behaviorism continues to build upon the original foundations of behaviorism. The scientific method, which structured early behavioral research, continues to guide cognitive behavioral therapy, and the same basic concepts of reinforcement and associational learning apply equally well to thoughts and behavior. Bandura's social learning theory looks at the interaction of person, behavior, and environment, acknowledging the role of cognition in mediating environment–person interactions. The OT practice framework and most of the occupation-based models described in Section II explain occupational performance in much the same way—as the result of the interaction of multiple systems and contexts. Figure 13-1 describes Bandura's model for learning within one's social context.

Some of Bandura's major contributions to cognitive behavioral theory follow: modeling and observational learning, the hierarchy of reinforcement, the role of self-control and self-regulation, self-awareness, self-efficacy, and insight.

Observational Learning

Observational learning helps us to understand how learning occurs continually throughout life in ways that we may not be aware. This becomes important in OT when clients fail to progress because of unacknowledged social observations. For example, in the novel *Blindsided*, a well-known television producer newly diagnosed with multiple sclerosis (MS) refused to use a cane in the studio despite multiple falls due to poor balance. Upon reflection, he acknowledged several social learning interactions that shaped this behavior: a father who continued to work despite MS, a close friend who was turned down by the Navy because of a chronic condition, and a relative who was ridiculed for attempting to do outrageous things from a wheelchair (Cohen, 2004). For him, the cane symbolized weakness, failure, and a diminished self-image.

Modeling

Modeling is a form of teaching by example. A young child may imitate behaviors of an older sibling, especially if the behaviors bring positive consequences. Children learn both positive and negative behaviors in this way. For example, if one student gets away with cheating on a test, other students may follow suit. Persons select behaviors to imitate based on perceived consequences. Imitation is more

Figure 13-1. Bandura's Social Learning Interaction.

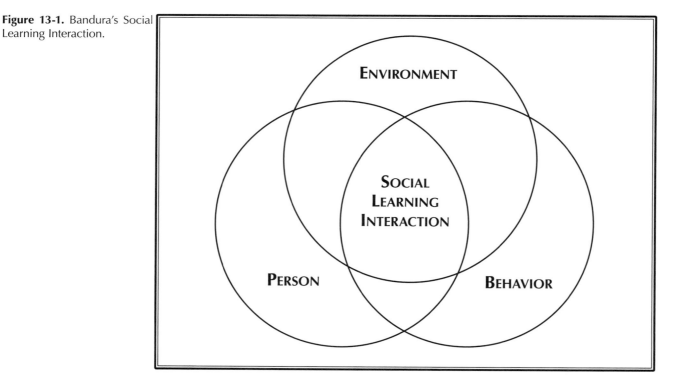

Table 13-1

Bandura's Hierarchy of Reinforcement

- *Initial:* external (money, food, social approval)
- *Symbolic:* internal images of success and failure
- *Social contract:* self-control because of knowledge of social consequences
- *Personal satisfaction:* self-produced (feeling competent is the best reward)

likely when positive consequences are observed in others, the basis for many of today's advertisements. In OT, we use modeling to demonstrate the steps of a task or to suggest a possible solution to a problem. Modeling in groups, such as role playing difficult situations, is a powerful tool to use in therapy.

Hierarchy of Reinforcement

The hierarchy of reinforcement expands the original behavior modification concept of using external reinforcement to shape behavior (Table 13-1). In moving along a continuum from concrete external rewards toward the internal satisfaction with a job well done, Bandura acknowledges the role of cognition in facilitating self-direction and self-control.

Self-Control amd Self-Regulation

Self-control and self-regulation are desired outcomes of therapy. A variety of techniques have sprung from this aspect of Bandura's work, such as the management of stress, anger management, and emotion regulation. For example, biofeedback has been used by Stein and Smith (1989) to monitor and facilitate the self-regulation of autonomic signs (pulse, heart rate, body temperature) associated with stress while practicing relaxation techniques. Self-regulation refers to the ability to direct one's own life by setting goals, creating strategies for achieving them, and building self-reinforcement into one's schedule. Goals serve as guidelines for self-regulation when they are observable and measurable (Bandura, 1985).

Self-Efficacy

Self-efficacy refers to the belief in one's own ability to interact effectively with the environment. Self-efficacy involves the cognitive ability to anticipate consequences. When 6-year-old Peggy is presented with a task, for example, swimming in a pool, she first relies on previous experiences to develop a general approach. If she has learned to swim and has felt fairly comfortable in the water in the past, she will enter the pool with confidence in her own ability. Self-efficacy changes with each situation, and may involve the observation of others, coaching, or demonstration

(modeling) to learn what skills or behaviors might be needed or expected when facing unfamiliar tasks or situations. Self-efficacy has also been cited in several other frames of reference.

Self-Awareness

Self-awareness is another important concept in several frames of reference. In the cognitive–behavioral frame of reference, self-awareness involves a realistic understanding of one's strengths and weaknesses and the realization of the effect of one's own behavior on others. Self-awareness also serves as the basis for insight.

Insight

Insight as a cognitive behavioral concept, involves an understanding of the changes in one's own abilities and disabilities as the result of a health condition. In OT, we encourage client narratives of the illness experience as a possible means of developing insight. Insight also involves acknowledging one's own internal barriers and sources of motivation for behavior. Cognition is needed to set realistic goals, to understand consequences, and to accurately interpret reality. Insight has a different meaning in the psychodynamic frame of reference (see Chapter 20).

Beck's Cognitive Therapy

Beck (1970, 1976) has focused much of his work on the treatment of depression. In his clinical work with clients, he noticed that emotions associated with depression often resulted from cognitive distortions and automatic thoughts. Beck developed the ABC method (A = stimulus situation, B = beliefs or thoughts by which clients interpret the situation, and C = response or behavior). Beck uses the scientific method with clients to further investigate their beliefs or assumptions. Following is a summary of Beck's contributions to this frame of reference.

Cognitive Distortions

Cognitive distortions are exaggerations or misinterpretations of an environmental interaction. For example, a woman with depression observes that her husband often comes home late from work. She interprets this as a sign that he does not love her anymore and even surmises that he is having an affair with someone from work. Beck teaches the client to use the scientific method to investigate the accuracy of her assumptions. He role plays the questions she might ask her husband to determine why he does not come home earlier and how he sees their relationship. He helps her to develop strategies to determine how her husband really feels by planning to do some activities together that they both enjoy. He instructs the client to devise experiments to prove or disprove her assumptions by gathering evidence and taking notes in a journal that she will bring to the next therapy session for discussion/analysis.

Automatic Thoughts

Automatic thoughts are thoughts that reflect habitual errors in logic. Beck concludes that psychological disturbances frequently stem from these habitual errors in thinking. For example, a male client complains that his boss is setting him up to fail by giving him too much work and is constantly "looking over his shoulder." Further discussion reveals that he has felt the same way in many other situations, and therapist and client make a list of all the specific situations in his life that have made him feel "victimized." The therapist teaches the client to apply logic to each situation, and together, they re-examine the patterns of automatic thinking. Again, experiments can then be devised to test alternate interpretations of the stimulus situations.

Using the Scientific Method of Therapy

Beck uses the scientific method when structuring the therapy session. He begins with the client identifying an "agenda" or a set of problems that will be the focus of therapy. Each problem is defined very specifically, including creating operational definitions of the variables, forming hypotheses, and devising methods for collecting data or evidence. Beck often assigns homework that includes discussions with individuals, field visits, social participation, gathering information, and keeping track of thoughts and emotions.

The Socratic Method

In his demonstrations of cognitive therapy, Beck often uses the Socratic method, asking the client questions that guide the investigation of their beliefs and assumptions. For example, Beck might ask the client to describe the specifics of a situation, for example, a telephone call from the client's husband telling her he was not coming home for dinner. He will ask for the exact words that were used, and the tone of voice, the specific timing of the call. He will ask the client to pinpoint the exact moment that she began to feel depressed or angry or to question whether her husband was telling her the truth. This method encourages the client to re-examine the beliefs and assumptions that caused the emotional response.

Albert Ellis's Rational Emotive Therapy

Ellis (1983) built on Beck's technique, expanding it to the ABCD method. D stands for "disputing" irrational beliefs. Ellis's style is different from Beck's. For example, he often uses humor and exaggeration to help clients to discover "crooked thinking." Ellis developed a technique called cognitive restructuring, a step by step process for disputing irrational beliefs (Ellis & Harper, 1975). The steps of cognitive restructuring are as follows:

1. Acknowledging our responsibility for creating our own problems

2. Accepting our ability to change

3. Recognizing that emotional problems stem from faulty thinking

4. Clearly perceiving our beliefs

5. Rigorously disputing beliefs

6. Working hard to change beliefs

7. Continued cognitive monitoring and restructuring

Ellis's cognitive restructuring can be understood as reframing the problem—that is, looking at it from a different perspective. Like Beck's cognitive therapy, the goal of rational emotive therapy (RET) is to develop a scientific or logical approach to solving one's own life problems.

Contemporary Cognitive Behavioral Therapy: Relevance for Occupational Therapy

Duncombe (2005) discusses many similarities between contemporary cognitive behavioral therapy (CBT) and the OT Practice Framework (AOTA, 2002). She compares occupation-based models with the principles of traditional CBT outlined by Vallis (1991).

- *Phenomenology* refers to the critical role of the client's perspective about the problems he or she brings to therapy. A detailed description of the client's subjective experiences (the illness experience) becomes the key factor in developing intervention strategies. This view is consistent with the client-centered approach proposed in the OT Framework.

- *Collaboration* is another "cornerstone" of both cognitive behavioral therapy and the OT client-centered approach. As occupational therapists become more client centered, they will place increased importance on collaboration and use the skills in the therapeutic use of self (Chapters 1 and 2) in order to 1) understand how illness or injury impact occupational roles, 2) help the client to clarify his or her own issues and priorities, 3) better define the occupational problems, and 4) when necessary, facilitate a more realistic understanding of the impact of illness (i.e., develop insight).

- *Activity*, not just verbal interaction, is another shared principle of OT and cognitive behavioral therapy. Attention is focused on the behaviors that result from perceptions and information processing. "The strategic use of activity in a therapeutic context clearly differentiates the cognitive therapists from the psychoanalysts" (Duncombe, 2005, p. 191).

- *Empiricism* refers to use of the scientific method, emphasizing the client's ability to apply reasoning to situations in his or her own life. "The collaboration between the client and the therapist in this systematic discovery process ensures that the intervention process and outcomes are not imposed on the client" (p. 191).

- *Generalization* is another shared goal of OT and CBT. Both seek to apply the benefits learned in therapy to life in the client's real world. CBT gives "homework" as a way of bringing life issues into therapy sessions, as Beck did with his clients in the examples cited previously. OT group sessions include a discussion of "application" to help clients bridge the gap between therapy and the "real world" (Cole, 2005). Other approaches, such as Toglia's dynamic interactional approach (Chapter 15) and the motor learning/task-oriented approach (Chapter 19), have a similar objective of enabling the client to continue to apply strategies learned in therapy in a variety of real life situations.

The connection between OT and CBT has been officially acknowledged in the psychological literature (Duncombe, 2005). A group of psychologists, including Aaron Beck (Wright, Thase, Beck, & Ludgate, 1993), write as follows:

> *Occupational therapists who work in a psychiatric setting are primarily concerned with teaching skills to promote self-reliance and independence. These therapists have received extensive training on how to deal with actual physical, intellectual, or social deficits. In fact, they are probably better prepared than most psychiatrists, psychologists, or social workers to teach adaptive skills to persons with significant handicaps. Occupational therapists can augment the cognitive therapy program in a number of ways. First, they can provide a detailed assessment of functional capacity. This evaluation often gives more practical information than does extensive psychological testing. Can the patient manage daily activities of living, handle financial matters, or complete job-related tasks? Accurate data in this regard help the cognitive therapist to determine whether the patient's concept of self-efficacy is valid. With inpatients, there is a frequent admixture of true performance deficits and cognitive distortions about abilities.*

> *During the treatment phase of occupational therapy, there is a natural partnership between the occupational and cognitive therapist. Both are interested in reducing symptoms and improving coping skills. The occupational therapist uses psychoeducational procedures, demonstrations, and in vivo rehearsal to build functional ability and self-esteem. Socratic questioning may also be used to uncover the patient's cognitive responses to the occupational therapy exercises. The cognitively-oriented occupational therapist will be able to point out maladaptive cognitions and help the patient to develop more balanced thinking. In addition, the occupational therapist can assist the patient in carrying out specific assignments from individual or group cognitive therapy. (p. 79)*

FUNCTION AND DISABILITY

Function involves the ability to use cognitive processes to reason, test hypotheses, and develop accurate self-awareness and realistic perceptions of others and the environment. Functional individuals can control and manage their own thoughts, feelings, and behavior to cope with stress, manage time, and balance their life roles and occupations. Cognitive ability may be conceptualized as a continuum, which can be measured on many levels, including intelligence, problem-solving, mental status, appropriateness of social behaviors, and life satisfaction. In OT, we look at how cognitive limitations affect one's occupations and identify the specific problems that cause occupational disruption.

Disability is not defined by diagnosis or symptoms of illness but by the presence of maladaptive behaviors, which are presumed to have been caused by maladaptive learning. This frame of reference defines both function and disability in terms of characteristics of the person, task, and environment that can be observed and measured.

CHANGE AND MOTIVATION

Following the guidelines of learning theory, the fundamental change agent is *reinforcement*. Clients are motivated by both external and internal reinforcement in the cognitive behavioral frame of reference (see Bandura's hierarchy, Table 19-1). In addition to money or earned privileges, persons are motivated by their wish to fulfill their obligations or to meet the expectations of others, or conversely, by the wish to avoid social sanctions (social contract reinforcement). Motivation works best when clients have internalized the personal satisfaction the comes with mastery and achievement of occupational goals.

As in behavior modification, occupational therapists look at the contexts within which clients perform occupations to better understand why they behave as they do. In doing so, we look at what aspects of the environment are reinforcing the specific behaviors the client wishes to change. Often, the social or cultural contexts create barriers—for example, a client's spouse may not welcome the assertive behavior a client has learned in therapy. A parent may disapprove of an adolescent's independence in choosing his own clothing, which may not meet the family's cultural or social standards. Many subtle aspects of the environment can reinforce passivity and dependence (or other maladaptive behaviors), making therapeutic change difficult for even the most motivated clients.

Additionally, the cognitive aspects of this frame require that occupational therapists also look for internal thoughts as possible reinforcers of maladaptive behaviors. Clients carry with them the irrational lessons learned from negative experiences past, which have so impacted their self-image that they continue to reinforce behaviors (binge eating, suicidal gestures, substance abuse, phobias) that otherwise do not make sense. Cognitive behavioral psychologists have demonstrated the presence of irrational thoughts and the persistence with which they continue to reinforce maladaptive behaviors. Sometimes, progress toward occupational goals cannot be achieved until we assist clients in identifying and removing these barriers.

Many of the techniques derived from CBT can be useful in OT for helping clients to manage their anxiety or emotions, and to remove the barriers caused by distorted thinking. These include relaxation training, decatastrophizing, challenging absolutes, visualization, thought-stopping, and self-instruction.

- *Relaxation training* has been effectively used in dealing with client anxiety. There are a number of ways to do this, including deep breathing, progressive muscle relaxation, and the application of Eastern movement disciplines such as Yoga and Tai Chi. Relaxation is considered to be incompatible with stress or anxiety. We can teach clients self-initiated strategies to intentionally produce relaxation as a way to cope with stressful situations. Stein has used a form of relaxation training, incorporating biofeedback as a self-monitoring tool for teaching stress management (Stein & Smith, 1989; Stein & Cutler, 2002). See Table 12-2 for an example.

- *De-catastrophizing* comes from the work of Albert Ellis (1985). He contends, "We, as psychologists who have worked with many miserable people, can tell you almost to a T just what you do the make yourself desperately unhappy—and how to stop doing it" (Ellis & Harper, 1975, p. 76). Ellis typically uses exaggeration as a way of challenging catastrophic emotional responses (typical of persons with depression). He writes, "unhappiness in the sense that it involves *awfulizing, horribilizing,* and *catastrophizing,* seems crazy and illegitimate" (p. 80). Using the example of losing a spouse or a job as point A, (your *activating* experience), he writes:

  > You feel sorrowful or sad at point C (your emotional consequence) because you tell yourself at point B (your belief system), "I think it unfortunate that I have lost this person or thing" (a rational belief). However, your feelings of anxiety or depression … stem from you irrational belief, "I find it awful or horrible …" giving you the illusion that you absolutely cannot control it and that you must remain too weak to cope with the awful essence of the universe that creates such horror and insists on plaguing you with it … (1975, pp. 77–78)

- *Challenging absolutes* is a technique used by both Beck and Ellis as a way of uncovering irrational beliefs. Ellis calls this kind of irrational thinking "musterbation." He writes:

  > Once you profoundly believe, "People must always love me sincerely," not only do you prepare for yourself a bed of thorns in case they don't, but you also keep lying in the same thorny bed when they do, because you inevitably think, "Suppose they no longer love me tomorrow? How awful. What a worthless slob I would then find myself." (Ellis & Harper, 1975, p. 80)

Beck uses another approach, encouraging clients to use their ability to reason to create alternate assumptions. This enables clients to imagine the worst consequence (their worst fears), but use rational thinking to consider other, perhaps more realistic or plausible interpretations of life events. This technique is especially useful in OT groups, which often uncover distressing emotional issues clients face in the aftermath of illness or injury (Cole, 2005).

- *Visualization* refers to the use of mental imagery in dealing with anxiety and fear. Several psychological techniques incorporate mental imagery, including flooding (imagining clients' most feared situations as a way to reduce anxiety) and systematic desensitization (a common treatment for phobias such as fear of flying). In systematic desensitization, relaxation techniques are used while gradually invoking mental images that are graded from the least to the most anxiety-provoking situations (called successive approximation). Occupational therapists have used visualization effectively in augmenting relaxation, as in the *Range of Motion Dance* (Harlowe & Yu, 1997), which instructs clients to picture themselves moving in the warm water at a beach. Envisioning real life situations can be useful in OT for many different occupational goals, from teaching safety precautions (What would you do if a fire started in your oven?) to cognitive rehearsal preceding task performance (Imagine yourself transferring from the bed to the wheelchair without losing your balance).

- *Thought stopping* is a technique for preventing automatic thoughts. For example, it has been used in treating obsessive compulsive disorder, by teaching the client to yell "stop" as soon as he or she begins the familiar obsessive thinking that leads to compulsive behavior (as in the case examples at the end of this chapter). Wolpe (1958) devised a technique of exposure and ritual prevention, which have been applied in a self help workbook format by Hyman and Pedrick (1999). The person with OCD's typical images of future disastrous events can be "exposed" by writing them down or recording them on a tape recorder. Repeatedly re-reading or listening to these accounts desensitizes clients with OCD by habituating them to their own obsessive thoughts, a technique called imaginal exposure (1999). Once clients have learned to recognize the obsessional thoughts, they can use thought stopping to prevent the thought, thereby eliminating the need to perform compulsive acts.

- *Self-instruction* has been discussed in Chapter 14 and is one of the strategies used in Toglia's dynamic interactional frame of reference. It involves teaching the client to mentally talk him- or herself through a task as follows:

o Mentally rehearsing the movements or steps, "Feet apart, knees relaxed, get a good grip on the pot, use both arms when lifting, move slowly …"

o Sequencing a multi-step task, "What's next? Fold, sort, put away."

o Remembering to use specific cognitive strategies such as error detection, "Have I checked my work?" or relaxation, "Take a deep breath."

o Replacing "bad thoughts" with positive "self-talk" such as reminding oneself not to be discouraged if something does not work out, "If at first you don't succeed, try, try again."

Reinforcement, as we have seen, is a double-edged sword. While it can be a powerful tool to motivate learning and skill development, it can also unconsciously or consciously create barriers to participation in occupations and can keep clients from deriving satisfaction and a sense of well-being from the occupations in which they do engage. The cognitive behavioral frame of reference gives us many techniques for dealing with the negative aspects of reinforcement as well as some powerful tools for establishing more positive behaviors.

EVALUATION

Evaluation in the cognitive behavioral frame of reference focuses on thought processes in relation to emotions and behavior. Many evaluation tools have been published based on this frame of reference. Most self-report checklists and rating scales depend on the cognitive abilities of clients to communicate information about their own perceptions, emotions, abilities, and problems. In OT, we begin with the occupational profile, giving special importance to phenomenology, or our understanding the client's perceptions and subjective experiences that bring him or her to therapy. We use therapeutic use of self to help the client to identify specific occupational problems that will become the focus of intervention. The assessments we choose will focus on the problem areas. Some examples follow:

- Self-report tests, such as the Role Checklist (Oakley, 1984)

- Mental status tests, such as Folstein's Mini Mental Status (1975)

- Mood inventories, such as Beck's Depression Scale (1978)

- Anxiety scales, such as The Stress Management Questionnaire (Stein, 1986; Stein, Bentley, & Natz, 1999)

- Life satisfaction inventories (Neugarten, Havighurst, & Tobin, 1961)

- Cognitive level tests, such as Allen's Cognitive Levels Screening (Allen, 2000) or the Loewenstein OT Cognitive Assessment (LOTCA) (Katz, Itzkovich, Averbuch, & Elazar, 1989).

- Tests addressing specific problems with engagement in occupation, such as the Bay Area Functional Performance Evaluation (BaFPE) (Bloomer & Williams, 1982)

- Tests of activities of daily living (ADL), such as the Kohlman Evaluation of Living Skills (KELS) (Thompson, 1992) and the Barthel Index (Mahoney & Barthel, 1965)

Duncombe (2005) reviews both formal and informal assessment tools occupational therapists use in the cognitive behavioral frame of reference. While there are some excellent tools for data gathering, evaluation in OT is an ongoing process, and observation of the affective, cognitive, and behavioral barriers to occupational performance continues through the intervention process (Bruce and Borg, 2002).

GUIDELINES FOR INTERVENTION

As a general rule, cognitive behavioral approaches work best with clients who are capable of self-awareness and inductive and deductive reasoning. This is because they must apply logic in order to recognize and dispute irrational thinking habits. However, when the approach is conceptualized as a continuum, those with less cognitive ability need a more behavioral approach, while those at higher levels need a more cognitive approach (Cole, 2005). Four areas for intervention identified by Bruce and Borg (2002) for the cognitive behavioral frame of reference are context, thoughts and attitudes, knowledge, and skills. Collaboratively designed OT interventions work on collaboratively agreed upon behavioral goals and objectives. Some of the specific OT approaches based on this frame of reference will be reviewed, including psychoeducational groups, social and life skills programs and groups, self-regulation programs, and Williamson's coping model.

Psychoeducational Groups

Psychoeducational groups evolved in the 1980s as an approach in mental health. Duncombe (2005), in reviewing the literature for this approach, found many descriptions of its use for both inpatients and outpatients (Bradlee, 1984; Courtney & Escobedo, 1990; Fine & Schwimmer, 1986; Giles, 1985; Greenberg et al., 1988; Jao & Lu, 1999; Kaseman, 1980; Stein & Nicholic, 1989; Salo-Chydenius, 1996; and Tang, 2001). Occupational therapists play the role of educator-facilitator in designing educational and skill-training experiences for groups of clients with mental health issues, requiring them to use rational thinking to apply new knowledge and skills through group problem-solving. Examples of skill areas addressed in psychoeducational groups follow:

- Medication management
- Living on a budget
- Meal planning and preparation
- Care of clothing and personal items
- Money management (banking skills, paying bills)
- Using public transportation
- Household safety
- Parenting and caregiving skills
- Keeping relationships—how to manage anger

Social and Life Skills Groups

Social and life skills groups also use a psychoeducational approach, in that skills related to everyday social interactions and socially acceptable behaviors are learned through individualization, collaboration, practice activities, problem-solving, and generalization (Salo-Chydenius, 1996). The groups, while using specific skill training strategies, are organized around the needs and prioritized goals of individual group members.

Following are topic areas used in Liberman's (1990) Social and Independent Living Skills trainer's manual:

- Basic conversation skills (places where there are people to talk to, people who are willing to talk, topics to talk about)
- Verbal and nonverbal communication behaviors (go/no-go signals)
- Starting a friendly conversation (opening lines/topics)
- Keeping a friendly conversation going (active listening, asking questions)
- Ending a conversation pleasantly (knowing when to stop, what to say)
- Putting it all together (practicing skills in real life, using skills to have better relationships with everyone, helping to make new friends)

Self-Regulation Programs

Self-regulation programs use a cognitive, rational approach to problem behaviors. Stein's (Stein & Cutler, 2002) stress management program provides a good example. Stress management training models are cognitive behavioral strategies that have been used successfully with the following health conditions:

- Depression (Hollon & Beck, 1979; Stein & Smith, 1989)
- Schizophrenia (Stein, 1987; Stein & Nikolic, 1989)
- Pain (Engel & Rapoff, 1990; Turk, Meichenbaum, & Genest, 1983; Turk, Zaki, & Rudy, 1993)

- Substance abuse (Konkol & Schneider, 1988)
- Eating disorders (Stockwell, Duncan, & Levins, 1988)
- Attention deficit disorder with hyperactivity (Kwako, 1980)

Stein's model begins with his stress management questionnaire, a self-report instrument that gathers information about the physiological, cognitive, emotional, and behavioral symptoms of stress; the everyday situations that trigger stress; and the everyday activities that reduce or provide a means of coping with stress. He then provides guidelines for both individual and group stress management interventions with the following objectives:

- Education about the client's specific health condition and its relationship with stress
- Increasing awareness of how stressors cause symptoms
- Explaining the psychological mechanisms of stress
- Increasing knowledge about how occupations reduce stress
- Learning new ways to manage stress through relaxation
- Learning to use occupations as coping strategies
- Teaching prevention techniques and self-regulation strategies
- Appreciating the importance of self-regulation and self-initiated use of strategies

Some of the methodologies Stein suggests for use in stress management groups are arts and crafts, creative media, informational handouts and discussion, nutrition and health awareness, prescriptive exercise, progressive relaxation, role-playing, visualization, values clarification, and biofeedback. Groups may be organized to address specific health conditions or may focus on wellness and prevention. An application for wellness is outlined in Table 13-2.

Coping Model of Pediatric Occupational Therapy

The Coping Model in Pediatric OT emphasizes the child's use of coping resources to meet challenges posed by the environment. These resources are both internal and external.

Internally, the child's sensory reactions, developmental skills, and emotional state guide environmental exploration and self-initiated behaviors. Confidence level is based on previous experiences and preferences. Through building on successful coping experiences, the child develops a unique coping style (Zeitlin, Williamson, & Szczepanski, 1988).

Externally, the family provides material resources (equipment, toys) and support (organization and controls in the task environment) as well as physical and emotional safety. Parents and primary caregivers provide the child's most

Table 13-2	
Self-Regulation for a Restful Night's Sleep	
Do	**Don't**
Set a specific bedtime and time to arise. Your body energy will become conditioned.	Sleep too late on weekends. Varying times for arising will disturb the sleep-wake cycle.
Exercise in the morning or before dinner.	Exercise within 2 hours of bedtime.
Meditate for 10-15 minutes twice a day.	Take naps during the daytime.
A warm bath calms you.	A shower tends to be alerting.
Eat a light snack, to avoid nighttime hunger. Consider medication effects on stomach.	Drink caffeine within 6 hours of bedtime (coffee, soda, chocolate, caffeinated tea).
Maintain a cool temperature in bedroom	No alcohol within 2 hours of bedtime.
Use visualization of pleasant experiences.	Begin conversations about upsetting issues.
Engage in occupations that calm you: reading, listening to music, watching television	Forget to lock doors, turn off lights and appliances, set alarm clock if needed.

Adapted from Stein, F., & Cutler, S. (2002). Psychosocial occupational therapy: A holistic approach (2nd ed., p. 438). Canada: Delmar, Thompson.

significant support for coping by buffering the child's exposure to stress, making demands, modeling coping behaviors, encouraging coping efforts, and giving feedback (Williamson & Szczpanski, 1999). This approach uses the following strategies to facilitate effective coping:

- Grade environmental demands to match the child's adaptive capacities.
- Design intervention activities that promote the development of self-efficacy.
- Give timely and explicit positive feedback to support coping efforts.
- Encourage child-initiated activities that extend and elaborate emerging coping skills. Many cognitive behavioral researchers have described the coping process (Antonovsky, 1979; Lazarus & Folkman, 1984; Moos & Billings, 1982).

Cognitive Orientation to Occupational Performance Model in Pediatric Occupational Therapy

The Cognitive Orientation to Occupational Performance (CO-OP) model, developed for children with developmental coordination disorder (DCD), views cognition as bridging the gap between inherent ability and actual performance (Polatajko & Mandich, 2005). In its focus on motor tasks of the child's own choosing, this approach also uses the principles of motor learning theory described in Chapter 19. The therapist encourages the development of global or domain-specific cognitive strategies through a process of "guided discovery" (p. 243). By asking children questions during task performance (tying shoes, getting on a swing), the therapist helps them pay attention to key features of the task and environment in order to solve problems whenever they get stuck. The authors describe seven guidelines for using this approach:

1. Client chooses the goals and/or tasks.
2. Therapist does a dynamic performance analysis by watching child attempt the tasks.
3. Cognitive strategies are encouraged through global problem-solving and domain-specific strategies such as verbal guidance, body positioning, or attention to doing.
4. Guided discovery through sequencing, questioning, and coaching
5. Enabling principles, such as making it fun, promoting learning, and generalization
6. Involving parents and/or significant others
7. Structuring the intervention

A dynamic performance analysis also has specific guidelines, which were developed by Polatajko, Mandich, & Martini (2000). The therapist, in observing and interacting with the child during a performance attempt, looks for the following:

- *Motivation:* does the child want to do the task?
- *Knowledge:* does the child know how to do the task?
- *Ability:* can the child do the task competently?
- *Breakdown:* what are the problems with performance?
- *Task demand:* what adaptations can/should be made?

- *Environment:* what supports are needed; what barriers can/should be removed?

This approach has been well researched. A clinical trial (Polatajko, Mandich, & Miller & Macnab, 2001) provided evidence of greater long-term maintenance of motor skills, cognitive strategy use, and parent satisfaction with use of the CO-OP model.

RESEARCH

The cognitive behavioral frame of reference, while drawing upon research in the field of psychology to validate its basic concepts, has also been well documented in the OT literature. Duncombe (2005) has recently published a review of these, most of which have been cited previously in this chapter. Cognitive behavioral theory may be considered a continuation of basic behavioral theories. See Chapter 12 for a review of research on behavioral theories.

LEARNING ACTIVITIES

1. Do the Behavioral Goals and Objectives Learning Activity in Chapter 12 (see p. 146). Consider one of these goals when developing a focus for this assignment.

2. Think about a habit you have that you would like to change or a new habit that you would like to form. Write a short-term goal addressing this habit, making sure that it is observable and measurable. The time frame for achieving this goal is approximately 2 weeks, so make sure that your goal is something that could realistically be achieved in that time frame. Examples include changing eating habits, stopping procrastination, cutting down on television watching or telephone time, learning the habit of daily exercise, and incorporating a stress management strategy into your daily routine.

3. Identify your hierarchy of reinforcement. Think about things that give you pleasure and support. What rewards can you build into your routine to keep you motivated? List five self-reinforcements, in the order of their importance for you. List five negative events that will deter you from straying from your plan.

4. Devise the steps needed to accomplish your goal. Specify exactly what you will do and when you will do it. Make a daily checklist to record your progress. Use a calendar to write the actions you will take each day. Specify when and where the actions will occur. Your checklists and calendar with your daily recordings will be handed in at the end of the 2 weeks, along with your report.

5. Incorporate a self-reinforcement schedule. Use interval reinforcement to keep yourself motivated (i.e., a favorite snack after exercising or a 10-minute call to a significant other after resisting dessert or snacking for an entire day). You must also consider the consequences of failure to achieve your goal. What penalty could you give yourself for failure to live up to your daily plan (be honest, no fibbing allowed)? Record your rewards and penalties on your calendar.

6. Choose a partner to act as monitor. This can be anyone you choose, but he or she must be willing to encourage you on a daily basis. Your monitor's role is as follows: listen to your daily progress reports, give you permission to reward yourself, or assign you a penalty for failing to accomplish your plan. Specify who your monitor is and when and where you will contact him or her each day.

7. After 2 weeks, write a short report evaluating your progress. Did you accomplish your short-term goal? What did you learn from this exercise? How did it feel to succeed/fail? What would you have done differently to increase your chances of success (and/or future successes)? How could you use self-management strategies in the future?

Cognitive Case Assignment

Directions: There are four parts to this assignment, each worth 25%. Cases are assigned by *last* name as follows:

- A to C: Case 1
- D to J: Case 2
- K to S: Case 3
- V to Z: Case 4

Part 1: Occupational Profile

Write an occupational profile on your case according to the following outline, using titles in italics as shown. Limit 2 pages, single spaced, 1-inch margins. Be selective and concise.

- *Identifying data:* Write one sentence including name, age, gender, place of residence, persons sharing residence, and date of admission to OT treatment.
- *Problem definition:* What are the primary reasons the client has sought help? Identify five occupational areas causing problems for this client. Define each problem in a separate paragraph, stating relevant details, client perception of cause of problem, and affect on occupational functioning.
- *Occupational status:* Identify client's primary roles and occupations. Include career or job, student or volunteer roles, family roles and responsibilities,

home-related occupations, and current and past patterns of time use. What are client skills, training, and educational level? What are client's plans for possible future roles or changes in occupational patterns?

- *Social participation:* What are the client's important relationships with others? Identify three persons with whom the client maintains close relationships or frequent contact. What occupations are associated with each role/relationship? How do the occupational problems identified previously affect these relationships.

- *Occupational contexts:* What are the primary contexts in which the client performs occupations? What are physical, cultural, and social expectations connected with the client's primary roles? Choose two different physical contexts to describe more fully. What is the temporal context, such as developmental life stage, or self/others expectations appropriate for the client's age? To what extent does virtual context play a part?

Part 2: Understanding the Health Condition for the Case

All of the cases represent anxiety disorders. Look up the disorders in Sadock and Sadock (2003), and summarize the main symptoms in one narrative paragraph.

In a second paragraph, look up the health condition on the Internet, and summarize the suggested approaches for treatment. Write down Web sites you use as references.

Part 3: Preparing for Intervention

Using principles of behaviorism, write one overall goal for each of the five occupational problems or concerns identified in Part 1. Goals are desired outcomes chosen by the client with the guidance of the occupational therapist. Overall goals should identify these desired outcomes as visualized by client and therapist together.

Write five behavioral objectives addressing each goal, making sure they are observable and measurable. The time frame for achieving this goal is approximately 4 weeks, so make sure that your objectives could realistically be achieved in that time frame.

Part 4: Self-Management Intervention Plan

Look up self-management on the Internet to get ideas for this part (e.g., techniques for changing habits at http://www.habitchange.com). Many resources exist in disability-related websites, such as OCD and eating disorders, which use cognitive behavioral approaches. Think about how the techniques described might be helpful to you or to the clients described in your cases. The approach should include the following:

- Training in identifying external triggers for problem behaviors. Discuss what client needs to be aware of and record in log/check sheet.

- A check sheet for keeping track of problem incidents or situations (separate sheet)

- Training in at least one strategy to stop problem thinking and/or prevent ritual (e.g., thought stopping, disputing beliefs, self-talking, self-monitoring, self-distracting, visualization, relaxation techniques, and meditation). Describe what this training will consist of; give details related to specific case.

- Reinforcement schedule. Identify your client's hierarchy of reinforcement. Think about things that give him or her pleasure and support. What rewards can you build into the client's routine to keep him or her motivated? List five self-reinforcements, in the order of their importance for your case. What possible negative events may result from failure to change? How might client's desire to avoid negative consequences deter him or her from straying from the plan?

- A check sheet or calendar for keeping track of successes and slip-ups, and resultant reinforcements (separate sheet, room for comments by client regarding feelings, etc.)

Your plan must be specific and detailed. You will need to create several worksheets for your case, including check sheets and calendar sheets.

Case Study 1: Sally

Sally is a 32-year-old mother of two girls, ages 3 and 6 years. When she first got married, she continued her job as a nursing supervisor. The birth of her first child coincided with her move from Maine to Georgia, where her husband, Will, was transferred. Will works as a chemist for a large pharmaceutical firm, and he received a substantial promotion in his new position. At that time, a decision was made that Sally would not seek employment but would become a stay-at-home mom.

The family lives in a three-bedroom brick home in an upper-middle–class neighborhood. At first, Sally enjoyed socializing with neighbors at their community clubhouse, which included a large playground and a pool. However, as the girls grew older, Sally became less sociable, depending upon church, schools, and mothers day out programs to provide playmates and activities for her daughters. Sally's occupations centered around their care and with organizing things around the house.

Sally has always been a good mother, convinced that she would not make the same mistakes her parents made. She felt that she did not get enough discipline growing up, and that made her feel neglected and unloved, as her mother worked full-time during most of her childhood. Soon, Sally became obsessed with every aspect of her children's care and especially with keeping them clean and safe. She cooks nutritious meals and reads to her daughters often.

As an occupational therapist, you make a home visit at 9:00 a.m. on a Monday. You hear voices inside, but no one answers the door for 5 full minutes. Sally opens the door a crack and asks if you would mind coming in through the garage. You squeeze past piles of empty boxes and bags of what appears to be trash, leaving little room for the Toyota van parked in the middle of the oversize garage. Sally asks you to take your shoes off in the laundry room, then disappears. You step past multiple laundry baskets overflowing with dirty laundry and enter the kitchen, also cluttered with unwashed dishes, pots, pans, toys, and empty food containers. However, the open dishwasher is full of clean dishes. Six-year-old Patty greets you in a school uniform, lunch box in hand. She tells you she has been waiting for an hour for mommy to take her to school, and now she is late. She informs you that Sarah has missed breakfast at her nursery school. Sarah sits in a high chair in only a diaper, playing with some dry cereal and an empty yogurt container.

"Where's your mommy now?" you ask Patty.

"She's supposed to be getting Sarah dressed, but first she has to check the bedroom."

Sally has been referred to you for help with occupational problems caused by OCD. Her symptoms are mostly of the "checker" type. Checkers live with an excessive, irrational sense of being held responsible for possible dangers and catastrophes that may befall others as a result of the checkers' imperfect actions. In Sally's case, she scans each room for small objects that Sarah might swallow and choke on and checks all clothes for lint, objects in pockets, etc.

Assessing the situation, you offer to ride with Sally while she drops off the girls at their respective schools. After waiting 10 minutes while Sally checks and re-checks the contents of each girl's lunch box, school bags or backpacks, etc., Sarah and Patty are safely strapped in their car seats. On the way, Sally apologizes for the confusion and tells you Mondays are always harder than other days. She exchanges affectionate hugs with each girl as she drops them off at private school.

Case Study 2: Lawrence*

Lawrence took at least an hour to finish a meal because he had to chew each bite of food 32 times. At one time, he walked up and down a flight of stairs for 8 hours until he "got it right." He had also informed me that if he did not get himself dressed in a specific fashion, his wife would "grow horns." Lawrence had prominent and severe OCD symptoms that were very handicapping to him. His response style was marked by a great deal of ambivalence, self-doubt, and a need to quantify everything. This paralyzed his ability to complete tasks.

Lawrence was always organized, neat, punctual, and a valued employee at a local dairy. He basically led a normal life, had two sons, enjoyed yard work, and played the organ. When he retired at age 65, he became depressed, was hospitalized for 3 weeks, and was treated successfully with antidepressant medication. In the hospital, he began to count things, and experienced obsessional associations. Two years later, he was hospitalized again and diagnosed with OCD. By then, he was unable to carry out many ADL at home. This time, he is started on Paxil (an antidepressant) and referred for outpatient rehabilitation.

As an occupational therapist in an outpatient clinic, you interview Lawrence and his wife together. Although Lawrence's wife, Betty, suffers from severe arthritis, she has taken over much of the household responsibility. She expresses a wish that her husband help more with the housework the way he used to do: "He used to do the yard work every weekend, and he'd help me by moving furniture while I vacuumed. I can't stand an untidy house and yard, but we can't afford to pay someone to come in. I wonder if we should sell the house and move into an assisted living facility."

You assess Lawrence's self-care activities with standardized tests and find that he has no problem carrying out tasks in the clinic. Physical tests reveal no limitations and a better-than-average endurance for someone his age. However, he expresses little interest in any leisure activities. Betty confirms his tendency to get "hung up" on certain tasks and "take forever" to complete them. "We don't do anything for fun any more. He used to play the organ and we'd sing. We'd have friends over or go to church socials, and they'd be clamoring for him to play for them. I go sometimes by myself, but it isn't the same. It's easier to just stay home and watch TV," Betty laments.

Lawrence, too, expresses regret that he is unable to do fun things with his wife. "It's no picnic having OCD," he says. "But I can't control it." You try out having Lawrence and his wife play a simple card game together. Surprisingly, you find that when you give Lawrence a repetitive, predictable, decisive, and controlled activity, Lawrence can do it with minimal disruption from symptoms. It is making decisions about what to do and when to do it that raises his anxiety and brings on the rituals.

Case Study 3: Harlow*

Harlow, a 30-year-old librarian, comes to your clinic escorted by his wife. "I have to get my life back together. I have been out of work for nearly a month, and if it weren't for my wife, I wouldn't be here now," he says.

*Adapted from Mabus. (1988). *Obsessive compulsive disorder: A case study.* Occupational Therapy Forum, 3(21), 1–4.

*Adapted from Sadock, B., & Sadock, V. (2003). Kaplan & Sadock's synopsis of psychiatry (9th ed., pp. 603–604). *Philadelphia, PA: Lippincott, Williams & Wilkins.*

About 4 months ago, while attending a family picnic, he had suddenly become "nervous." His heart began to race "a mile a minute," and he began to perspire profusely, felt nauseated, experienced a tightness in his chest, and felt he was suffocating, "as if someone was smothering me with a pillow." The attack came for no apparent reason and continued for about 15 minutes. It terrified him ("I thought that I was going to die"), so much so that he asked his wife to drive for fear that he might have another attack while driving. Later that day, he experienced a second attack while sitting on the porch with a neighbor.

During the next 3 weeks, he underwent numerous examinations by different specialists (cardiologists, endocrinologists, gastroenterologists, and so forth), but the results of all tests were negative.

The attacks continued at a rate of two or three a week. Harlow noticed that the attacks were more likely to occur in trains, although they did not always occur in that situation. He had already stopped driving to work and needed the train to get to work. He began to take early trains (6:00 a.m.) and late trains (7:00 p.m.) to and from work to avoid crowds that might block his escape route. Also, he would limit himself to local trains since they made more stops, and therefore, the doors open more frequently. The anxiety experienced in anticipation of having an attack was almost as intense as the attacks themselves. Soon, he could no longer bear the extreme discomfort of riding in a train and, consequently, took a leave of absence from work. In addition, his fear generalized to all crowded places (stores, banks, offices, streets) to the extent that he needed his wife to accompany him whenever he left the house.

When seen in the clinic, he was experiencing three or four attacks a week, was essentially housebound, and was in constant fear of having a fatal episode. The physician diagnosed Harlow as having panic disorder with agoraphobia. With an antipanic drug, Harlow could tolerate situations in which panic is likely.

OT testing showed that he had no difficulty performing high-level cognitive tasks and that he was a good creative problem solver. He is referred to OT for cognitive behavior therapy to provide a structure for anticipating probable panic situations, learning relaxation techniques to use in concert with the medication, and keeping track of disruptions (thoughts of panic) during task performance. A schedule of activities (occupations) that is sequenced according to intensity of fear of panic needs to be developed with Harlow.

Case Study 4: Alice*

Alice, age 21, has an 8-year history of bulimia. Overweight at 15, she missed making the cheerleading

team. Other stresses included the death of her grandfather, with whom she was close, and several good friends moving away. Additionally, her parents gave away her pets, citing that they were too much trouble. Alice, determined to lose weight, learned self-induced vomiting. That was one thing she could control. By senior year, she was purging four times per week, had stopped eating with the family, and developed the habit of late night eating binges followed by purging.

Alice dropped out of college after a year for lack of interest. After that, she held a series of jobs in stores, a deli, a donut shop, and a clothing store. She lost all of these because of taking too much time off for eating rituals. She left home and moved in with her boyfriend, with whom she shared a very steady and stable relationship. He supported her while entering an eating disorders program.

In the hospital, Alice reported frequent crying spells, insomnia, and total preoccupation with thoughts of food. She participated in a multidisciplinary program including group therapy, individual therapy, and OT. She learned to verbalize feelings of emptiness, loneliness, and a sense of inadequacy and came to understand their connection as triggers for binges. Response prevention techniques were used to stop binging and vomiting, and she responded well to the structured setting. She also was started on Prozac.

In OT follow-up, self-management techniques were recommended to help Alice to maintain control over rituals after leaving the 4-month program. Alice lived with her boyfriend, and got accepted to an evening educational program in fashion merchandizing, an interest she had developed in high school. She worked part-time in a clothing store to help pay for her education.

When interviewing Alice, you are impressed with her motivation to maintain normal weight, look good in her clothes, and feel good about herself. While encouraging, these are also factors that place her at risk for relapse. OT will be scheduled 2 times per week for 4 weeks to establish a self-management program. This will include a check sheet for recording incidents causing anxiety or thoughts of binging. She will need to learn strategies for calming herself and distracting herself during these times. Visualization and self-reassurances are needed in situations of extreme anxiety. Finally, Alice needs help in establishing a self-reinforcement schedule including rewards for preventing binge eating and consequences for the occasional slip-ups she is bound to have.

*Adapted from Sadock, B., & Sadock, V. (2003). Kaplan & Sadock's synopsis of psychiatry (9th ed., p. 748). Philadelphia, PA: Lippincott, Williams & Wilkins.

REFERENCES

Allen, C. A. (2000). Allen Cognitive Level Screen (ACLS) Test Manual (Copyright Allen Conferences, Inc.). Colchester, CT: S & S Worldwide.

American Occupational Therapy Association. (2002). The occupational therapy practice framework: Domain and process. American Journal of Occupational Therapy, 56, 609–639.

Antonovsky, A. (1979). *Health, stress, and coping.* San Francisco, CA: Jossey-Bass.

Bandura, A. (1977). *Social learning theory.* Engelwood Cliffs, NJ: Prentice Hall.

Bandura, A. (1985). Model of causality in social learning theory. In M. Mahoney & A. Freeman (Eds.), *Cognition and psychotherapy* (pp. 81–99). New York. NY: Plenum.

Beck, A. T. (1978). Beck Inventory. Room 602, 133 South 36th St. Philadelphia, PA, 19104: Center for Cognitive Therapy.

Beck, A. T. (1970). Cognitive therapy: Nature and relation to behavior therapy. *Behavior Therapy, 1,* 184–200.

Beck, A. T. (1976). *Cognitive therapy and emotional disorders.* New York: Penguin Books USA, Inc.

Beck, A. T. & Weishaar, M. (1994). Cognitive therapy. In R. Corsini & D. Wedding (Eds.). Current psychotherapies, Fourth edition (pp. 285–320). Itsaca, IL: Peacock.

Bloomer, J., & Williams, S. (1982). The Bay Area Functional Performance Evaluation. In B. Hemphill (Ed.), *The evaluative process in psychiatric occupational therapy.* Thorofare, NJ: SLACK Incorporated.

Bradlee, L. (1984). The use of groups in short term psychiatric settings. *Occupational Therapy in Mental Health, 4,* 47–57.

Bruce, M. A., & Borg, B. (2002). *Psychosocial frames of reference: Core for occupation-based practice.* Thorofare, NJ: SLACK Incorporated.

Cohen, R. (2004). *Blindsided: Lifting a life above illness.* New York: HarperCollins.

Cole, M. (2005). *Group dynamics in occupational therapy: A theoretical basis and practice application of group intervention* (3rd ed.). Thorofare, NJ: SLACK Incorporated.

Crist, P. (1986). Community living skills: A psychoeducational community-based program. *Occupational Therapy in Mental Health, 6,* 51–64.

Courtney, C., & Escobedo, B. (1990). A stress-management program: Inclient-to-outclient continuity. *American Journal of Occupational Therapy, 44,* 306–310.

Duncombe, L. (2005). The cognitive-behavioral model in mental health. In N. Katz (Ed.), *Cognition & occupation across the life span: Models for intervention in occupational therapy.* Bethesda, MD: American Association of Occupational Therapy.

Ellis, A., & Harper, R. (1975). *A new guide to rational living.* Hollywood, CA: Wilshire Book Company.

Ellis, A. (1985). Expanding the ABCs of rational emotive therapy. In M. Mahoney & A. Freeman (Eds.), *Cognition and psychotherapy.* (pp. 81–99). New York: Plenum.

Engel, J. M., & Rapoff, M. A. (1990). Biofeedback assisted relaxation training for adult and pediatric headache disorders. *Occupational Therapy Journal of Research, 10,* 283–299.

Fine, S. & Schwimmer, P. (1986). The effects of occupational therapy on independent living skills. *AOTA Mental Health Special Interest Section Newsletter, 9*(4), 2–3.

Folstein, M. F. (1975). The Folstein Mini-Mental Status Exam (MMSE). *Journal of Psychiatric Research, 12,* 196–197.

Giles, G. (1985). Anorexia nervosa and bulimia: An activity oriented approach. *American Journal of Occupational Therapy, 39,* 510–517.

Greenberg, L., Fine, S., Cohen, C., Larson, K., Michaelson-Bailey, A., Rubinton, P., et al. (1988). An interdisciplinary psychoeducation program for schizophrenia clients and their families in an acute care setting. *Hospital and Community Psychiatry, 39,* 277–282.

Harlowe, D., & Yu, P. (1997). *The ROM dance: A range of motion exercise and relaxation program.* Madison, WI: Uncharted Country Publishing.

Hollon, S. D., & Beck, A. T. (1979). Cognitive therapy of depression. In P. C. Kendall & S. D. Hollon (Eds.), *Cognitive-behavioral interventions.* New York, NY: Academic.

Hyman, B., & Pedrick, C. (1999). *The OCD workbook: Your guide to breaking free from obsessive-compulsive disorder.* Oakland, CA: New Harbinger Publications.

Joa, H. P., & Lu, S. J., (1999). The acquisition of problem solving skills through instruction in Siegel and Spivack's problem solving therapy for chronic schizophrenia. *Occupational Therapy in Mental Health, 14,* 47–63.

Kaseman, B. (1980). Teaching money management skills to psychiatric outclients. *Occupational Therapy in Mental Health, 1,* 59–71.

Katz, N., Itzkovich, M., Averbuch, S., & Elazar, B. (1989). Loewenstein Occupational Therapy Cognitive Assessment (LOTCA) battery for brain injured clients: Reliability and validity. *American Journal of Occupational Therapy, 43,* 184–192.

Kendall, P. C. (1993). Cognitive-behavioral therapist with youth: Guiding theory, current status and emerging developments. *Journal of Consulting and Clinical Psychology, 61,* 235–247.

Konkol, B., & Schneider, M. (1988). Treatment of substance-abuse and alcoholism. In D. W. Scott & N. Katz (Eds.), *Occupational therapy in mental health: Principles in practice.* London, UK: Taylor & Francis.

Kwako, R. (1980). Relaxation as therapy for hyperactive children. *Occupational Therapy in Mental Health, 1,* 29–45.

Law, M., Missiuna, C., Pollock, N., & Stewart, D. (2005). Foundations for occupational therapy practice with children. In J. Case-Smith (Ed.), *Occupational therapy for children* (5th ed.). St. Louis, MO: Elsevier Mosby.

Lazarus, R. S. & Folkman, S. (1984). *Stress, appraisal, and coping.* New York: Springer.

Leew, J. (2001). Passport to learning: A cognitive intervention for children with organizational difficulties. *Physical and Occupational Therapy in Pediatrics, 20,* 145–160.

Liberman, P. (1990). *Social and independent living skills: Basic conversation skills module.* Los Angeles, CA: Clinical Research Center for Schizophrenia & Psychiatric Rehabilitation.

Mabus. (1988). Obsessive compulsive disorder: A case study, OT Forum, 3, 21, 1-4.

Mahoney, F. I., & Barthel, D. (1965). Functional evaluation: The Bartel Index. *Maryland State Medical Journal, 14,*56–61. Available at Internet Stroke Center, http://www.strokecenter.org.

Martini, R., & Polatajko, H. (1998). Verbal self-guidance as a treatment approach for children with developmental coordination disorder: A systematic replication study. *Occupational Therapy Journal of Research, 18,* 157–181.

McCormick, C. B., Miller, G., & Pressley, M. (1989). *Cognitive strategy research: From basic research to educational applications.* New York, NY: Springer-Verlag.

Meichenbaum, D. (1977). *Cognitive-behavioral modification: An integrative approach.* New York, NY: Plenum Press.

Moos, R. H., & Billings, A. G. (1982). Conceptualizing and measuring coping resources and processes. In L. Goldberger, & S. Breznitz (Eds.) *Handbook of stress: Theoretical and clinical aspects* (pp. 212–230). New York: Free Press.

Neugarten, B. L., Havighurst, R. J., & Tobin, S. S. (1961). The measurement of life satisfaction. *Journal of Gerontology, 16,* 134–143.

Oakley, F. (1984). *The role checklist.* Bethesda, MD: National Institutes of Health, Dept. of Rehabilitation Medicine.

Polatajko, H., & Mandich, A. (2005). Cognitive orientation to daily occupational performance with children with developmental coordination disorder. In Katz, N. (Ed.), *Cognition and Occupation across the lifespan: Models for intervention in occupational therapy* (2nd ed.). Bethesda, MD: American Occupational Therapy Association.

Polatajko, H., Mandich, A., & Martini, R. (2000). Dynamic performance analysis: A framework for understanding occupational performance. *American Journal of Occupational Therapy, 54,* 65–72.

Polatajko, H., Mandich, A., Miller, L., & Macnab, J. (2001). Cognitive orientation to daily occupational performance: Part II: the evidence. *Physical and Occupational Therapy in Pediatrics, 20,* 83–106.

Sadock, B., & Sadock, V. (2003). *Kaplan & Sadock's synopsis of psychiatry* (9th ed.). Philadelphia, PA: Lippincott, Williams & Wilkins.

Salo-Chydenius, S. (1996). Changing helplessness to coping: An exploratory study of social skills training with individuals with long-term illness. *Occupational Therapy in Mental Health, 8,* 21–30.

Stein, F. (1986). *Stress management questionnaire.* Vermillion, SD: University of South Dakota, Author.

Stein, F. (1987). Stress and schizophrenia. *Alberta Psychology, 16,* 10–11.

Stein, F., Bentley, D., & Natz, M. (1999). Computerized assessment: The Stress Management Questionnaire. In B. Hemphill (Ed.), *Assessments in occupational therapy mental health: An integrative approach.* Thorofare, NJ: SLACK Incorporated.

Stein, F., & Cutler, S. (2002). *Psychosocial occupational therapy: A holistic approach* (2nd ed.). Canada: Delmar, Thompson.

Stein, F., & Nikolic, S. (1989). Teaching stress management techniques to a schizophrenic patient. *American Journal of Occupational Therapy, 43,* 162–169.

Stein, F., & Smith, J. (1989). Short-term stress management programme with acutely depressed inpatients. *Canadian Journal of Occupational Therapy, 56,* 185–191.

Stockwell, R., Duncan, S., & Levins, M. (1988). Occupational therapy with eating disorders. In D.W. Scott, & N. Katz (Eds.), *Occupational therapy in mental health: Principles in practice.* London, UK: Taylor & Francis.

Tang, M. (2001). Clinical outcome and client satisfaction of an anger management group program. *Canadian Journal of Occupational Therapy, 68,* 228–236.

Thompson, L. (1992). *The Kohlman evaluation of living skills* (3rd ed.). Bethesda, MD: American Occupational Therapy Association.

Turk, D., Meichenbaum, D., & Genest, M. (1983). *Pain and behavioral medicine.* New York: Guilford Press.

Turk, D., Zaki, H., & Rudy, T. (1993). Effects of intraoral appliance and biofeedback/stress management alone and in combination in treating pain and depression in patients with temporomandibular disorders. *Journal of Prosthetic Dentistry, 70,* 158–164.

Vallis, T. M. (1991). Theoretical and conceptual bases of cognitive therapy. In T. Vallis, J. Howe, & P. Miller (Eds.). *The challenge of cognitive therapy: Applications to nontraditional populations* (pp. 3–21). New York, NY: Plenum

Williamson, G. G., & Szczepanski, M. (1999). Coping frame of reference. In P. Kramer & J. Hinojosa (Eds.), *Frames of reference for pediatric occupational therapy* (2nd ed.). Philadelphia, PA: Lippincott, Williams & Wilkins.

Wolpe, J. (1958). *Psychotherapy by reciprocal inhibition.* Stanford, CA: Stanford University Press.

Wright, J., Thase, M., Beck, A., & Ludgate, J. (1993). *Cognitive therapy with inpatients: Developing a cognitive milieu.* New York, NY: Guilford.

Zeitlin, S., Williamson, G. G., & Szczepanski, M. (1988). *Early coping inventory.* Bensenville, IL: Scholastic Testing Service.

Chapter 14

BIOMECHANICAL AND REHABILITATIVE FRAMES

"Occupational performance is a descending hierarchy of roles, tasks, activities, abilities and capacities."

– CATHERINE TROMBLY (1995, P. 961)

The biomechanical frame of reference was identified by recent graduates in occupational therapy (OT) as the most frequently used in practice, and rehabilitation frames were among the top five (National Board of Certification in OT [NBCOT], 2004). The biomechanical frame of reference applies the principles of physics to human movement and posture with respect to the forces of gravity. Many health professionals use biomechanical principles in their practice. Occupational therapists are unique in applying them to clients' engagement in the tasks of everyday life. In OT, the principles of movement, including range of motion (ROM), strength, endurance, ergonomics, and the effects or avoidance of pain, must be considered within the context of occupation.

WHY A COMBINED APPROACH?

We have combined these approaches to illustrate a continuum of OT intervention beginning with establishing or restoring functional skills (remediation) and continuing with modifying the task or the environment (adaptation and compensation) in order to enable continued occupational performance within the constraints of a more chronic or ongoing disability. While rehabilitation may often be associated with a medical model of recovery, the term remains relevant as long as occupational therapists continue to work in rehabilitation environments (Sabari, 2008) and/or as members of rehabilitation teams (Yasuda, 2008; Forwell, Copperman, & Hugos, 2008). Also noteworthy is the continued inclusion of rehabilitation as a category of research in both the *American Journal of Occupational Therapy* and the *World Federation of Occupational Therapy Bulletin*, and the *International Classification of Function, Disability, and Health* (ICF) repeatedly refers to the use of its guidelines in determining or describing rehabilitation outcomes (WHO, 2001). The biomechanical frame of reference is typically identified with remediation, or improvements in strength,

ROM, or endurance. However, the principles include the management of weight-bearing against gravity and, thus, guide the design of splints, adaptive seating, and the design and use of prosthetic devices. For example, Colangelo (1999) uses biomechanical principles for positioning children with motor and postural difficulties to enable their engagement in the normal occupations of childhood. The same applies to adults with Cerebral Palsy (Figure 14-1).

The rehabilitative approach is described by Trombly (2002) as "aim(ing) at making people as independent as possible in spite of any residual impairment" (p. 13). As such, it consists mainly of environmental adaptation and compensatory strategies. Trombly includes wheelchair selection and high technology adaptations to compensate for disability or aging. More recently, Trombly (2008) describes rehabilitation in the context of her occupational functioning model (OFM), which begins with the proposition that "to engage satisfactorily in a life role, a person must be able to do the tasks that, in his or her opinion, make up that role" (p. 2). She suggests beginning with the roles and tasks clients choose and taking a close look at the contexts within which preferred tasks will be performed. Colangelo (1999) describes the use of biomechanical principles to create compensatory devices for movement and positioning in the absence of voluntary movement or postural control.

While a traditional view of the rehabilitative approach addresses mainly physical disabilities, occupational therapists now recognize the need to consider both physical and mental features of occupational performance. An updated understanding of a rehabilitative approach in OT recognizes the need to view occupational performance holistically. Mosey's theory is included here to illustrate the importance of combining both physical and psychosocial aspects in an OT rehabilitative approach.

In psychosocial rehabilitation, Mosey (1988) defined a "role acquisition" approach to address those individuals whose disability has stabilized and who continue to have

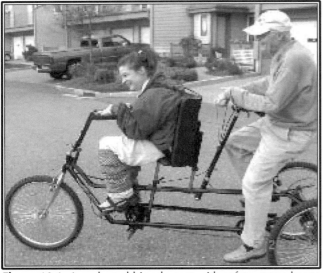

Figure 14-1. An adapted bicycle seat with safety straps keeps Heather in a functional position for pedaling while dad does the steering.

Table 14-1	
Mosey's Role Acquisition Theory: Basic Skills	
Task Skills	**Interpersonal Skills**
Willingness to engage in tasks	Initiate, respond to, and sustain verbal interaction
Adequate posture for tasks	Express ideas and feelings
Physical strength and endurance	Be aware of needs and feelings of others
Gross and fine motor coordination	Participate in cooperative and competitive situations
Interest in the task	Compromise and negotiate
Rate of performance	Assert self
Follow oral, written, pictorial or demonstrated directions	Take on appropriate group roles
Use tools and materials	
Acceptable level of neatness	
Attention to detail	
Solve problems	
Organize task in logical manner	
Tolerate frustration	
Self-direct	

Adapted from Mosey, A. (1988). Role acquisition: An acquisitional frame of reference. In S. Robertson (Ed.), Mental health focus. Rockville, MD: American Occupational Therapy Association.

difficulty in performance of life roles. Mosey identifies the basic skills common to all social roles as task skills and interpersonal skills. These basic skills sustain the major domains of occupational performance: activities of daily living (ADL), instrumental ADL (IADL), education, work, play, leisure, and social participation (American Occupational Therapy Association [AOTA], 2002). See Table 14-1 for a list of Mosey's task and interpersonal skills.

The client's mental and physical functions work together in creating problems with occupational performance, and both need to be considered when using a rehabilitation approach. For example, persons with chronic back pain have different levels of frustration tolerance when faced with limitations in physical capability. Some may be willing to alter the way they perform a task (adaptation), while others may resist the use of compensatory strategies such as wearing a back brace or asking for help with heavy lifting. This illustrates the need for a client-centered and systems-oriented approach when using the biomechanical and rehabilitative frames of reference.

FOCUS

Occupational therapists often use the biomechanical approach with deficits in ROM, strength, and endurance, whatever the cause. The OT practice framework calls these *body functions*. Areas of practice using this frame of reference include musculoskeletal disorders, cumulative trauma, such as back injuries or carpal tunnel syndrome, hand injuries, work hardening, ergonomics, and prevention. The OT practice domains include performance areas for application, analysis of task demand when using occupation as a means

of providing graded exercise (Trombly, 2002), and consideration of contexts as they impact task performance.

THEORETICAL BASE

Range of Motion

ROM involves the angles and direction of human movement, including extension, flexion, abduction (away from the body), adduction (toward the body), and rotation. Occupational therapists are particularly concerned with ROM when injury or illness causes extended periods of immobility (e.g., in paraparesis caused by a stroke), or when neurological disorders produce specific excessive movements that create an imbalance in muscle development (e.g., in cerebral palsy). Therapists may create regular programs of passive ROM (PROM) to prevent contractures due to disuse. A good example of an active ROM (AROM) strategy is the ROM Dance, a technique of visualization and exercise created to maintain flexibility and to prevent reduced ROM for persons with rheumatoid arthritis (Van Dusen & Harlowe, 1987).

Kinematics

Kinematics addresses the amount, direction, speed, and acceleration of human movement. Researchers have used advanced technology to analyze human movement through quantitative descriptors addressing the underlying forces that cause motion and maintain stability (Luttgens & Hamilton, 1997; Soderberg, 1997). These studies combine ROM, strength, endurance, and effort, which OT researchers have begun to apply to a variety of occupations of daily life.

Torque

Torque is the effectiveness of a force in causing rotary movement, which depends on the amount of force (strength), the amount of resistance (weight of limb and object and position with respect to gravity), and the distance of the force from the axis (joint). Without giving details of calculation, the importance of this principle involves OT minimizing client effort of movement (strength needed) through reducing resistance (weight of object to be lifted) and by placing the object closer and more central to the body. For example, lifting a heavy pitcher of lemonade from the center of the table takes more effort than sliding the pitcher close to the edge of the table before lifting it.

Strength

Strength refers to both stability and motion produced by muscle tension. Normal daily activity consists of combined muscle groups either moving or stabilizing the body in well-learned patterns or sequences (standing, sitting, walking). Additionally, work tasks may require more specialized or skilled patterns (driving a truck, mowing the lawn, using a computer). Stabilization is achieved through muscle co-contraction, also called postural control. Stability in various positions is necessary in order for skilled movement to occur.

Endurance

Endurance involves the ability to sustain muscular activity. This is more complex than strength or ROM because it involves other body systems, such as the cardiopulmonary system. Endurance may also be dependent on a person's general state of health. For example, the presence of infection or the lack of sleep are likely to temporarily decrease endurance.

FUNCTION AND DISABILITY

Function involves maintaining strength, endurance, and ROM within normal limits for one's age, gender, and physical characteristics. Function may also relate to the knowledge and use of good body mechanics and ergonomics in one's daily occupations to prevent the likelihood of injury or cumulative stress syndrome.

Disability is identified whenever a restriction in joint ROM, strength, or endurance interferes with everyday occupations. Conditions that adversely affect biomechanical functioning include orthopedic injury, edema, pain, skin tightness (burns, scars), spastic (excess contraction) or flaccid (too little) muscle tone, or immobilization (disuse) over extended periods of time. Biomechanical disability is often related to the inability to perform specific tasks, such as using a computer or working in a factory. In this instance, OT creates behavioral goals and objectives with regard to the task, situation, and specific contextual factors.

CHANGE AND MOTIVATION

Some of the ways people can change their biomechanical abilities involve changes in positioning; exercises or graded tasks involving stretching, lifting, and moving; repetition and practice; and the manipulation of environmental conditions within which therapeutic activities are performed. Jackson, McLaughlin, Gray, and Zemke (2002) have organized principles of therapeutic change according to the following goals: 1) maintain or prevent limitations in ROM, 2) increase ROM, 3) increase strength, and 4) increase endurance. The use of physical agent modalities (PAMs) in facilitating movement or passive stretch and in minimizing the effects of pain may also be included within this frame of reference.

1. Maintaining or preventing limitations in ROM may be accomplished through three methods:
   - Compression (wrapping with elastic strip) reduces edema associated with limitations in ROM.
   - Positioning through therapist handling (as in neurodevelopmental therapy [NDT]), bracing or splinting in ways that facilitate functional movement.
   - Movement through the full ROM, either actively (AROM) or passively (PROM); twice daily is recommended.
2. Increasing ROM can be accomplished through the following:
   - Passive stretching in ways that create tension on the muscles and tendons but do not injure them may be accomplished through therapist handling or external devices. Occupational therapists perform passive stretching prior to engagement in therapeutic activity.
   - Active stretching is best accomplished through the use of occupations so that clients perform stretching movements within the context of meaningful tasks.

- Proprioceptive neuromuscular facilitation (PNF) techniques may be used to facilitate active movement (Brody, 1999; Voss, Ionta, & Myers, 1985).

3. Strength may be increased through the following:

   - Exercise that stresses muscles to the point of fatigue. When clients are motivated to exercise regularly, exercise itself may be considered an occupation.

   - Other daily occupations may be analyzed and structured to provide strengthening exercise (walking or running to work, housecleaning or gardening tasks, lifting and carrying objects).

   - Either type of strengthening program uses grading principles of increased resistance (weight) and repetition through isometric (moving) or isotonic (nonmoving) exercise.

4. Endurance may be increased through the following:

   - Light resistive exercise that increases repetitions of less than maximum movements

   - Grading and gradually increasing time spent in identified occupations

   - Grading of cardiovascular aspects of activities and alternate period of rest

   - Use of interest-sustaining tasks in which client is motivated to participate (such as board games or sports activities)

5. Incorporating PAMs (Bracciano & Earley, 2002):

   - Superficial heat agents facilitate biomechanical treatment by reducing pain or increasing pain tolerance, increasing blood supply to specified areas, enabling metabolic processes that encourage tissue repair and pain reduction, and increasing collagen elasticity, which reduces joint stiffness.

   - Superficial cold agents (cryotherapy) serve to reduce edema and inflammation following trauma and lower the temperature of body tissue, thereby reducing external or internal bleeding.

   - Therapeutic ultrasound applies deep heat through acoustic energy. Different types of ultrasound have been used to relieve pain, facilitate movement, and aid the healing process. Use of ultrasound requires specialized training.

   - Electrotherapy stimulates nerves and muscles to prevent atrophy, alleviate pain, manage spasticity, and facilitate nerve regeneration. Electrical stimulation devices should not be applied or modified without specialized training.

EVALUATION

Range of Motion

ROM is usually measured with a dynamometer recording the degrees of movement at the axis of each joint. Latella and Meriano (2003) provide excellent guidelines for students in measuring ROM and muscle strength.

Strength

Strength, defined as the maximum tension produced under voluntary effort, may be measured with a dynamometer (grip strength, pinch strength) by manual muscle testing, and by more sophisticated devices such as the Baltimore Therapeutic Exercise (BTE) machine or other work simulators. Most people are familiar with gym equipment such as Cybex, which measures or selects the amount of weight to be moved by each specified muscle group.

Endurance

Endurance is usually measured by determining the duration of activity or the number of repetitions of a specified movement before fatigue occurs.

Pain

Occupational therapists are concerned with pain because it frequently represents a barrier to the use of biomechanical capacities (ROM, strength) for occupational performance. Evaluating pain involves more complex processes and requires a more subjective form of measurement. Clients vary widely in their perception of and tolerance for pain. The location of pain may be reported by the client through pointing to the affected area, by verbal expression during passive or active movement or manipulation, or by marking the areas on a diagram of the body. Intensity of pain may be rated by the client on a numerical scale, such as 0 to 10, with 0 being no pain and 10 representing excruciating pain.

Additionally, occupational therapists distinguish themselves from physical therapists by using a rehabilitative approach to assessment. While the above evaluations are shared with physical therapists, occupational therapists evaluate these body functions within the context of client occupations. Trombly (1995) suggests that biomechanical activity analysis be focused on functional movements using purpose of a task to organize the movements required. Functions such as lifting, carrying, grasping, and reaching have meaning for clients in terms of functional goals, as opposed to traditional biomechanical terminology.

GUIDELINES FOR INTERVENTION

OT interventions focus on the client's identified roles and priorities for task performance. Methods of intervention include activity adaptation, application of compensatory strategies or technologies, and physical reconditioning.

Activity Adaptation

Activity adaptation involves changing the activity demand to reduce or increase biomechanical requirements. Trombly (1995) suggests that in using activity as a means of establishing or restoring ROM, strength, or endurance, the attributes of a task may be modified by the following:

- Positioning the task
- Adding weights or other devices that provide graded resistance
- Modifying the tools to increase or decrease demands
- Changing the materials or size of objects used
- Changing the method of accomplishing the task

When the client's goal is to accomplish a task (activity as end), the task demand can be reduced to adapt to musculoskeletal limitations. The previous strategies used to increase task requirements may be graded to decrease task requirements. Additionally, environmental factors are considered. Following are examples of actions that can be taken to reduce task demand:

- Changing client's position for doing the task to minimize stress or fatigue, for example, sitting versus standing
- Organizing frequently used objects or supplies within easy reach
- Training in and using adaptive equipment, such as reachers or stabilizers
- Applying positioning devices, such as bolsters or splints, to compensate for the effects of gravity
- Eliminating steps of the task, such as using garlic powder instead of fresh
- Changing the tools used, such as an electric instead of a manual can opener
- Changing the weight or size of objects, such as smaller bags of groceries
- Educating clients in use of good body mechanics and avoidance of repetitive movements that cause cumulative trauma
- Using rolling devices such as hand trucks for heavy objects, rolling carts for household tasks, and rolling briefcases or backpacks for books and laptop computers

Energy Conservation Techniques

Many clients find it difficult to modify the way they have always done tasks despite acquired biomechanical dysfunction. Occupational therapists work with clients to modify tasks and environments in ways that conserve a limited amount of energy. Strategies for reducing fatigue include the following:

- Planning activities around client's unique patterns of high or low energy
- Modifying positions for doing tasks to compensate for weakness or pain
- Planning ahead by organizing one's supplies and equipment before beginning task
- Clustering similar tasks, such as doing several errands while out
- Alternating active and passive tasks to give the body a chance to recover
- Accepting assistance from others for less important tasks
- Prioritizing and conserving one's energy for the most meaningful tasks

Work Hardening

This term usually refers to physical attributes of work tolerance, such as sitting tolerance, standing tolerance, and endurance for sustained lifting or use of heavy equipment. Sophisticated work simulators can imitate the movements required for specific work tasks and can assist occupational therapists in evaluating complex skilled movements. Work reconditioning requires repetition of the required movements for increased amounts of time. Jacobs (1985) identifies a variety of work behaviors related to work hardening:

- *Work tolerance:* physical endurance for remaining at work
- *Staying on the job:* remaining at one's work station or area
- *Sitting tolerance:* physical ability to sit for specified work sessions
- *Attending to the task:* physical and mental ability to sustain focus on work tasks
- *Task completion:* ability to adequately perform work tasks within a reasonable time
- *Quality:* work can be completed within quality requirements
- *Following instructions:* ability to follow general work rules and problem-solve complex tasks

- *Flexibility:* ability to work cooperatively with others, accept feedback from supervisors, and adapt to required changes in work requirements

Ergonomics and Prevention

Ergonomics is the science of fitting workplace conditions and job demands to the capabilities of the working population (National Institute for Occupational Safety and Health [NIOSH], 1997; Noack, 2005). The benefits of OT ergonomic interventions in the workplace include the following (Bloswick, Villnave, & Joseph, 1998):

- Reduced occupational illness and injury
- Reduced workers' compensation costs
- Reduced absenteeism
- Increased productivity
- Increased worker comfort and satisfaction on the job

Ergonomic assessments and interventions may be applied to a wide variety of work settings and include an analysis of the tools and equipment, the tasks to be performed, and the physical workstation and environment. An example of good ergonomic guidelines for office workers using computers to avoid injury follow:

- Working posture includes seating with head, neck, and trunk facing forward with upper arms and elbows close to the body.
- Seating provides support for the lower back and armrests that do not interfere with movement.
- Keyboard and mouse are used at a comfortable height without reaching.
- Top of monitor is at or below eye level and located directly in front of user.
- Bifocals or trifocals, if used, do not require bending head down or back when reading computer screen.
- Duration of repetitive motions may be limited with rest breaks or by varying work tasks to decrease the risk of cumulative trauma (e.g., carpal tunnel syndrome).

Worker education can dramatically reduce the risk of occupational injury. For construction workers, education in skillful lifting might involve the following:

- Plan your movements ahead of time, eliminate obstacles, and estimate effort needed.
- Place one foot firmly alongside the load, the other slightly behind the load.
- Position the heavy object close to the body before lifting.
- Set muscles of legs, hips, and back ready to take the strain.
- Get a firm grip with fingers under the load.
- Lift heavy objects using primarily legs and thighs, avoiding bending from hips.

- Lift gradually, avoiding jerky, twisting motions (turn feet to rotate object).
- Put down the load by reversing the process.
- Avoid reaching as you lift.
- Do not maintain stressful positions for extended periods of time.
- Know your limits, and never lift beyond your strengths and abilities.

Back injuries are a common complaint of those involved in physical work. Risk factors for back injury are poor posture, faulty body mechanics, stressful living and work habits, loss of flexibility, and general decline in physical fitness. Preventive education can substantially reduce the risk of back injuries and includes the following precautions:

- Maintain normal spinal curves with balanced upright posture.
- Sit upright with the lower back supported and head in neutral position.
- While sitting, feet should be supported on floor or foot rest.
- Avoid twisting back when relaxing or doing ordinary tasks.
- Avoid lifting with the back; use legs and arms instead (assisting with arms when getting up from bed, kneeling with one leg to pick up a small child).
- Avoid slumped shoulders and a forward head posture (such as leaning over bathroom sink while shaving or applying make-up, or leaning over counter while eating or preparing food).
- Use lumbar support (pillow) while driving or riding in a car.

Rehabilitation

Traditional rehabilitation approaches tend toward adaptation and compensation. As such, the approach may be understood as beginning where remediation of skills has leveled off. Adaptation of tasks and environments in order to compensate for lost physical body structures and functions, include splinting, the use of slings, positioning aides, and all types of adaptive equipment that facilitates engagement in occupations by compensating for lost skills or body functions. The reader is referred to Randomski & Trombly (2008) for a more complete description of compensatory strategies used in OT.

RESEARCH

Dunn (2000) reviewed the evidence for OT biomechanical approaches in pediatrics. She concludes that most of the research has involved small samples of children with severe and/or multiple disabilities. Children with movement

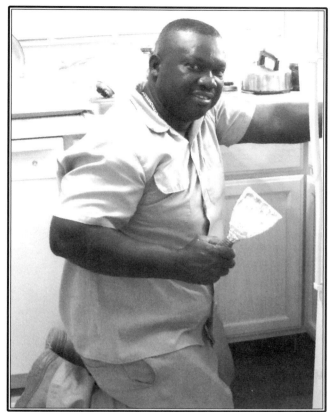

Figure 14-2. Cecil on the job.

disabilities perform better when orthotics are fabricated using biomechanical principles (Daniels, Sparling, Reilly, & Humphry, 1995).

Most of the research on this approach comes from interdisciplinary sources (Jackson et al., 2002). Morrissey, Harman, and Johnson (1995) found that strengthening programs that resemble desired occupations in terms of positions, speed, and contractions yield the best results. This reinforces the importance of using the biomechanical frame of reference in the context of specific, client-chosen occupations.

LEARNING ACTIVITY

Case Study: Cecil

During a recent visit to Freeport, Bahamas, I (M. Cole) had occasion to hire a contractor to install new cabinets in the kitchen of my condo which was damaged by Hurricane Jeanne. Cecil had a regular construction job during the week and planned to install my new kitchen on two consecutive weekends (Figure 14-2). As Cecil worked to remove the old cabinets, he complained of pain shooting down his right leg whenever he bent over. I watched him bend from the hip to lift the heavy cabinets and twist to carry them out the door on his way

to the dumpster. Finally, I could no longer stand to see his face contorted in pain. I handed him a bottle of beer, and we sat on the patio in the shade. He slouched in the chair and kicked off his shoes, dangling his feet in the pool. "Have you seen a doctor about your back pain?" I asked.

"It ain't my back, it's my leg," Cecil replied. "The doctor gave me these." He pulled a pill bottle from his pocket, which appeared to be a heavy dose of codeine. "Only trouble is, if I take 'em, I can't work. So I only take one when I'm done for the day."

By now I had guessed that the pain in his leg likely emanated from an impingement of the sciatic nerve caused by herniated disc in his lumbar spine. I should add here that health care in the Bahamas does not compare with the United States. There are no rehabilitation centers and no practicing occupational therapists. Cecil has a national health care plan that covers only occasional doctor visits. Unemployment compensation and medical leaves of absence are not options, and he is married with several small children to support. We discussed his work during the week, which he admitted caused similar pain.

Theory Application

Create an intervention plan for Cecil, using three different techniques from the biomechanical/acquisitional/rehabilitative frame of reference.

Biomechanical Wellness Activity

Directions: Everyone wants to become more physically fit these days. As part of a healthy lifestyle, they might join a gym or jog a few miles before work or school. In OT, we often suggest that our clients get their exercise by doing an activity rather than just exercise. To fully understand how to do this, we try it out on ourselves.

Following are some examples of biomechanical goals for daily exercise:

- Stretch all major muscle groups.
- Sustain moderate aerobic activity 30 minutes each day.
- Strengthen abdominals with 3 sets of 10 repetitions.
- Strengthen back extensors with 3 sets of 10 repetitions.
- Lift 20 pounds bilaterally using correct body mechanics, 10 repetitions.

1. For each goal, suggest one everyday occupation that incorporates at least some the required movements, positions, and/or endurance. Everyday occupations can involve ADL (self-care), IADL (life maintenance tasks such as grocery shopping, doing laundry, and cleaning), work, education, play, leisure, and/or social participation.

2. Choose two goals for yourself, and define the following for each:

- What specific task could you do each day to accomplish the goal?

- How would you structure and sequence the task?

- What is the purpose or meaning of the task for yourself and/or others?

- How could you motivate yourself to do this task on a daily basis?

REFERENCE

American Occupational Therapy Association. (2002). The occupational therapy practice framework: Domain and process. *American Journal of Occupational Therapy, 56,* 609–639.

Bloswick, D., Villnave, T., & Joseph, B. (1998). Ergonomics. In P. King (Ed.), *Sourcebook of occupational rehabilitation.* New York, NY: Plenum.

Bracciano, A., & Earley, D. (2002). Physical agent modalities. In C. Trombly, & M. V. Radomski (Eds.), *Occupational therapy for physical dysfunction* (5th ed.). Philadelphia, PA: Lippincott, Williams & Wilkins.

Brody, L. (1999). Mobility impairment. In C. M. Hall, & L. T. Brody (Eds.), *Therapeutic exercise: Moving toward function.* Philadelphia, PA: Lippincott, Williams & Wilkins.

Colangelo, C. (1999). Biomechanical frame of reference. In P. Kramer, & J. Hinojosa, (Eds.), *Frames of reference for pediatric occupational therapy* (2nd ed.). Philadelphia, PA: Lippincott, Williams & Wilkins.

Daniels, L., Sparling, J., Reilly, M., & Humphry, R. (1995). Use of assistive technology with young children with severe and profound disabilities. *Infant, Toddler Intervention, 5,* 91–112.

Dunn, W. (2000). *Best practice occupational therapy in community service with children and families.* Thorofare, NJ: SLACK Incorporated.

Forwell, S., Copperman, L. & Hugos, L. (2008). Neurodegenerative diseases. In M. V. Radomski & C. Trombly Latham (Eds.), *Occupational therapy for physical dysfunction* (6th ed.). (pp. 618–641). Philadelphia: Lippincott, Williams & Wilkins.

Jackson, J., McLaughlin Gray, J., & Zemke, R. (2002). Optimizing abilities and capacities: Range of motion, strength, and endurance. In C. Trombly & M. V. Radomski (Eds.), *Occupational therapy for physical dysfunction* (5th ed.). Philadelphia, PA: Lippincott, Williams & Wilkins.

Jacobs, K. (1985). *Occupational therapy: Work-related programs and assessments.* Boston, MA: Little-Brown.

Latella, D., & Meriano, K. (2003). *Occupational therapy manual for evaluation of range of motion and muscle strength.* Clifton Park, NY: Delmar.

Luttgens, K., & Hamilton, N. (1997). *Kinesiology: Scientific basics of human motion* (9th ed.). Madison, WI: Brown & Benchmark.

Morrissey, M. C., Harman, E. A., & Johnson, M. J. (1995). Resistive training modes: Specificity and effectiveness. *Medicine and Science in Sports and Exercise, 27,* 648–660.

Mosey, A. (1988). Role acquisition: An acquisitional frame of reference. In S. Robertson (Ed.), *Mental health focus.* Rockville, MD: American Occupational Therapy Association.

National Board for Certification in Occupational Therapy. (2004). A practice analysis study of entry-level occupational therapist registered and certified occupational therapy assistant practice. *OTJR: Occupation, Participation, and Health, 24,* (Suppl 1).

National Institute for Occupational Safety and Health (NIOSH). (1997). *Elements of ergonomics programs: A primer based on workplace evaluations of musculoskeletal disorders* (DHHS publication N. 97–117). Cincinnati, OH: Author.

Noack, J. (2005). Development of an employer-based injury-prevention program for office workers using ergonomics principles. *Occupational Therapy Practice, 10,* CE1–CE8.

Radomski, M. V., & Trombly, C. (2008). *Occupational therapy for physical dysfunction* (6th ed.). Philadelphia: Lippincott, Williams & Wilkins.

Sabari, J. (2008). Optimizing functional skills using task related training. In M. V. Radomski & C. Trombly Latham (Eds.), Occupational therapy for physical dysfunction, 6th Edition (pp.618-641). Philadelphia: Lippincott, Williams & Wilkins.

Soderberg, G. L. (1997). *Kinesiology: Application to pathological motion* (2nd ed.). Baltimore, MD: Williams & Wilkins.

Trombly, C. (1995). Occupation: Purposefulness and meaningfulness as therapeutic mechanisms. *American Journal of Occupational Therapy, 49,* 960–972.

Trombly C. (2002). Conceptual foundations for practice. In C. Trombly & M. V. Radomski (Eds.), *Occupational therapy for physical dysfunction* (5th ed.). (pp. 1–35). Philadelphia, PA: Lippincott, Williams & Wilkins.

Trombly C. (2008). Conceptual foundations for practice. In M. V. Radomski & C. Trombly (Eds.), *Occupational therapy for physical dysfunction* (6th ed.). (pp. 1–20). Philadelphia: Lippincott, Williams & Wilkins.

Van Deusen, J., & Harlowe, D. (1987). The efficacy of the ROM dance program for adults with rheumatoid arthritis. *American Journal of Occupational Therapy, 41,* 90–95.

Voss, D. E., Ionta, M. K., & Myers, B. J. (1985). *Proprioceptive neuromuscular facilitation: Patterns and techniques* (3rd ed.). Philadelphia, PA: Harper & Row.

World Health Organization. (2001). *International classification of function, disability, and health.* Geneva: Author.

Yasuda, Y. L. (2008). Rheumatoid arthritis, osteoarthritis, and fibromyalgia. In M. V. Radomski & C. Trombly Latham, Eds. *Occupational therapy for physical dysfunction* (6th ed.). (pp. 618–641). Philadelphia, PA: Lippincott, Williams & Wilkins.

Chapter 15

TOGLIA'S DYNAMIC INTERACTIONAL APPROACH

"Cognition is defined as a person's capacity to acquire and use information to adapt to environmental demands."

– LIDZ (1987)

Joan Toglia's dynamic interactional approach to cognitive rehabilitation (2005) has undergone several name changes as it continues to evolve. First introduced in the early 1980s, Toglia and Abreu (1987) developed a cognitive rehabilitation approach for the treatment of traumatic brain injury (TBI). Toglia continued her research in the area of generalization of learning and, in the 1990s, renamed her approach "multi-contextual," implying that cognitive strategies may be generalized and applied to a broader range of life situations if each strategy is applied in multiple contexts during therapy. Kielhofner (2004) continues to call Toglia's approach "cognitive perceptual," while Bruce and Borg (2002) call it "the dynamic interactional model."

FOCUS

This approach has been used with all types of acquired brain injury as well as some mental health and developmental disability populations. The goal is to restore functional performance for persons with cognitive dysfunction. Domains of concern have previously been identified as orientation, attention, visual processing, motor planning, cognition, occupational behaviors, and effort.

THEORETICAL BASE

This approach has its foundation in *neuroscience* and its application guidelines within the theory of occupation. Some key terms from neuroscience are as follows:

- *Cognition* involves a person's capacity to acquire and use information to respond to activity demands, including information processing, learning, and generalization.

- *Information processing* begins with sensory input and continues to organize, assimilate, and integrate new

information with previous experiences. Processing occurs in three stages:

1. Registration of the stimulus event (sensory perception)

2. Analysis (interpretation and organization of raw sensory information)

3. Hypothesis formation (comparing the stimulus with experiences in long-term memory and relating the stimulus to an overall purpose or goal)

- *Systems approach:* current evidence shows that cognition works as a system and cannot be divided into separate sub-skills.

- *Brain plasticity* may be demonstrated in the way the brain forms new neural pathways to relearn the skills of daily living in spite of injury. In other words, there is more than one way to accomplish the same task. Cognition changes with interaction with the external world and may be influenced by guided intervention.

- The brain's *structural capacity* is limited and can process only a limited amount of information at one time. The brain's *functional capacity* demonstrates the ability to use a limited capacity efficiently.

Toglia (2005) has consistently updated her theory, currently integrating occupation-based concepts of person, activity, and the environment. Performance in occupations is based on the ability to perceive and evaluate sensory information and the ability to conceive of, plan, and execute purposeful action. Occupational therapy (OT) concepts that form the basis of the dynamic interactional approach include aspects of the person, the activity, and the environment.

The Person

- *Personal context* includes a person's coping styles, emotional states, expectations, motivations, beliefs, values, and lifestyle. These can significantly influence the way new information is processed. For example, depression or anxiety can interfere with effort toward recovery. Meaningfulness and relevance of an activity influences one's effort to adapt or compensate by using new cognitive strategies.

- *Self-knowledge* is the relatively stable awareness of one's own cognitive ability, strengths, and weaknesses as part of one's self-concept or sense of self.

- *On-line awareness* refers to metacognition, such as judging task demand, anticipating problems, monitoring, regulating, and evaluating one's own performance. Unlike self-knowledge, on-line awareness changes during one's occupational performance.

- *Processing strategies* are small units of behavior that can be used as interventions to increase the effectiveness and efficiency of occupational performance.

- Strategies may be *surface level*, such as memorization, or *deep level*, such as relating new information with old to reflect on meaning and develop a conceptual understanding of something.

- Strategies may be *internal*, such as self-cues and mental repetition, or *external*, such as aids, timers, or environmental cues.

- Strategies differ in their range of application. Some apply to only *specific* situations, such as rehearsing a sequence of steps in doing a task. Other strategies apply to many situations, such as pacing oneself or visualizing consequences, and these may be called *nonspecific*.

The Activity

- *Activity demand* from a cognitive perspective refers to what cognitive capacities and skills are required to do the task. More complex tasks require more time and effort to process and may involve the use of multiple strategies.

- Tasks that are *familiar* and predictable (preparing a favorite recipe) and performed in one's natural environment (one's own kitchen) will be performed with greater efficiency and speed than under other circumstances.

- Regardless of difficulty, activities should be analyzed in contexts within which they will be performed in order to discover or understand the conditions that cause occupational performance to break down.

- *Transfer of learning* may be increased by practicing cognitive strategies in situations that gradually move away from original learning.

The Environment

- *Social context* may facilitate cognitive functioning by structuring and mediating the learning environment to facilitate learning (as a teacher does in a classroom).

- The *zone of proximal development* (Vygotsky, 1978) refers to the distance between unaided performance and guided performance, also called *learning potential* (Feuerstein, 1979), *region of potential restoration of function* (Baltes et al., 1992, 1995), and *zone of rehabilitation potential* (Cicerone & Tupper, 1996). These studies highlight the importance of involving family members, caregivers, and teachers in the rehabilitation process.

- *Cultural context* influences the cognitive recovery process through attitudes about expression of emotion, role expectations, and level of support for client functioning.

- *Physical context* provides a backdrop of potential facilitators or barriers to occupational performance. Environmental conditions, objects, tools, and resources may be organized in logical and familiar ways to provide cues for task performance.

FUNCTION AND DISABILITY

Cognitive functioning requires the ability to receive, elaborate, and monitor incoming information and the flexibility to use and apply one's analysis of information across task boundaries. Traditional OT interventions address attention, memory, and perception. Katz and Hartman-Maeir (2005) include the higher-level cognitive skills necessary for performing occupations, also called metacognitive skills or *executive functions*:

- *Anticipatory awareness*, which allows the person to anticipate problems and plan strategies for compensation

- *Intellectual awareness*, which encompasses a realistic knowledge of one's own deficits, also known as insight

- *Intention*, which includes forming the idea of doing something, motivation, and initiation (Lezak, 1995)

- *Planning*, which includes identification and organization of steps needed to reach a goal, the capacity for sustained attention (concentration), to control impulses, and to choose among alternatives (flexibility and decision-making)

- *Monitoring*, which includes the ability to continually judge one's own performance during purposive action, to self-correct, and to regulate the intensity, tempo, and other qualitative aspects of performance (Lezak, 1995)

Table 15-1

High-Level Cognitive Functions Necessary for Daily Tasks

- Self-awareness
- Goal selection
- Planning steps to achieve a goal
- Initiation of behavior toward implementing the plan
- Inhibiting behavior that would interfere with goal achievement
- Monitoring and evaluating performance in relation to goals
- Strategic problem-solving in the face of obstacles

Adapted from Ylvisaker, M., Szekeres, S. F., & Feneey, T. J. (1998). Cognitive rehabilitation: Executive functions. In M. Ylvisaker (Ed.), Towards brain injury rehabilitation: Children and adolescents (Revised ed.). Boston, MA: Butterworth-Heinemann.

Performance of executive functions includes solving novel problems, modifying behavior within a changing environment, generating strategies, and sequencing complex actions (Elliot, 2003). An operational definition of executive functions in daily occupations (Ylvisaker, Szekeres, & Feneey, 1998) appears in Table 15-1.

Cognitive disability, as summarized by Toglia (2005), involves core deficiencies in the following abilities:

- To select and use efficient processing strategies to organize and structure incoming information
- To anticipate, monitor, and verify the accuracy of performance
- To access previous knowledge when needed (memory)
- To flexibly apply knowledge and skills to a variety of situations (generalization)

These areas of vulnerability or weakness may apply to specific domains, such as visual processing or motor planning, or may occur over a broader range of functioning. People with brain injury often display inflexible and inefficient use of cognitive strategies, decreased awareness, distractibility, and difficulty prioritizing and breaking tasks into steps (Toglia & Golisz, 1990). These issues cause problems not only with task performance but with social participation as well. Thus, cognitive dysfunction is approached from a systems perspective, focusing on the general strategies that interfere with occupational functioning in a variety of areas. Toglia's definition of cognitive dysfunction includes not only deficiencies within the individual but environmental factors and activity parameters as well.

CHANGE AND MOTIVATION

Cognitive change depends upon one's ability to learn and generalize. Self-awareness and processing strategies determine how individuals will be influenced by OT interventions. As part of assessment, occupational therapists need to try out cues and guidance strategies in order to observe client responses to different types of assistance. To observe client learning, it is imperative to observe occupational performance of both familiar and unfamiliar tasks. For example, a client may be able to make a peanut butter and jelly sandwich when provided with all the necessary supplies, but the same client may be unable to prepare lunch when presented with a free choice of food items, working in a normally cluttered kitchen, and simultaneously dealing with unexpected interruptions.

Self-Awareness

Intervention includes helping clients adjust to cognitive changes that have occurred. Clients with brain injury are often unaware of their limitations in cognitive ability and are, therefore, unable to make good judgments about what tasks they should or should not attempt. Skills in the *therapeutic use of self* described by Cole (2005) may be necessary when dealing with barriers to self-awareness. Additionally, structured logs or journals of daily activities can increase self-awareness through reflection and learned self-observation. The effectiveness of journals is increased through review and discussion with the occupational therapist or therapist feedback.

Enabling Transfer of Learning

Transfer of learning is increased through practice of cognitive strategies within multiple contexts. When therapists teach skills embedded in one context, the skills may not be accessible or used in other real-life situations. In a *multicontextual approach*, treatment progresses along a "horizontal continuum that gradually places more demands on the ability to transfer and generalize use of the targeted strategies" (Toglia, 2003). This continuum begins with similar situations (near transfer), moving to somewhat similar activities (intermediate transfer), to physically different activities (far transfer), and ends with very different applications (very far transfer) that include situations of everyday life. The multicontextual approach involves a careful analysis of treatment tasks to determine which parameters will change and which will remain the same. The underlying strategy to be practiced stays constant across the spectrum of intervention activities. Some examples of parameters that can change are number of items or steps, degree of detail, rules or guidelines, number of possible choices, degree of distraction in the environment, types of stimuli, and unpredictability or unfamiliarity of the environment.

Self-Directed Strategies

In this dynamic approach, no distinction is made among establishing or restoring function, making adaptations, or utilizing compensatory strategies. The emphasis on learning effective strategies motivates clients to recognize and overcome cognitive difficulties (e.g., distractibility, disorganization, inattention to one side of the environment, tendency to over-focus on parts of a task, or losing sight of the original goal). Occupational therapists teach clients to be self-directed in checking their own performance, shifting emphasis away from actual task outcome, and focusing on their ability to apply cognitive strategies. Clients also learn to identify and monitor task demands that create cognitive difficulties and environmental conditions under which problems are most likely to emerge. Adaptations and/or compensations are planned collaboratively with the client to prevent the recurrence of problems or difficulties.

EVALUATION

Cognitive impairments can be hidden and not readily observed by others (Golisz & Toglia, 2003). In addition to assessing basic activities of daily living (ADL), instrumental ADL (IADL) beyond the clinical setting and unstructured social, work, and community situational problem-solving may need to be observed by the therapist in order to fully understand the cognitive issues of individual clients.

Learning of self-awareness and processing strategies occurs within the context of occupational performance. Therefore, use of psychological assessments and standardized tests that measure separate cognitive abilities do not accurately reflect the client's cognitive potential.

Dynamic assessment does not refer to a specific procedure or technique, but describes a wide range of methods (Toglia, 2005). In comparison to static assessments, dynamic assessments provide guided assistance to facilitate changes in performance. Toglia suggests that an OT assessment begin with observation of the client's engagement in actual tasks, and include the following components:

- Self-perception of performance and abilities prior to task performance (client is asked to anticipate perceived difficulties and to predict own performance)

- Facilitating changes in performance during the task through cues or strategy teaching and changing the parameters of the task or environment

- Self-perceptions of performance during and after the task (general questioning, estimation, and strategy investigation) (Toglia, 2005, p. 41)

Some published assessment tools created by Toglia are the Contextual Memory Test (CMT) (1993); the Toglia Category Assessment (TCA) (1994), used for assessment of both categorization and deductive reasoning; and the Dynamic Object Search test of visual processing (Toglia & Finkelstein, 1991).

GUIDELINES FOR INTERVENTION

In the dynamic interactional approach, assessment and intervention often cannot be separated. Self-awareness develops within the context of engagement in occupations, and clients often learn to improve task performance through therapist cues and strategies applied during the dynamic interactional assessment. Intervention begins with identifying the specific task parameters within which the client can function (baseline).

Some cognitive strategies for increasing self-awareness (Toglia, 2005) include the following:

- Anticipation of problems or obstacles in proposed task

- Self-prediction about difficulty of the task and own ability to do it

- Self-checking and self-evaluation through checklists or interval monitoring

- Self-questioning using key questions to address client's unique cognitive difficulties, such as "Do I understand the problem?" or "Am I getting sidetracked with irrelevant details?"

- Monitoring time, such as estimating the time limits of a task or interval checking of one's progress with use of a timer

- Role-reversal, in which therapist demonstrates client dysfunctional behaviors during task performance, and client identifies errors/lapses

Some strategies used to improve task performance follow:

- Verbal mediation, which is talking self through steps of a task

- Underlining, circling, or highlighting critical details of instructions

- Stimuli blocking, such as covering parts of reading matter already read

- Visual imagery, which is visualizing self performing task successfully

- Verbalization of object characteristics, prior to making a decision about it

- Categorization, such as arranging items in meaningful clusters (grocery list; contents of drawers, shelves, or closets)

- Task segmentation as a method of simplifying a complex task by breaking it down into smaller steps (cleaning one's house, throwing a party)

- Re-arrangement of items, such as placing cosmetics in the order of their use

Table 15-2		
Near, Intermediate, Far, and Very Far Transfers		
Analyses of Tasks	**Examples to Follow**	**Choose a Strategy and Fill In**
Cognitive strategy to be practiced	Visual scanning top left to bottom right	
Beginning application	Finding your account number on an electric bill	
Near transfer	Finding the phone number of your hairdresser in the yellow pages of a telephone book	
Intermediate transfer	Finding the butter in the refrigerator	
Far transfer	Finding garlic powder in a grocery store	
Very far transfer	Finding a specific address while driving in a car	

- Looking at the whole before focusing on details (scan table of contents of book before beginning to read it)

Applying the Multicontextual Approach

Once a strategy is identified, clients practice using the strategy in a series of different situations. Tasks may be collaboratively chosen but sequenced by the therapist through careful activity analysis. Intervention begins with tasks and environmental conditions that are similar. For example, sorting silverware into piles of similar items on a table, then sorting the same items and putting them into different sections of a drawer. This is a *near transfer* of the sorting strategy. In *intermediate transfer*, the client takes dishes out of a dishwasher and puts similar items on shelves in a cabinet. Selecting colored tiles in preparation for making a tile trivet represents a *far transfer* of the same sorting strategy. Matching socks from a laundry basket represents a *very far transfer*, a daily living task that is very different from previous applications of the sorting strategy. In designing a multicontextual intervention, occupational therapists need to be sure that the cognitive strategy remains constant throughout all the transfer activities. The parameters that make a task more difficult will depend on the skills and constraints of individual clients. Toglia does not specify the number of parameters that must change in differentiating near, intermediate, far, and very far categories, as they are intended only as a general guideline. Use Table 15-2 to practice the grading of activities using Toglia's guidelines. Choose one of the cognitive strategies from the preceding list as an example and fill in the right hand column in Table 15-2.

Using a Memory Notebook

A memory notebook/journal is a cognitive strategy that compensates for deficits in attention and short-term memory. When initiating the use of a journal to assist with remembering or analyzing and reflecting on occupational performance, clients need instruction in when to write notes and how to structure them. First, the client and therapist set a collaborative goal. For example, the goal in using a memory notebook may be to assist in remembering the details of problem situations or to remember facts, things to do, names and telephone numbers of specific people (family members, classmates, people who do home repairs), or monthly bills to pay. Second, intervals for entering information need to be set (e.g., daily or each evening after dinner). Third, identify what information should be written, such as date, name of task, event, or category (problems during grocery shopping, meeting with my study group, cleaning supplies I need to buy) depending on the goal. Some clients with brain injury need to carry a memory notebook with them throughout each day to write the details of activities or experiences they might otherwise forget. In training a hospitalized client to use the notebook, the therapist can assign the client specific information to be written, such as the lunch special in the cafeteria or the price of specific items in the gift shop, and specific things to remember to do (call your mother at 2:00 p.m., write your name on a card and tape it to my door by 6:00 p.m.). Caregivers need to participate in reminding client to use/read notebook to help reinforce its use. Notes may be written in sequence with dates, marking the place with a post-it, and the notebook may be sectionalized and color-coded for different types of information. The occupational therapist should set aside therapy time for reviewing, discussing, and analyzing

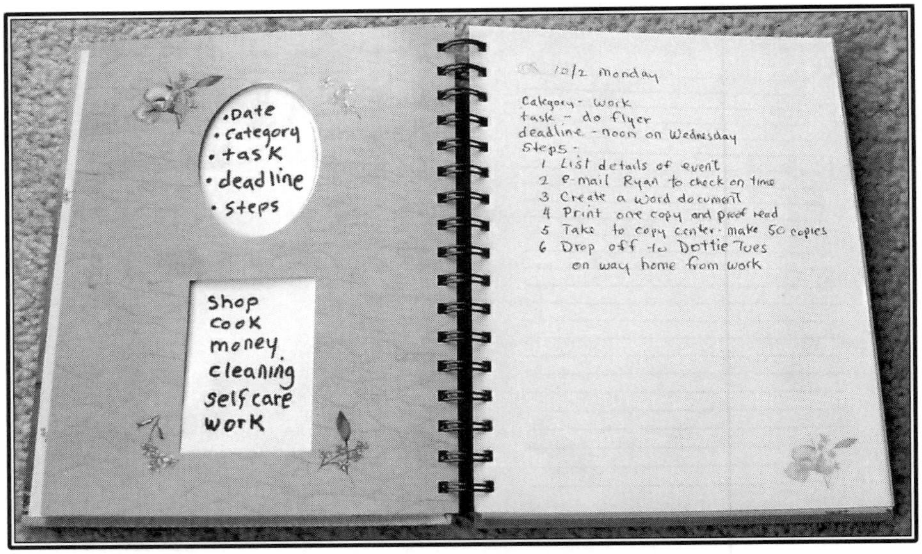

Figure 15-1. Memory notebook with guidelines and categories.

information in the notebook to reinforce its use. Toglia (2004) suggests giving a "notebook quiz" to assist clients in monitoring use of this strategy by asking the following:

- What did you write in the book?
- When did you write in the book?
- What are the different sections for?
- When do you re-read your notes?
- If you want to check your schedule for the day, where do you look?

The questions can be modified to meet different client goals. Techniques for periodic updates to note taking (reducing number or type of entries) and discarding information no longer needed are useful as a client's memory improves. Figure 15-1 shows an example of notebook structure for someone having trouble with planning ahead and meeting deadlines.

Individual Versus Group Intervention

Some cognitive strategies are best learned individually, while others are more appropriately learned within group interventions. Individual OT intervention may be indicated when clients have cognitive difficulties within a specific environment, such as home, school, or work settings. Clients usually need to begin with individual sessions in order to set goals and priorities, establish a baseline of occupational functioning, and choose appropriate cognitive strategies.

In group intervention, members often practice different cognitive strategies or work on individualized goals within the same group session. Activities involving group problem-solving and role-playing offer an opportunity to practice cognitive strategies in realistic social contexts. Some examples of group interventions using the dynamic interactional approach follow:

- Learning and using cognitive strategies along the multicontextual transfer of learning continuum
- Tasks that require cooperative effort, planning, and organization
- Role-playing problem situations to practice understanding different points of view and to consider alternative solutions
- Tasks to increase self-understanding and self-monitoring of cognitive or memory problems
- Tasks that promote attention, memory, and executive functioning
- Tasks that require communication in a variety of sensory areas, such as giving directions to an unfamiliar location through use of a map, visual landmarks, or sequenced verbal directions
- Self-discovery tasks using group feedback to promote insight
- Comparison of different cognitive strategies for doing the same task

RESEARCH

Studies validating this frame of reference include case reports (Landa-Gonzalez, 2001; Toglia, 1989, 1991), and the effectiveness of strategy training. Here is a summary of cognitive strategies that have been researched:

- Verbal mediation (Cicerone & Giacino, 1992; Kray, Eber, & Lindenberger, 2004)
- Self-instruction procedures (Stuss, 1991)
- Mental rehearsal and visual imagery (Driskell, Cooper, & Moran, 1994; Niemeier, 1998)
- Pacing and task reduction methods (Cicerone, 2002)

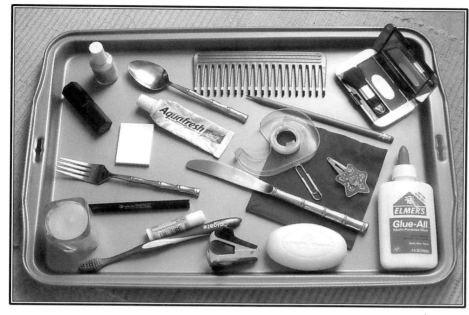

Figure 15-2. Memory tray of 20 items. (Photo courtesy of M. Cole)

- Memory and self-monitoring (Freeman, Mittenberg, Dicowden, & Bat-Ami, 1992)
- Memory retrieval through retrospection and self-questioning (Deelman, Berg, & Koning-Haanstra, 1990)
- Organizational and planning strategies including categorization (Nelson & Lenhart, 1996)
- Problem solving through task reduction, definition of steps, alternate solutions generation, and self-checking (Cicerone, Dahlberg, Kalmar, et al., 2000; Levine et al, 2000)
- Visual imagery strategies for unilateral neglect (Nemeier, Cifu, & Kishore, 2001)

Toglia (2005) concludes that most studies of strategy training report greater success when clients have awareness of goals and the ability to self-monitor. Similar results were found for strategy use in educational settings (Pressley, 1995). Toglia and Kirk (2000) have defined the critical role of awareness to rehabilitation outcomes using the dynamic interactional approach.

LEARNING ACTIVITIES

Group Activity

Materials: Place 20 small common objects on a plain-colored tray or box top so that they can be viewed and identified easily. See example in Figure 15-2. Cover the tray with a cloth so that objects cannot be seen. The leader needs a stopwatch or clock with a second hand. Each group member needs a pencil and paper.

Directions: "I would like to help you develop an awareness of your ability to remember things. I'm going to show you a tray with 20 common items on it. You may get up to

look at it silently for 1 minute, and then go back to your seat and write down as many items as you can remember. To demonstrate your current self-awareness, I'd like each of you to predict how many items you think you will remember in this exercise. Write your name at the top of the paper and, next to it, the number you predict you will remember."

Answer any questions the group may have.

"You may stand in a circle so that you have a good view of the objects. Let me know when you are ready to begin." The leader uncovers the items on the tray, making sure they do not overlap. Time the viewing for exactly 60 seconds. Then, immediately cover the tray again with the cloth. "Now please return to your seats and write down as many of the items as you can remember. You have 2 minutes to write your answers." Time 2 minutes. "Please put your pencils down."

Discussion

1. How many got all 20 items? 19? Etc.?
2. Did you correctly predict your score? Discuss.
3. What mental strategies did you use to remember (clustering, etc.)? Discuss.
4. What might be some everyday occupations where you might need this skill?

Wellness: Dynamic Interactional Approach

Directions: Identify one task from the following list that you might find difficult, and answer the questions:
- Sorting through 2 weeks worth of mail following a vacation

- Clearing out and cleaning your refrigerator after 2 weeks of neglect
- Figuring out your average monthly income and expenses
- Washing 2 weeks worth of laundry, sorting, and putting it away
- Planning a surprise birthday party for your best friend (20 people)

1. What meaning does this task hold for you? Describe the specific environmental conditions and task demands that apply to you when performing this task.
2. Analyze your chosen activity by listing separate steps. Estimate the time you would take to accomplish each step.
3. What executive functions does this task entail? List at least three.
4. With what part of this task would you anticipate having difficulty? Explain.
5. What cognitive strategies or guidelines would you use to accomplish this task?
6. What conditions or task parameters create barriers for you in doing this task?
7. How could you change your daily routine, the environment, and the task parameters to make this task easier in the future?

Using Generalization of Learning

Directions: Use Toglia's concept of generalization of learning by choosing a cognitive strategy to help you do something better. Design a study with the following steps:

- Write a goal for the specific strategy you will practice. For example, increasing your time management by accurately predicting how long tasks will take to complete.
- Describe the steps for applying the strategy. For example, before starting to read an article, write down how long you think it will take you, record how long it actually takes, possibly stop yourself part way through to note the time and revise your prediction.
- Using a multicontextual approach, list five different tasks/scenarios within which you will practice the cognitive strategy.
- Create a form to record your progress. For example, your time predictions, your actual times, and the discrepancies.

- Describe a method to measure outcome. For example, create a pretest/post-test, looking at quality and quantity of occupational performance.

Guideline: 2 pages, single spaced, and sample form for recording progress/outcome.

Case Study 1: Jerry

Jerry, an adolescent with attention deficit disorder (ADD), loved to play "spider solitaire" on his computer. He complained that he always got scores around 140. The therapist suggested a "stop and think" strategy. Instead of impulsively starting to play the game each time the cards were dealt, he should first think of three possible first moves and decide which move would produce the most new moves. When half the cards were dealt, or when he reached a score of 50, he should stop again and predict whether he would win or not and how many more moves it would take for him to win. When he reached a score of 100, he should stop again and revise his prediction. The strategy had several benefits. First, he learned that he could control his impulsiveness by saying "stop and think" to himself, a strategy that could also be used when answering questions in class or on tests. Second, he refocused his goal from getting a better score in the card game to making an accurate prediction.

Reflection

How could Jerry use his newly learned skill in predicting to help him succeed in other aspects of life? What other life situations might he use the "stop and think" strategy to control his impulses? What effect do you think the use of strategies might have on his sense of self-efficacy?

Case Study 2: Julie

Julie sustained a closed head injury during a multi-car collision, resulting in cognitive deficits in attention, organization, and short-term memory. At the time she was a teaching assistant in her fourth year of medical school. Unable to attend classes because of severe neck pain and fatigue, Julie made the difficult decision to drop out of school and worked at home as an editor of medical textbooks. While using a notebook computer, Julie was able to support her neck with pillows in bed and work with the computer on her lap, taking breaks every half hour. Distractabity prevents her from participating in maintaining her apartment, following through with social plans, and meeting deadlines. Her roommate, a fellow medical student, refers her to OT.

Theory Application

Create an intervention plan for Julie using three different cognitive strategies from the dynamic interactive frame of reference.

REFERENCES

Baltes, M. M., Kuhl, K. P., Gutzmann, H., & Sowarka, D. (1995). Potential of cognitive plasticity as a diagnostic instrument: A cross-validation and extension. *Psychology and Aging, 10,* 167–172)

Baltes, M. M., Kuhl, K. P., & Sowarka, D. (1992). Testing for limits of cognitive reserve capacity: A promising strategy for early diagnosis of dementia? *Journal of Gerontology, 17,* 165–167.

Bruce, M., & Borg, B. (2002). *Psychosocial frames of reference: core for occupation-based practice.* Thorofare, NJ: SLACK Incorporated.

Cicerone, K. D. (2002). Remediation of "working attention" in mild traumatic brain injury. *Brain Injury, 16,* 185–195.

Cicerone, K. D., Dahlberg, C., Kalmar, K., Langenbahn, D. M., Malec, J. F., Bergquist, T. F., et al. (2000). Evidence-based cognitive rehabilitation: Recommendations for clinical practice. *Archives of Physical Medicine and Rehabilitation, 81,* 1596–1615.

Cicerone, K. D., & Giacino, J. T. (1992). Remediation of executive function deficits after traumatic brain injury. *NeuroRehabilitation, 2,* 12–22.

Cicerone, K. D., & Tupper, D. E. (1986). Cognitive assessment in the neuropsychological rehabilitation of head-injured adults. In B. P. Uzzell & Y. Gross (Eds.), *The clinical neuropsychology of intervention* (pp. 59–84). Boston: Martines Nijhoff.

Cole, M. B. (2005). *Group dynamics in occupational therapy* (3rd ed.). Thorofare, NJ: SLACK Incorporated.

Deelman, B. G., Berg, I. J., & Koning-Haanstra, M. (1990). Memory strategies for closed-head injured patients: Do lessons in cognitive psychology help? In R. Wood & I. Fussy (Eds.), *Cognitive rehabilitation in perspective.* London, UK: Taylor & Francis.

Driskell, J. E., Cooper, C., & Moran, A. (1994). Does mental practice enhance performance? *Journal of Applied Psychology, 79,* 481–492.

Elliott, J. (2003). Dynamic assessment in educational settings: Realizing potential. *Educational Review, 55,* 15–32.

Feuerstein, R. (1979). *The dynamic assessment of retarded performers: The learning potential device, theory, instruments, and techniques.* Baltimore, MD: University Park Press.

Freeman, M. R., Mittenberg, W., Dicowden, M., & Bat-Ami, M. (1992). Executive and compensatory memory retraining in traumatic brain injury. *Brain Injury, 6,* 65–70.

Golisz, K. & Toglia, J. (2003). Perception and cognition. In E. B. Crepear, E. S. Cohn, & A. B. Schell (Eds.), *Willard and Spackman's occupational therapy* (10th ed.). Philadelphia, PA: Lippincott, Williams & Wilkins.

Katz, N., & Hartman-Maeir, A. (2005). Higher-level cognitive functions: Awareness and Executive functions enabling engagement in occupation. In N. Katz (Ed.), *Cognition and occupation in rehabilitation: Cognitive models for intervention in occupational therapy.* Bethesda, MD: American Occupational Therapy Association.

Kielhofner, G. (2004). *Conceptual foundations of occupational therapy* (3rd ed.). Philadelphia, PA: FA Davis.

Kray, J., Eber, E., & Lindenberger, U. (2004). Age differences in executive functioning across the lifespan: The role of verbalization in task preparation. *Acta Psychologica, 115,* 143–165.

Landa-Gonzalez, B. (2001). Multicontextual occupational therapy intervention: A case study of traumatic brain injury. *Occupational Therapy International, 8,* 49–62.

Levine, B., Robertson, I. H., Clare, L., Carter, G., Hong, I., Wilson, B. A., et al. (2000). Rehabilitation of executive functioning: An experimental clinical validation of goal management training. *Journal of the International Neuropsychological Society, 6,* 299–312.

Lezak, M. D. (1995). *Neuropsychological assessment.* New York, NY: Oxford University Press.

Lidz, C. S. (1987). Cognitive deficiencies revisited. In C. S. Lidz (Ed.), *Dynamic assessment: Evaluating learning potential* (pp. 444–478). New York: Guilford.

Nelson, D. L., & Lenhart, D. A. (1996). Resumption of outpatient occupational therapy for a young woman five years after traumatic brain injury. *American Journal of Occupational Therapy, 50,* 223–228.

Niemeier, J. P. (1998). The lighthouse strategy: Use of a visual imagery technique to treat visual inattention in stroke patients. *Brain Injury, 12,* 399–406.

Niemeier, J. P., Cifu, D. X., & Kishore, R. (2001). The lighthouse strategy: Improving the functional status of patients with unilateral neglect after stroke and brain injury using a visual imagery intervention. *Topics in Stroke Rehabilitation, 8*(2), 10–18).

Pressley, M. (1995). More about the development of self-regulation: Complex, long-term, and thoroughly social. *Educational Psychologist, 30,* 207–212.

Stuss, D. T. (1991). Disturbances of self-awareness after frontal system damage. In G. P. Prigatano & D. L. Schacter (Eds.), *Awareness of deficit after brain injury.* New York, NY: Oxford U. Press.

Toglia, J. (1991). Generalization of treatment: A multicontext approach to cognitive perceptual impairment in adults with brain injury. *American Journal of Occupational Therapy, 45,* 505–516.

Toglia, J. (1993). *Contextual memory test.* San Antonio, TX: Psychological Corp.

Toglia, J. (1994). *Dynamic assessment of categorization skills: The Toglia category assessment.* Pequannock, NJ: Maddak.

Toglia, J. (2003). Multicontext treatment approach. In E. Crepeau, E. Cohn, & B. Boyt Schell (Eds.), *Willard & Spackman's occupational therapy.* Philadelphia, PA: Lippincott, Williams & Wilkins.

Toglia, J. (2005). A dynamic interactional approach to cognitive rehabilitation. In N. Katz (Ed.), *Cognition and occupation in rehabilitation: Cognitive models for intervention in occupational therapy.* Bethesda, MD: American Occupational Therapy Association.

Toglia, J. (1989). Approaches to cognitive assessment of the brain-injured adult: Traditional methods and dynamic intervention. *Occupational Therapy Practice, 1,* 36–57.

Toglia, J. (2004). *Dynamic assessment and unilateral neglect. Unpublished doctoral dissertation.* New York: Columbia University.

Toglia, J., & Abreu, B. (1987). *Cognitive rehabilitation.* New York, NY: Authors.

Toglia, J., & Finkelstein, N. (1991). *Test protocol: The dynamic visual processing assessment.* New York, NY: New York Hospital Cornell Medical Center.

Toglia, J., & Golisz, K. (1990). Cognitive rehabilitation: Group games and activities. Tucson, AZ: Therapy Skillbuilders.

Toglia, J., & Kirk, U. (2000). Understanding awareness deficits following brain injury. *NeuroRehabilitation, 15,* 57–70.

Vygotsky, L. S. (1978). *Mind in society: The development of higher psychological processes.* Cambridge, MA: Harvard University Press.

Ylvisaker, M., Szekeres, S. F., & Feneey, T. J. (1998). Cognitive rehabilitation: Executive functions. In M. Ylvisaker (Ed.), *Towards brain injury rehabilitation: Children and adolescents* (Revised ed.). Boston, MA: Butterworth-Heinemann.

Chapter 16

ALLEN'S COGNITIVE LEVELS FRAME

"We believe that occupational therapy should be driven by the (client's) best ability to function."

– ALLEN, BLUE, & EARHART (1995, P. 3)

Claudia Allen began working on the cognitive levels at Eastern Pennsylvania Psychiatric Institute during the late 1960s; I (M. Cole) was privileged to work with her as a student and entry-level therapist. The cognitive levels, as observed in clients with chronic mental illness, were originally based on Piaget's theory (1972) of intellectual development and further developed from the foundations of neuroscience in the works of Russian physiologist Alexandr Luria (1966). The six clinically defined cognitive levels and 52 cognitive modes offer occupational therapists some of the best detailed guidelines for assessing, assisting, and adapting environments for persons with cognitive disabilities. Use of Allen's frame of reference grew rapidly in mental health settings during the 1980s (Allen, 1982; Allen, 1985; Allen & Allen, 1987; Allen, 1987). As new evidence in cognitive neuroscience and cognitive psychology has emerged, Allen's cognitive disabilities frame of reference has been updated by Levy and Burns (2005) and renamed the cognitive disabilities reconsidered model (Burns & Levy, 2006; Levy & Burns, 2005). For the most part, this new evidence validates the original six levels and coincides with the "trajectory of dementing diseases" and the cognitive limitations that can be observed during performance of routine tasks for older adults with dementia (Burns & Levy, 2006).

LEVELS OF WELLNESS

While Allen's use of the term disabilities is currently unpopular, the approach is designed to promote a client's best ability to function despite limitations. However, that is not the only reason I (M. Cole) use this term. Each person uses different levels of cognitive effort in going about his or her daily activities. I have asked my students to identify examples of daily tasks they perform at each of the Allen cognitive levels (ACLs). They almost always use sleeping for ACL 1; ACL 2 is walking to class, climbing the stairs, taking a seat, jogging on the treadmill, and so

forth for every level up to ACL 6, taking an exam, writing a paper, or creating a study schedule. As a wellness model, my students have used Allen guidelines to reorganize their task environments for greater efficiency and have applied the principle of brain conservation to simplify their daily routines (thereby reserving higher level cognitive skills for processing and learning new information in class).

FOCUS

ACLs apply to all performance areas of the framework domain (American Occupational Therapy Association [AOTA], 2002), including activities of daily living, instrumental activities of daily living, education, work, play, leisure, and social participation. This frame of references focuses on the role of cognition (a process skill), the role of habits and routines, the effect of physical and social contexts, and the analysis of activity demand. Types of health conditions that include cognitive deficits are dementias, acquired head injuries, chronic mental illness, chronic diseases affecting the nervous system, and developmental disabilities. Limitations in cognitive ability create predictable safety issues in daily occupations and have been used to guide decisions regarding the client's ability to live independently, demonstrate autonomy in being self-directed, and show competence in managing one's own affairs.

THEORETICAL BASE

Allen defines a *cognitive disability* as "a global incapacity to do universal human activities. A biologically determined lack of attention impairs awareness of environmental cues but may spare memories of prior knowledge" (Allen, 2002). Occupational therapists familiar with the attributes of the six ACLs can observe limitations in routine task behavior that clearly demonstrate the client's level of cognitive disability.

The concept of *brain conservation* explains why people with normal or unimpaired cognitive ability sometimes function at lower ACL levels in doing daily tasks (Allen, 1985). The brain tends to expend only the amount of energy necessary to adequately perform a task. When the steps of a task are familiar and practiced routinely, as many self-care tasks are (e.g., brushing one's teeth, taking a shower), people perform these tasks in the range of ACL 3 (i.e., in a habitual way that does not require much awareness). This is the brain's way of conserving energy for more difficult or complex tasks.

Allen uses the concept of *task equivalence* to identify daily life activities that have similar physical and cognitive demands based on task analysis. For example, the ACL screening (ACLS) assessment uses leather lacing stitches, which have been researched and found to be "equivalent" to various daily tasks. *Task analysis* is a method of determining the complexity of an activity by separating the activity into steps and determining the physical and cognitive functional capacities required to perform each step. Analysis of a variety of crafts has been accomplished in the Allen Diagnostic Module (ADM) (available from S & S Worldwide [Colchester, CT] [1-800-642-7354]), an alternate assessment of ACLs that can be administered in groups, with specific task behaviors defined at each level and mode.

The *task demand* includes the materials, equipment, instructions, assistance, and skills necessary to accomplish a task. This concept coincides with the AOTA Practice Framework's "activity demands" category, which includes the objects, space, social demands, sequencing and timing, required actions, and body functions and structures necessary to do the activity (AOTA, 2002). The demands of the task or activity are derived from the task analysis together with contextual factors. They become important when it becomes necessary or appropriate to adapt the demands of a task in order to facilitate occupational performance. Task demand changes when clients have prior experience with the activity because they can rely on procedural memory to substitute for working memory.

The *task environment* is the setting in which the task is performed, including furniture and seating, lighting, temperature, placement of supplies, equipment available, positioning of clients, assistance available, and other relevant attributes affecting occupational performance. Allen (1985) provides specific guidelines for structuring the task environment at each cognitive level and mode to optimally facilitate a client's best ability to function. The portion of the environment of which clients are aware at different cognitive levels is described in Figure 16-1. Generally, as cognitive levels increase, awareness of the environment expands.

Figure 16-1. Allen's usable task environments at different cognitive levels. (Adapted from Allen, C. K. [1985]. *Occupational therapy for psychiatric diseases: Measurement and management of cognitive disabilities [p. 99].* Boston, MA: Little, Brown & Co.)

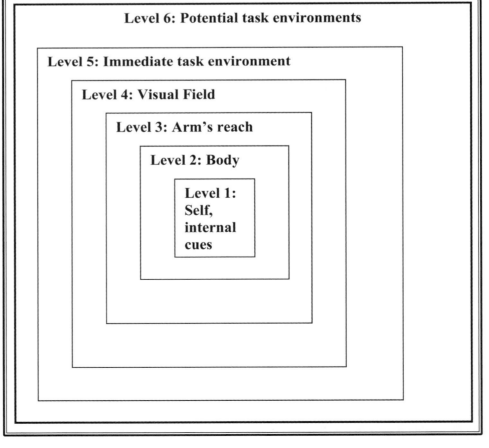

Just Right Challenge

In selecting activities for evaluation and intervention, task demand is matched to the individual's current capacity to function. This provides a sense of well being and motivation for the client to stretch his or her own cognitive resources. This process requires activity analysis and synthesis. Allen makes this easy for occupational therapists by providing assessment tools using both crafts and activities of daily living, with rating guidelines that approximate the cognitive level of the client.

Information Processing Model: Extrinsic and Intrinsic Factors

Extrinsic Factors

Extrinsic factors are those things that we can observe. Occupational therapists make assumptions about clients' ability to process information by observing how they respond to environmental cues and the behaviors they demonstrate during task performance.

- *Cues* are objects or conditions in the environment that stimulate the senses. In the context of tasks, objects, supplies and tools, demonstrations, verbal or written instructions, and a completed sample to follow provide cues that facilitate task performance.

- *Attention* changes as cognitive level increases. Figure 16-1 gives some general guidelines for what parts of the environment clients are likely to pay attention to. For example, at ACL 4, clients are most tuned in to visual cues. This means they learn best by visual demonstrations and by seeing a completed sample of the goal. This does not mean that a client functioning at level 4 does not hear verbal instructions or cannot read written instructions. It simply means that visual cues are the most efficient way for him or her to learn.

- *Motor action* or activity provides another way for therapists to observe information processing. For example, we tell a client to rinse the paint brush in water before using another color paint. If the client acts on our suggestion, we might assume that he can attend to verbal instruction (probably close to ACL 5). If the client ignores the instruction, Allen would suggest that we try another type of cue, such as demonstration. When adding a visual cue results in the desired motor action (i.e., client washes his brush), we assume that he is currently functioning at ACL 4.

- *Speed* or pace of activity can reflect the efficiency with which clients process information.

Intrinsic Factors

Intrinsic factors of the information processing model are internal processes that can only be implied or interpreted through assessments and observations.

- *Visual spatial* information processing, often attributed to the right brain, includes creativity, imagination, and the ability to see the big picture or holistic view.

- *Verbal propositional* information processing, often attributed to the left brain, includes reasoning and language/communication ability, understanding of cause and effect, classification, timing, and sequencing.

- *Memory's* role in information processing has changed in light of recent research. Memory includes what one is doing now and what one has learned in the past. The *working memory model* expands our understanding of attention or awareness as the initial step in processing information. The working memory processes new information and temporarily stores it in *short-term memory*. Learning requires the transfer of short-term memory to *long-term memory*.

Levy's Cognitive Disabilities Reconsidered Model

Linda Levy (2005) updates Allen's cognitive disabilities frame of reference in two important ways: 1) by revising the interactions and categorizations of memory within the information processing model, and 2) by grounding the ACLs within occupational performance and best practice (Burns & Levy, 2006). First, Levy cites new findings from neurocognitive research on three interconnected memory systems: sensory perceptual memory, working memory, and long-term memory.

Sensory Perceptual Memory

Sensory perceptual memory includes information gathered from the environment. Much of the information is filtered out and only what is "deemed relevant" is retained for further processing. Much of the screening process is automatic and below the level of consciousness. Sensory impairments in older adults can limit the amount of information coming into the system. For example, persons with low vision will not take note of changes within the visual field, relevant or not. Citing the process of late-stage dementia (ACLs 1 and 2), Levy notes that when deficits exist, little information is transmitted to working memory for processing. Some dementia research has suggested that deficits in visual and auditory perception are related to the severe perceptual distortions of hallucinations and delusions that often occur in severe stages of the disease (Leiter & Cummings, 1999). Accurate perceptions are necessary in order for a client to respond to environmental cues. A caregiver cues the client by telling him or her the next step of a task, "now its time to put on your socks" or "you need to rinse the shampoo out of your hair before you get out of the shower." Verbal cues can only be followed if they make it through the sensory perceptual memory screening process and are relayed to working memory, where they can be recognized as familiar concepts.

Figure 16-2. Levy's cognitive disabilities reconsidered model. (Reprinted with permission from Levy, L. L. & Burns, T. [2005]. Cognitive disabilities reconsidered: Rehabilitation of older adults with dementia. In N. Katz [Ed.], *Cognition & occupation across the life span: Models for intervention in occupational therapy* (pp. 347–388). Bethesda, MD: American Occupational Therapy Association.)

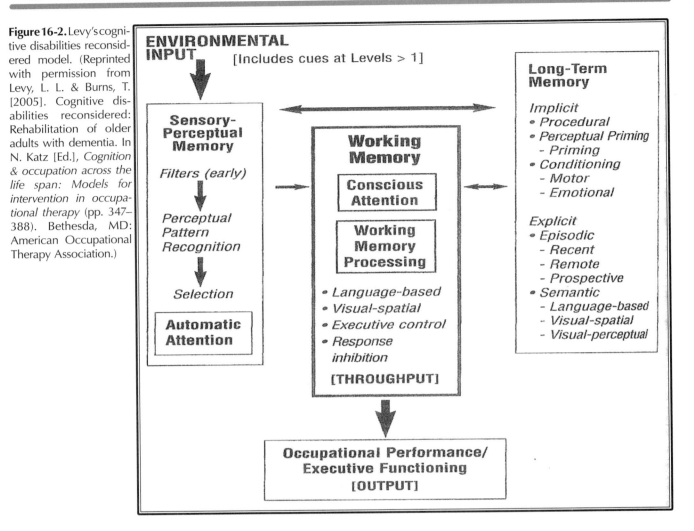

Working Memory

Working memory is an exceedingly complex concept. As noted in Figure 16-2, it coordinates perceptions with long-term memory. Intact working memory retrieves relevant information stored in long-term memory, while at the same time screening out distracting sensory information so that a person can focus on a task. Working memory provides all of the information needed for performing occupations. Additionally, working memory allows the person to perform executive functions such as planning, setting goals, and problem-solving. Allen level 6 problem solving requires a well-functioning working memory. This concept replaces the concept of short-term memory as a necessary first step in new learning. When Allen talked about new learning being unlikely at level 4, she was referring to deficits in working memory, which Levy concurs become obvious by ACL 4.

Long-Term Memory

Long-term memory includes two general categories: explicit and implicit.

Explicit Memory Stores

Levy describes two memory stores in this category: semantic and episodic. Semantic memory involves what we generally refer to as knowledge. This has also been called declarative memory, and it is the most stable type, showing a slower rate of decline with increased age. Speaking and understanding language is an example of semantic memory. Episodic memories are tied to a specific event or circumstance. Allen (1999) uses the example of teaching a client safety precautions. This type of memory must be formed at higher cognitive levels and is easier to recall if episodic (such as learning kitchen safety while performing kitchen tasks). Deficits in episodic memory for newly learned situations is typically one of the earliest and most diagnostic symptoms of Alzheimer's disease (Duchek, Cheney, Ferraro, & Storandt, 1991; Levy & Burns, 2005).

Implicit Memory Stores

Implicit memory stores are things people have learned without being aware of it. There are three types: procedural memory, perceptual priming, and conditioning. *Procedural memory* includes skills and habits for doing things. Using this type of memory typically does not require conscious thought. Examples of activities that rely on procedural memory are walking, talking, driving, knitting, keyboarding, and playing the piano. When occupational therapists work with clients who have acquired cognitive dysfunction, such as a stroke, procedural memory helps to explain what they can still do in terms of self-care. Clients at ACL 5 and 6 may have enough short-term memory for new learning, but at ACL 4 and below, they do not. At the lower cognitive levels, therapists rely on procedural memories and work on providing cues that help clients retrieve the habits of self-care and doing activities that were already stored in long-term memory prior to the onset of illness. *Perceptual priming* is an unconscious process by which prior exposure to a stimulus activates association networks. This automatic association helps to explain the concept of subliminal learning and can have implications for some instantaneous affective responses to stimuli. *Conditioning* is the most automatic form of memory. Allen uses classical conditioning to describe learning at the lower cognitive levels. For example, constantly cueing a client at ACL 3 seems to facilitate task completion without conscious awareness.

FUNCTION AND DISABILITY

Allen defines six cognitive levels and 52 modes of performance to define the range of cognitive function and disability (scale of 0.8 to 6.8). Below level 1 is basically comatose, and above level 6 is considered normal functioning. Allen (1999) has identified ACL 4.6 as minimal for living independently with the condition that dangerous items in the environment are removed or disabled and some supervision is available.

The six ACLs will be reviewed here as general categories of function and dysfunction. It is recommended that students purchase and use *Understanding Cognitive Performance Modes* (Allen, Blue & Earhart, 1995) (available from Allen Conferences, Inc. [Ormond Beach FL] [1-800-853-2472 or http://www.allen-cognitive-levels.com]). The modes further define each whole level.

Table 16-1 outlines the information processing parameters for each whole cognitive level (not modes). The categories in the table will be used as a guide to describe each level. All the ACLs and modes have names that describe a defining feature of that level.

Table 16-1

Allen's Cognitive Levels: 1 to 6

	ACL 1. Automatic Actions	ACL 2. Postural Actions	ACL 3. Manual Actions	ACL 4. Goal-Directed Actions	ACL 5. Exploratory Actions	ACL 6. Planned Actions
Attention to Sensory Cues	Subliminal	Proprioceptive	Tactile	Visible	Related (all senses)	Symbolic
Motor Actions						
Spontaneous	Automatic	Postural	Manual	Goal-directed	Exploratory	Planned
Imitated	None	Approximations	Manipulations	Replications	Novelty	Unnecessary
Conscious Awareness						
Purpose	Arousal	Comfort	Interest	Compliance	Self-control	Reflection
Experience	Indistinct	Moving	Touching	Seeing	Inductive reasoning	Deductive reasoning
Process	Habitual or reflexive	Effect on body	Effect on environment	Several actions	Overt trial and error	Covert trial and error
Time (attention span)	Seconds	Minutes	Half-hours	Hours	Weeks	Past/future
OT Activities	Sensory stimulation	Gross-motor, games, dance	Simple, repetitive tasks	Several-step tasks	Concrete tasks	Conceptual and complex tasks

Level 1: Automatic Actions

Picture someone coming out of a coma moving his or her fingers and toes, blinking his or her eyes with the bright light, and perhaps moaning or making sounds to indicate he or she is uncomfortable. Attention to *sensory cues* is subliminal (i.e., from within a person's own body, such as hunger, thirst, pain, or temperature). *Motor actions* are mainly reflexive and the blankness of his or her eyes implies that not much information processing is occurring. Therapy might be done for the purpose of arousal using sensory stimulation activities. A bright colored balloon might capture the client's attention for a few seconds; pop the balloon and the client demonstrates a startle response to the sound. Level 1 is the lowest end of the cognitive disability scale and consists of the following modes:

- *ACL 1.0:* Withdrawing from stimuli: Edge of consciousness
- *ACL 1.2:* Responding to stimuli
- *ACL 1.4:* Locating stimuli
- *ACL 1.6:* Moving in bed
- *ACL 1.8:* Raising body parts

Level 2: Postural Actions

Clients at level 2 respond best to *proprioceptive cues.* Moving a client's arm to reach for a railing or taking the client's hand and leading him or her to the dining room are examples of proprioceptive cues. Persons at level 2 are not always physically disabled, but one of their main concerns is body comfort and stability. At the midrange of level 2, clients are able to imitate movements. However, their *imitations are approximate,* not exact. I once designed a feeding program for an elderly client functioning at level 2. He sat in an adapted wheelchair with a tray to eat. His left side was weak because of a stroke, but he had good strength and flexibility in his right arm. I provided an adapted bowl with suction cups to keep it from sliding and filled the bowl with applesauce. To cue him, I placed his fingers around the spoon handle and moved his arm through the motions of scooping a spoonful of applesauce and bringing it to his lips. The movements of self-feeding are stored in procedural memory for most people, but retrieval of the movements requires cuing, proprioceptive cues in the case of this client. Once begun, he repeated the motion and fed himself the rest of the applesauce. This small step will not make him an independent eater. With each part of his meal, a caregiver will need to set up his bowl and cue him.

Clients at level 2 can attend to an activity for several minutes at a time. However, they may not sit for an entire meal. They are *motivated by comfort* and will rock in a rocking chair, for example, because it makes them feel good. At the beginning of level 2, clients need a great deal of physical assistance and guidance. As they move toward level 3, OT activities involving postural movements, simple exercises, motor games such as batting a balloon or kicking a beach ball, or simple dances to music are possible.

Modes of performance within level 2 include the following:

- *ACL 2.0:* Overcoming gravity
- *ACL 2.2:* Standing and using righting reactions
- *ACL 2.4:* Walking
- *ACL 2.6:* Walking to identified location
- *ACL 2.8:* Using railings and grabbing bars for support

The Lower Cognitive Levels Test is nonstandardized and seems to discriminate between ACLs 2 and 3. Directions are as follows: Get the client's attention. Say, "Watch what I do, and then you do the same thing. Okay?" Clap your hands loudly three times at eye level. Say, "Now you do it." If the client can copy three audible claps and stop, he or she is probably at level 3. Clients at level 2 will give approximate imitations, such as clapping silently or doing more or less than three claps. This may be a useful test when identifying clients who will be able to participate in groups, engage in craft projects, or perform the ACLS test, all of which begin at ACL 3.

Case: Theis

My (M. Cole) mother, Theis, now age 91, lived with me until she reached ACL 2, which is equivalent to stage 7, severe dementia (Alzheimer's). Now in a nursing home, she remains at level 2 (Figure 16-3). She feeds herself 50% of

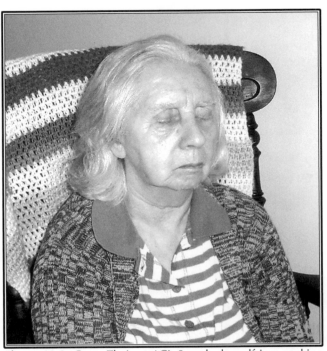

Figure 16-3. Case: Theis at ACL 2 rocks herself in a rocking chair.

meals; walks behind a wheelchair, holding on for support and balance; and still attends daily exercise groups, where she imitates the leader and has been observed tapping her toes to the music. She does not speak and does not recognize me any more. I can get her attention by gently shaking her arm, and recently when I placed a piece of chocolate mint on her tongue, she opened her eyes and seemed to say "thanks, my favorite."

(I will continue this example through each ACL level.)

Level 3: Manual Actions

Manipulation of objects is necessary to accomplish most self-care tasks. While clients at level 2 can only assist caregivers, some self-care can be done independently at level 3. Therapists may capture the client's attention with *tactile cues* (in addition to proprioceptive cues), and the client will *imitate manual actions that are demonstrated*. At this level it is important to give tactile cues for self-care tasks that are stored in procedural memory. Many ordinary tasks are culture-specific (i.e., the client previously had a set way of doing them, and recall will be dependent on familiar cues). New learning is not in place at level 3; therefore, clients need frequent cues when performing unfamiliar tasks.

At level 3, clients will be motivated to do simple craft projects that involve manipulating interesting objects and textures. In doing a craft project, they will need the steps demonstrated one at a time. Clients can concentrate for up to 30 minutes and will continue repeating a step until they reach the end (leather lacing) or all the materials are used up (e.g., stringing beads, stuffing envelopes, folding laundry).

Level 3 includes the following modes of performance:

- *ACL 3.0:* Grasping objects
- *ACL 3.2:* Distinguishing among objects
- *ACL 3.4:* Sustaining acts on objects
- *ACL 3.6:* Noting the effects of actions on objects
- *ACL 3.8:* Using all objects and sensing completion of an activity

Case: Theis, Continued

My mother got into a lot of trouble at level 3. She liked to walk, but could not find her way back home. On one occasion, a health care worker who was not paying attention left the front door ajar. An hour later, I found my mother half a mile down Main Street on her way to visit her parents (who had died many years ago). We got her a "safe return" bracelet after that (her name, our address, and my phone number etched on it).

Precaution: Persons at ACL 3 should not be left alone.

At ACL 3, my mother was no longer oriented to time. She would get up in the middle of the night, turn on lights, and see what she could manipulate. Sometimes I heard her, but often she did not wake me up. One morning, I found

her at the breakfast table surrounded by pieces of a radio she had somehow taken apart. It was still plugged in!

Precaution: Caregivers need to child-proof areas that may be accessed during the night or any other time person may be momentarily unsupervised.

Persons at ACL 3 tend to pick up whatever looks interesting. One unfortunate home health aid left her purse on the counter while she made a phone call. We found it several hours later under my mother's bed, along with stacks of pilfered mail that included several overdue bills.

Precaution: Do not leave important (fragile, dangerous) items out in plain view.

On a positive note, my mother and her pet Chihuahua, Crissy, were inseparable. She carried that dog everywhere, even to bed. Crissy kept my mother out of trouble for many hours and offered her own brand of warm, tactile comfort. However, at ACL 3, Theis was not aware of the needs of a pet. I had to feed Crissy and take her out for walks, usually under my mother's protest. Even then, Crissy wet the bed almost every night.

Precaution: Clients at level 3 should not be responsible for the care of pets!

Level 4: Goal-Directed Actions

There is a vast difference between levels 3 and 4, and that difference is goal-directedness. In activities of daily living, it marks the change from being dependent on others to being self-directed. Many self-care tasks can be performed independently at level 4. Working memory functions longer in the immediate situation, making it possible for the client to recall a sequence of steps toward a goal. *Visual cues* work best with ACL 4 (in addition to proprioceptive and tactile cues). The focus on vision allows the client to see errors when comparing his or her own project with a sample. Demonstrations are still necessary for performing unfamiliar tasks, but the occupational therapist can now demonstrate *several steps at a time*. In craft activities, a sample that is the exact match of the client's project can serve as a visual goal. Longer term activities up to 1 hour in length can be done.

The visual field is very significant at level 4 because things that were not noticed at level 3 now become distractions. When working in a cluttered environment, it is difficult for clients at level 4 to select relevant or needed items, and their occupational performance will be slow and inefficient. Best ability to function may be seen when only items needed to do the task are visible. In home environments, occupational therapists advise caregivers to simplify task environments by getting rid of clutter and to facilitate self-care tasks by placing needed items in plain view (e.g., laying out clothing items on the bed or keeping all bathing items in a basket next to the tub).

Modes of performance at level 4 are as follows:

- *ACL 4.0:* Sequencing self through steps of an activity

- *ACL 4.2:* Differencing among parts of an activity
- *ACL 4.4:* Completing a goal
- *ACL 4.6:* Scanning the environment
- *ACL 4.8:* Memorizing new steps

Special importance is given to ACL Mode 4.6 because it is the lowest level at which clients should be left alone. However, at this level, they still need a great deal of protection and supervision. Allen describes the change from 4.4 to 4.6 as follows: "At 4.4 you can see all the way to the edge of the table and a little bit of your neighbor in front of you. At 4.6 you pick your head up and look around the room" (1999, p. 98). She gives the example of a client smelling coffee and wanting some. The clients at 4.4 will ask, "Where's the coffee pot?" At 4.6, they will get up and help themselves.

Case: Theis, Continued

My mother's level 4 stage gave me a good education about level 4 thinking. When people have dementia, their cognitive level declines in some predictable ways, and one way is losing an understanding of things you cannot see. One day I had a landscaper come over to trim the shrubs. It was late spring, and I simultaneously took the house plants, which stayed on a table in the breezeway all winter, and put them in planter pots out on the patio. This disturbed my mother, who thought something just did not look right. I noticed her collecting the clippings from the shrubs, and when I came into the breezeway, my mother had "planted" the clippings in cans and empty boxes, so that the table looked much as it had before I moved the house plants outside. Her understanding of how things grow, an abstract concept, was lost.

The loss of abstract thought became painfully clear when I found a bottle of Pine Sol in the refrigerator (she thought it was apple juice). "Didn't you read the label?" I asked. She could read the words but their meaning was lost. Likewise, I had prepared a chicken casserole for dinner, and she decided to embellish it by adding a layer of dog food. My mother had lost the ability to distinguish between things that look similar. Written words also represent abstract concepts that are no longer understood.

On another occasion, I awoke to find her inserting neatly stacked orange cocktail napkins into the toaster. Electricity was an abstract concept she could no longer understand.

Precaution: Disable or remove electric appliances and lock up cleaning materials. Do not depend on labels to distinguish the use or purpose of items. Putting things out of sight usually works because if a level 4 client cannot see them, they do not exist for the client.

Level 5: Exploratory Actions

As the title implies, thinking at level 5 is inductive, or trial and error. An understanding of three dimensions begins at this level. It is interesting to watch clients at level 5 start a woodworking project. Without assistance, they will skip the instructions and immediately begin to fit the pieces together, using a trial-and-error approach. Unfortunately, they use a similar strategy to see if the iron is hot. *Overt trial and error* means they have to actually do it to know if it works. They are *unable to anticipate* or plan ahead. This explains why ACL 5 clients have been called impulsive or accident prone. Spontaneous actions are exploratory because level 5 clients like to try new things and create unique or individualized projects (not following the sample). In OT, we always give them choices. Persons at level 5 can learn by *relating all types of cues* up to and including *verbal instructions*. Longer-term projects that last for more than one session are possible, and learning carries over from one weekly session to the next. Occupational therapists often use ongoing projects to encourage the ability to anticipate and plan, which is difficult for clients at level 5. At level 5, clients have issues with self-control, and precautions need to be taken for clients to adhere to safety guidelines when doing activities.

Modes of performance at level 5 are:

- *ACL 5.0:* Learning to improve effects of actions
- *ACL 5.2:* Improving the fine details of actions
- *ACL 5.4:* Engaging in self-directed learning
- *ACL 5.6:* Considering social standards
- *ACL 5.8:* Consulting with other people

Working with clients at level 5 always involves making decisions and judgments (what color combination looks best, or how long does the paint take to dry?). Level 5.6 has special significance because it is the point at which clients begin to have insight and become aware of the social as well as physical consequences of their actions (Allen, 1999). This makes an understanding of the perceptions of others possible. Relationships with friends and family members have far less turmoil after this level, although there may still be verbal conflicts and a win/lose perception of disagreements with others.

Some occupations of daily living that require anticipation are menu planning, shopping, budgeting, planning or packing for trips, cleaning out closets, planning a daily or weekly schedule, entertaining others, and caring for children. All are difficult for a person at level 5 ACL.

Case: Theis, Continued

In recalling the first signs of my mother's dementia, I can attribute many incidents to trial-and-error thinking and my mother's failure to plan ahead. Like the time I got the call from the security office at the mall, informing me that my parents had lost their car in the parking lot. It is a big parking lot and could happen to anyone. This did not seem a big deal to me until, on another occasion, I arrived home from a weekend away to find that the car was gone. Neither of my parents knew where the car was, but my father (who was blind) remembered that a policeman had driven them home. The police told me the car had gone off the road in the snow and was stuck in a ditch. My mother apparently had not considered the dangers of driving in a snowstorm.

Precaution: Persons at level 5 do not anticipate problems or dangers.

Financial management is a predictable area of difficulty at level 5. My father, who remained at ACL 6 despite two strokes (causing his blindness), relied on my mother to pay bills by writing checks and mailing them. One evening, my father asked me to read him a certified letter that my mother did not understand. It said the electricity would be shut off because they had not paid the bill for 3 months. On another occasion, I found a certified letter folded up in the pocket of my mother's cardigan. This one said the contents of their safe deposit box would be confiscated because the fee had not been paid.

My mother was unconcerned about these consequences and no longer able to handle finances. I took over helping my father with financial matters after that.

Precaution: Clients at ACL 5 need supervision with finances.

Another issue that alerted me to my mother's decline was the laundry. One day, my father asked me to call someone to come and fix the washing machine. I investigated and found that it worked fine; my mother had forgotten how to use it. Dirty clothes were being hung back up in the closet, and there was no longer a routine for washing clothes. Other areas of housekeeping had also declined. I hired someone to come in once a week to clean and do their laundry.

Precaution: Occupational therapists need to check the routine household tasks for persons functioning at level 5. While most clients can still perform these tasks, they need help with organizing and structuring them to avoid unpleasant consequences.

Level 6: Planned Actions

At level 6, people are not geniuses, but they do not have a cognitive disability. Normally, people can think *deductively* (i.e., they can generalize or think on an abstract level). *Covert trial and error* means that these people can visualize how the pieces of the woodworking project will fit together without actually trying to do it. This allows them to anticipate problems and to take steps to avoid them. Understanding the highest level of functioning clarifies what those below that level cannot do. Persons at level 6 can attend to symbolic cues. As I tell my students, at level 6, you should be able to learn to program your VCR by reading the instruction book. *Symbolic cues* include the written word. *Anyone below a level 6 cannot be counted on to read or to follow written instructions.* People at level 6 can consider

the past, present, and future when making decisions and judgments. We can count on them to understand our OT recommendations and to apply them appropriately.

In summary, there are many scales that measure cognition. Table 16-2 summarizes and compares them with the ACLs. The Ranchos Los Amigos Head Trauma Scales were developed to measure recovery from traumatic brain injury. The Global Deterioration Scale was based on Reisberg's Fast Staging for Alzheimer's (1986; Reisberg, Franssen, Souren, et al., 2002), the most common form of dementia. Bayley's (1993) Infant Scales measure physical and cognitive development in children, and the Global Assessment of Functioning (GAF) Scale (Evans, Heaton, Paulsen, et al., 2003) is typically used in psychiatry when diagnosing the functional consequences of mental illness.

CHANGE AND MOTIVATION

Cognitive changes occur because of changes in brain chemistry, brain physiology, and brain plasticity. The ACLs and modes can assist therapists in monitoring change through observation of client engagement in daily activities. Occupational therapists can influence the client's ability to engage in occupations through instructions, cues, and assistance and by adapting the environment.

Assistance

Cognitive assistance from another individual can facilitate task performance. Assistance involves the following:

- *Observing:* looking for signs of client information processing and attempts at problem solving to understand what cues might be helpful

- *Cueing:* offering sensory input during task performance to prompt the client to begin next step, check for errors, or change the methods he or she is using

- *Probing:* asking questions that guide the client's thought process, such as, "How is your lacing stitch different from mine?" or "What happens when you touch the paint before it dries?"

- *Rescue:* when clients become overwhelmed with frustration, the best move is to correct the error or do the next step for them.

Adapting the Task Environment

Changes in the physical and social contexts can greatly affect occupational performance within the limits of one's cognitive capacities. Allen defines the usable task environment differently for each cognitive level (see Figure 16-1).

Table 16-2									
Allen's Comparison of Various Scales for Cognition									
ACL	**Medicare Cognitive Assist. %**	**Medicare Physical Assist. %**	**Rancho Head Trauma**	**GDS**	**FIM ADL**	**FIM Eat**	**GAS**	**GAF**	**Age**
0.8	100	100	I			1			0 to 1 mo.
1.0	99*		II						1 to 5 mo.
1.2	98*		III						4 to 8 mo.
1.4	96*	75				2			4 to 10 mo.
1.6	92*								
1.8	88*	50				3			6 to 12 mo.
2.0	84*	25	IV	7					9 to 17 mo.
2.2	82*	15							10 to 20 mo.
2.4	78*	10			1		1 to 10		
2.6	75					4			12 to 23 mo.
2.8	70*							1 to 10	
3.0	64*		V				11 to 20	11 to 20	18 to 24 mo.
3.2	60*						21 to 30		
3.4	54*			6	2		31 to 40	21 to 30	
3.6	50				3	5	41 to 50		3 yr.
3.8	46*				4			31 to 40	
4.0	42*	8*	VI	5	5	6 to 7	51 to 60		4 yr.
4.2	38*				6 to 7				5 yr.
4.4	34*						61 to 70		6 yr.
4.6	30*		VII	4				41 to 50	
4.8	25						71 to 80		
5.0	22*	6*							7 to 10 yr.
5.2	18*	4*					81 to 90		11 to 13 yr.
5.4	14*	2*		3				51 to 60	14 to 16 yr.
5.6	10	0	VIII	2			91 to 100	61 to 80	17 yr.
5.8	6*							81 to 90	
6.0	0			1				91 to 100	18 to 21 yr.

Percentages added to Medicare Guidelines to correspond to ACL scores

Reprinted with permission from Allen, C. K. (1998). Cognitive disabilities: How to make clinical judgments. In N. Katz (Ed.) Cognitive rehabilitation: Models for intervention in occupational therapy (p. 248). Rockville, MD: American Occupational Therapy Association.

EVALUATION

Several assessments have been designed specifically for the ACL frame of reference. The ACL Screen (ACLS) (Allen, 2002) and Large ACLS (LACLS) are task-focused and all of the others are occupation-based. Although there are 52 modes of performance, these assessments rate only even numbered modes, 26 in all. The ACLS uses leather lacing to assess the ability to learn. This standardized test has verbatim instructions, demonstrations, and questions to estimate the cognitive level and mode of the client. The ACLS test kits and instructions are available from S & S Worldwide in regular or large sizes for under $10.00 USD each. (The large version is preferable for older adults because the large print compensates for visual difficulty.) The ACLS is a quick screening (5 to 15 minutes) and serves

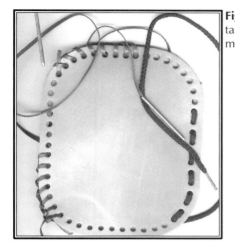

Figure 16-4. ACLS: A task-focused assessment tool.

Table 16-3	
Allen's Routine Task Inventory	
Activities of Daily Living	**Instrumental Activities of Daily Living**
Grooming	Housekeeping
Dressing	Getting food
Bathing	Spending money
Walking/exercising	Shopping
Eating	Doing laundry
Toileting	Traveling
Taking medications	Telephoning
Using adaptive equipment	Adjusting to change
Performing Major Role	**Communicating**
Spare time	Following instructions
Pacing/timing	Family activities
Exerting effort	Dependents
Judging results	Cooperating
Speaking	Supervising
Safety precautions	Keeping informed
Emergency response	Citizenship

Adapted from Allen C. K., Earhart, C., & Blue, T. (1992). Occupational therapy treatment goals for the physically and cognitively disabled. Bethesda, MD: American Occupational Therapy Association.

as a guide to OT individual and group interventions where assessment of cognitive level continues to be monitored. The ACLS set up after demonstration but prior to assessment is pictured in Figure 16-4 (see p. 199 for validity and reliability studies on the ACLs).

The Routine Task Inventory (RTI-2) (Heimann, Allen, & Yerxa, 1989; Allen, Earhart, & Blue, 1992) rates clients cognitive levels in activities of daily living, using three perspectives to validate scores: self-report, therapist observation, and caregiver report. All scores are estimates of the cognitive level, which are interpreted by the therapist according to specific guidelines. The tasks rated in the RTI-2 are listed in Table 16-3.

Cognitive Performance Test (CPT) was developed by Theressa Burns (Allen, Kehrberg, & Burns, 1992; Burns, Mortimer, & Merchak, 1994), using ACL guidelines in the performance of everyday activities. Each specific task specifies standard equipment and procedures. This assessment is also occupation-based. The tasks of the CPT are as follows:

- Dressing
- Shopping
- Making toast
- Telephoning
- Washing
- Traveling

This assessment has been updated by the author. Therapists who are not comfortable with leather lacing or crafts prefer this assessment of cognitive functioning using familiar daily tasks.

The Allen Diagnostic Module (ADM) uses standardized craft projects to assess the client's cognitive level (Earhart, Allen, & Blue, 1993). This assessment can be administered in groups, has a standardized format for setting up the environment, and craft kits that are standardized according to Allen's specifications. The ADM includes a manual containing guidelines and rating sheets for dozens of craft projects rated according to the range of cognitive levels for which they are appropriate. The kits are purchased/ordered separately. For example, the recessed tile box (cost about $5 USD per kit) may be used to evaluate ACL 3.0 to 4.8. Place mats (cost about $2 USD per kit) can rate ACL 3.0 to 4.6. The ADM introduces unfamiliar tasks that provide an opportunity to observe how new information is processed without the interference of well-learned habits.

The qualities of the ADM craft projects are carefully graded to meet the needs of each cognitive level. For example, a group of craft projects are specified for safety screenings at ACL 5. Coasters require the use of an iron, T-shirt designs require iron-on decals, and stencil cards require fine differences in pressure and the ability to judge just the right amount of paint for artistic effects.

Training videos are available for students and therapists to establish interrater reliability in doing the ACLS and the ADM (available from Allen Conferences, Inc. [1-800-853-2472]). Group guidelines and examples may be found in Cole (2005).

GUIDELINES FOR INTERVENTION

In using the ACLs, there is not a clear distinction between assessment and intervention. Both processes are simultaneous, dynamic, and observable through therapist–client interactions. The following guidelines may be applied with either individuals or groups. Groups using craft projects or everyday tasks may be organized by cognitive level, grouping clients with similar cognitive abilities together. The ADM gives examples of projects that might be suitable for ACL 3, 4, and 5. Each level requires a different way of setting up the task environment (see Figure 16-1).

Level 3 clients need the supplies for the task to be within arm's reach. However, they can do only one step at a time. Therefore, in doing a multistep task such as sanding, painting pieces, and gluing together a wood project, only the supplies for the first step should be set up before beginning the task. In assisting an ACL 3 client, each step will need to be demonstrated, and clients will need frequent cues to continue with the task (because they are not goal directed). The focus at ACL 3 will be initiating and completing each step and learning to detect and correct errors (such as sanding until all the edges are smooth [tactile cue]). The time limit for level 3 is 30 minutes.

In breaking down tasks in the home environment, therapists should follow guidelines from Table 16-1. Tasks can be structured for independence if the same step is repeated with a naturally occurring limit. For example, a client at ACL 3 can hand dry dishes or kitchen items that are placed in a drying rack. The process is repetitive, and the task ends when there are no more dishes in the rack to be dried.

Level 4 clients can concentrate for up to 1 hour and can do longer term tasks. Level 4 groups always needs a completed sample, which is an exact match of the task they will complete during the group. For individuals or groups, the therapist can demonstrate several steps at the beginning because ACL 4 clients are goal directed and can sequence themselves through more than one step. However, they also will need cues in order to correct errors and complete each step correctly. Remember, at ACL 4, what the client does not see does not exist. When painting a piece of wood, for example, they will need cues to turn the wood over in order to completely cover all the sides and edges. Supplies for a task should be visible but can be placed in the center of the table or on a nearby counter.

However, each group member needs his or her own tools and supplies during group implementation and should not be expected to share. Having clients gather their own supplies prior to starting can help them to organize the task and provides a model for learning to anticipate and plan ahead (a concrete form of a higher-level skill). Occupational therapists can refer clients to the completed sample (a visible cue) to remind them of the goal and to assist them with self-correction of errors.

Level 5 clients will need a different focus. The goal for them will be safety screening and a more abstract form of anticipation and planning. Verbal instructions will be adequate for the task, and they will begin to rely more on written directions or diagrams as reminders. The therapist's role will be directed toward making clients aware of impulsive behaviors and getting them to slow down and read or repeat instructions to make sure they understand all the steps in order to avoid the mistakes they will inevitably make when using a trial-and-error approach. The ADM uses crafts that purposely involve the use of iron-on designs so that members can demonstrate their use of the necessary safety precautions when handling a hot iron. Planning ahead is also required for stenciling, a craft process that involves judging the right amount of paint and pressure when applying layers of color. This is a skill that needs to be practiced, as students have often learned the hard way.

Clients with physical disabilities may find activities of daily living more meaningful than crafts. Cooking or baking, for example, might serve equally well when focusing on the safe use of appliances and the skill of planning ahead. Persons with mild head injuries, stroke survivors, and adolescents with attention deficit disorders make good candidates for ACL 5 groups.

Levy and Burns (2005) discuss the stepwise onset of cognitive difficulties when applying the cognitive disabilities reconsidered in working with clients with dementia. They stress the application of the Allen guidelines to alert caregivers as to when clients' ACLs decline and what safety precautions they are likely to ignore in their trial-and-error approach to everyday tasks. Following the Allen modes downward, precautions and guidelines for many routine daily tasks are provided at each ACL level and mode in the book *Understanding Cognitive Performance Modes* (Allen, Blue, & Earhart, 1995).

Home care is an important area for application of this frame of reference because of its extensive guidelines for caregivers at each mode of performance. The example of Theis, mentioned earlier, focuses on environmental adaptations that facilitate clients' best ability to function while keeping them safe. The same guidelines used for crafts can be used in the home setting for doing self-care tasks such as bathing, dressing, and grooming. Any client who demonstrates an ACL lower than 4.6 should not have access to appliances (e.g., stove, toaster) or machinery (e.g., car, lawn mower) and will need increasing amounts of supervision as their ACL decreases (as with dementia). Clients at levels 3 and 4 will often depend on procedural memory for doing familiar self-care and household tasks, and their already learned (cultural) way of doing things can be reinforced by the therapist and caregiver. This frame of reference easily applies to changes that need to be made in the home environment based on an understanding of how the client thinks.

Creating Safe Environments

David (1988) first focused our attention on the usefulness of Allen guidelines in adapting and creating safe environments. In working with caregivers in the home setting, the most important rooms to evaluate for safety are the kitchen, bathroom, and bedroom (Allen, 1994). As environments in which most self-care tasks will be performed, their contents and arrangements need to facilitate the client's best ability

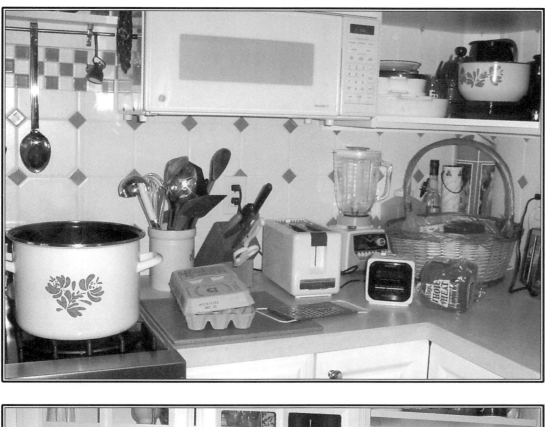

Figure 16-5. Cooking or meal preparation task environment to be adapted. (Photo courtesy of M. Cole)

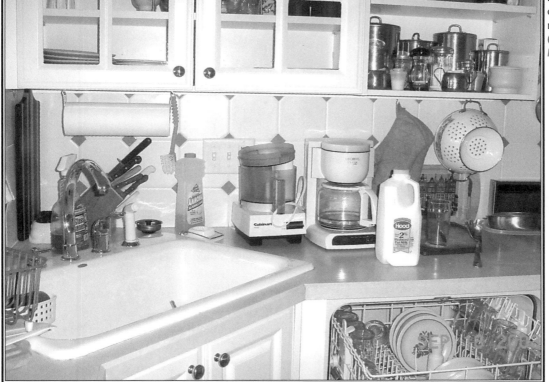

Figure 16-6. Kitchen cleanup task environment to be adapted. (Photo courtesy of M. Cole)

to perform valued tasks without creating safety issues for each specific Allen level of cognitive disability. Figures 16-5 through 16-8 represent nonadapted task environments. As a practice exercise, students can look at these photos and discuss how they should be adapted for the Allen midrange levels (3, 4, and 5) or for any of the cases at the end of the chapter. Allen guidelines described in Figure 16-1 may be applied in adapting each specific task environment.

Figure 16-7. Bathroom self-care task environment to be adapted. (Photo courtesy of M. Cole)

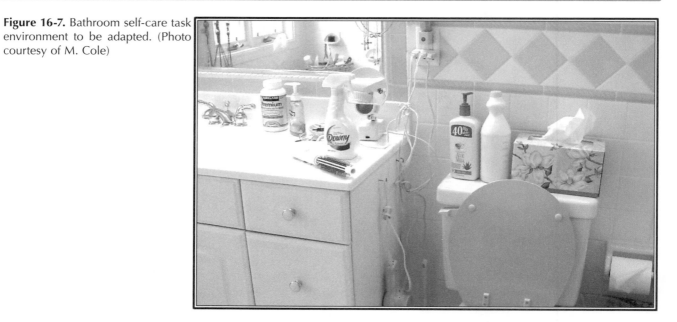

Figure 16-8. Dressing task environment to be adapted. The closet door may be closed to reveal a full length mirror mounted on the front of the door. (Photo courtesy of M. Cole)

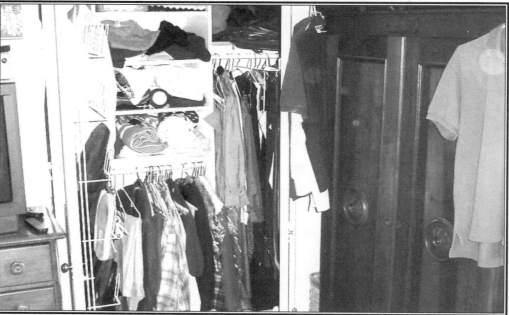

Discussion issues for Figure 16-5 meal preparation tasks include the following:

- What cooking and/or meal preparation tasks is the client able to perform or learn at ACL 3, 4, or 5?

- What items should be removed or added in order to perform a task?

- What adaptations need to be made for safety at ACL 3, 4, or 5?

- What parts of the task would require caregiver assistance/supervision and at what level?

- What cues could be given to facilitate the accomplishment of a task?

Discussion topics for Figure 16-6 kitchen cleanup tasks include the following:

- What cleanup tasks could the client be expected to perform at ACL 3, 4, or 5?

- What items should be removed or added to facilitate the task?

- What items should be removed or added for safety reasons?

- How could the cleanup area be better organized for task efficiency?

- What cues or assistance would be needed to accomplish cleanup tasks at ACL 3, 4, or 5?

- How could tasks be adapted for safety and function at ACL 3, 4, or 5?

- How could clients with different ACL levels routinely assist the caregiver with cleanup tasks?

Discussion issues for Figure 16-7 self-care task environment follow:

- What self-care tasks would be performed independently at ACL 3, 4, or 5?

- What items should be added or removed and why?

- What adaptations should be made for safety reasons?

- How should this environment be reorganized for task efficiency?

- What cues or assistance would be needed for specified tasks at ACL 3, 4, or 5?

- What adaptive equipment might be helpful for specific cases?

- How could independent functioning for specific tasks be facilitated at different ACL levels through adapting either task, environment, or both?

Discussion issues for Figure 16-8 dressing tasks are as follows:

- What steps would the task of dressing involve at ACL 3, 4, or 5?

- How could the items be stored for greater task efficiency at each ACL level?

- What adaptations would you make for each level?

- How could you work with caregivers to better organize the dressing and storage areas for greater client independence with dressing at each ACL level?

- What cues and/or assistance would be needed to accomplish various dressing tasks?

- What could be routinely done to help clients with cognitive disabilities to perform dressing tasks independently?

Levels of Wellness

Persons at ACL 6, who do not have a cognitive disability, can also apply Allen guidelines to their own daily living tasks and environments to make the best use of their cognitive abilities. The following are guidelines for persons at ACL 6:

- Conserve brain energy by learning as many routines as possible

- Organize task environments by eliminating visual or auditory "clutter" (distractions)

- Use best effort for true level 6 tasks (What are these?)

- Plan ahead for low-energy times

RESEARCH

Most of the research has been done on the assessment tools to establish reliability and validity. Mayer (1988) found high correlations between the ACLS test and the Wechsler Adult Intelligence Scale-Revised, establishing concurrent validity of the ACLS. Josman and Katz (1991) constructed a problem-solving version of the ACLS and concluded that both tests discriminated between normal and patient groups, as well as different levels within the patient groups. They concluded that both tests provide an accurate assessment of cognitive level. Katz and Heimann (1990) conducted a literature review of studies on the ACLs done in Israel. The patterns of cognition that were used to construct the levels originally paralleled the developmental theories of Piaget (1972), which was also the basis for the Riska Object Classification test. These two tests results have been highly correlated. Studies from 1983 to 1990 have established the ACL's reliability, content, and construct validity. Katz and Heimann's (1990) review resulted in the expansion of the ACLS scoring system (creating the decimals, currently called modes). The expansion created a cognitive ability measure that is highly sensitive to changes, making the ACL a good tool for monitoring the effects of medication and other advances or declines in cognition. Levy's updates bring this frame of reference into an occupation-based framework and incorporate new neurocognitive evidence substantiating many of the basic concepts of the ACLs and their use with older adults with dementia (Burns & Levy, 2006; Levy & Burns, 2005).

Research efforts continue to support both Allen's assessment tools and her guidelines for intervention. Sarah Austin (2006) presented a literature review in poster format at the World Federation of Occupational Therapy Congress in Sydney, Australia, citing over 50 studies published in professional journals, disability newsletters, or textbooks. These studies apply the Allen frame in evaluation and interventions with schizophrenia (Brown, 2000; Burke et al., 1995; Evans et al., 2003; Secrest et al., 2000) depression (Carmel, Katz, & Modai, 1996), deafness (Black & Glickman, 2006), adolescents (Shapiro, 1992), older adults (Bar-Yosef, Weinblatt, & Katz, 1999; Beiber & Keller, 2005; Hartman-Maier, Soroker, & Katz, 2001; Sevier & Gorek, 2000), and many others.

LEARNING ACTIVITIES

Allen Levels of Wellness Assignment

Directions: According to the cognitive disabilities frame of reference, the human brain conserves energy by performing tasks throughout the day using the lowest possible level of cognitive functioning. This implies that we all perform a variety of tasks across the range of cognitive levels on any given day.

Assessment

Using the Allen textbook as your guide, familiarize yourself with the six cognitive levels. Summarize each level and discuss two possible ways to assess a person functioning at each level. Several assessment instruments are described in the Allen text.

Task Demand

The demands of a task include the following: materials, equipment, instructions, tools, sample or standard of performance, choice, storage or placement of material objects, and steps necessary to accomplish the task.

1. List as many tasks as you can think of that you perform on a typical day (25). Categorize these tasks by the cognitive level you needed to use to perform them.
2. Choose one task from each level (2 to 6) to analyze. List the task demands (i.e., materials, tools, steps, etc.), and explain why you decided to list this task as an example of ACLs 2 to 6. For example, why did you choose level 3 for (task) instead of level 2 or 4?

Task Environment

The task environment is the setting in which the task was performed. It includes room or specific outdoor setting, lighting, temperature, placement of supplies, equipment available, positioning of person, furniture, assistance required or available, as well as cultural or social expectations.

1. For each of the tasks described in part B, describe the task environment. Take a photograph of each task environment, or have someone take a photograph of you performing the task in that environment. Do not take photos too close up; you should be able to see the whole area where the task takes place. Cameras may be borrowed if you do not have your own. (Attach each photograph to a separate page and describe the task you are doing below it.)
2. Evaluate each task environment. How well or efficiently could you perform the task in the specific environment you described? Using Allen's book and the principles of the usable task environment, describe three changes you could make to the environment so that your task performance could be accomplished better, faster, or more efficiently.

Intervention Plan Assignment: Using Allen's Diagnostic Module

The references are Cole (2005) and Allen, Earhart, and Blue (1999). The assignment has four parts: a project analysis, intervention goals, a group leadership plan, and a discharge analysis. Each part is worth 25%.

Four cases will be described on the next few pages. Assume that you are the occupational therapist who must lead a crafts group for these four clients. You may structure the group in one or two sessions. Any of the craft projects from the ADM can be adapted for this group.

The cases may either be assigned or selected.

Use specified headings when preparing written paper. Limit 10 pages, 1-inch margins, 10 to 12 point font. List title (case name) and ACL mode.

Section A. Project Analysis

1. After carefully reading your case, choose an appropriate first project from Allen's Diagnostic Module. Given the personal circumstances and preferences of the case, why is this project a good choice?
2. From Allen, Chapter 6, look up the craft processes for your client at the correct level and mode. List and describe 3 predictable problems your case may have with this project. Describe the cues you would provide and/or the assistance you would give to assist your client with these problems.

Section B. Intervention Goals

1. Using task equivalence, what problems can you predict this client will have with everyday functioning? Include at least one from each category: grooming and dressing, eating and/or meal preparation, work or leisure activity, social interaction, community participation, and home safety. Describe each briefly in a separate sentence.
2. Set goals for working with this client after discharge. List five realistic goals you would work on in OT. Utilize the activities of daily living analysis in the Allen text to determine these goals. Give your reasons for choosing each of these goals. Consider not only the cognitive level but also the case circumstances (i.e., availability of assistance from family, social roles, previously learned skills, preferences, etc.).

Section C. Group Leadership Plan

Assume you will be leading a group of all four of the cases in doing the project you selected in section A. All clients must work on the same project; you must adapt it for different cognitive levels. (This is not a formal ADM assessment). You will have a certified occupational therapist assistant (COTA) assisting with this group.

1. Describe the environment you would choose, what equipment should be available, and what preparations you would make before the group begins. Write instructions for the COTA on how to set up the furniture, seating, and supplies.

2. Draw a diagram of the group's task environment. If you are using two sessions for the project, draw one diagram for each session. Include seating arrangement, specific materials, and how they should be arranged on the table or elsewhere in the clinic. Draw a 6-inch square as your clinic. Use colored pencils or markers to draw a floor plan as well as arrange tables and counters.

3. List steps in your instruction of this craft project for your case only. Explain how these might be adjusted for the level of each client. How would you divide the assistance between yourself and the COTA?

Section D. Follow-Up Analysis

1. Write a brief report of your client's cognitive level, as you might explain it to a treatment team. Include what you know about the client's home environment from the case history. Explain why this client will need occupational therapy follow-up at home.

2. Assume that the client is continuing to live at home (where he or she was prior to the illness). What can you predict about the type of assistance this client will need? Discuss how you would advise the client's family members or caregivers regarding everyday management of the client at home. Include bathing/dressing, meals/budgeting, leisure/socialization, etc.

3. From what you know of this client's history, how would you adapt the home environment to support your client's best ability to function? Describe adaptations in these three areas: bedroom, bathroom, and kitchen.

Case Studies

Case Study 1: Clovis, ACL 3.8

Clovis is a 55-year-old married male, former construction worker who is 9-months post-traumatic brain injury. Socially inappropriate behavior landed him in the psychiatric ward.

Chief Complaint

"My wife says I drink too much."

History of Present Illness

Until 9 months ago, Clovis was working fairly steadily as an operator of heavy equipment. He was involved in a construction accident and a severe traumatic brain injury left him in a coma for several days. He has a residual partial paralysis on his left side and visual perceptual difficulties. Four months ago he was discharged from the rehabilitation hospital and was attending outpatient therapy for gait training and cognitive rehabilitation. His wife, who worked the evening shift at a hospital, looked after him during the day. She noticed alcohol on his breath on more than one occasion when she returned home from work. One week ago, he was arrested while drinking with a few buddies at a local bar. He was charged with sexual harassment by some of the waitresses. The judge sent him to the psychiatric ward for treatment of his social conduct disorder.

Medical/Psych

History of high blood pressure, two hernia operations. No psychiatric history.

Past History

Two years vocational school after high school. Married 29 years, no children. He and his wife once owned a cement mixing business, but it went bankrupt. Clovis used his training in construction for hourly work and was able to make a decent living. His wife is a licensed practical nurse and has worked for most of their marriage. They own a house, a truck, and two dogs. He was always a fun-loving guy and liked his drinks but was not a problem drinker prior to his injury. He treated his wife well and was fond of buying her gifts, often ones they could not afford. She was shocked by his arrest and his aberrant behavior, which seemed to be the result of his injury.

Occupational History

Since discharge from the rehabilitation center, Clovis has been very slow to recover. He finds it difficult to move around, and he spends most of his time on the couch in front of the television. He is able to follow his wife's instructions to take clothes out of the dryer and fold them or hang them up. He can make a peanut butter and jelly sandwich, if all the necessary supplies and tools are in front of him. His wife has to remind him to bathe, shave, and wash his hands; however, he uses the toilet independently. He cannot figure out how to organize tasks without specific instructions. Things he used to do easily, such as fixing a doorknob or replacing a window screen, are no longer possible. When friends drop over, he often has trouble following the conversation. He tells the same story over and over, forgetting what he has said. Sometimes his sexual humor is inappropriate.

Case Study 2: Joan, ACL 5.4

Joan is a 24-year-old, single female who was admitted to the psychiatric unit on June 1st. Her diagnosis is post-traumatic stress disorder. Joan was raped violently 1 year ago. On the 1-year anniversary date, she was flooded with memories and flashbacks. Out of desperation, she attempted to slit her wrists. She immediately called a friend. Her close friend, Susan, rushed her to the emergency room.

Joan presently lives alone in her own apartment in New Haven. She was recently fired from her job as a waitress because she had called in "sick" so many times. She did not complete high school but chose to start working at age 16. "I am a hard worker and I make good money on tips," she proudly reports to the therapist. She is very worried that she will be evicted from her apartment soon because she is already 2 months in debt.

Joan left home when she was 17, having worked hard for a year to earn money for rent. She reports that her relationship with her mother had deteriorated over a duration of 5 years and that they were constantly fighting about Joan's social life. Her mother never approved of her friends, believing that they were all addicted to drugs and sex. The more that Joan's mother tried to set limits and control her, the more angry and rebellious Joan became during adolescence. Joan admits to experimenting with drugs and alcohol and taking many risks like sleeping with guys she only met once at a bar. She tells the therapist that she is surprised that she has not contracted HIV yet. The therapist wonders if this is a death wish. She is an only child; her father left the family when she was 1 year old and was never to be seen again.

Joan loves to dance, and she has a beautiful voice. When she was 18, she stripped at a famous bar downtown. She made excellent money in tips because she is so physically attractive and so good at dancing. Joan quit the night that her close friend died from a drug overdose. She tries to forget about her experiences with stripping and feels guilty that she did not stop her friend from taking that last snort of cocaine in the dressing room.

Currently, the therapist is evaluating Joan's ability to live independently. While doing a kitchen task, she follows the instructions but spills water on the floor, which she does not bother to clean up. Then she forgets to set the timer and simply estimates the cooking time. She can bathe, dress, and eat independently. She burns her finger when testing the temperature of a cup of water taken from the microwave. She monopolizes the therapist's attention in a group and seems unaware of the needs of others. In her bedroom, soiled clothes lie everywhere, and the contents of her closet and bureau are jumbled and disorganized. She seems incapable of arriving anywhere on time.

Joan reports the following symptoms: anxiety and panic attacks, depressed mood, loss of appetite, low energy level, sleeplessness, forgetfulness, recent flashbacks, loss of interest in activities that previously gave her pleasure, low self-esteem, and guilt feelings. For example, Joan loved to socialize with friends, dancing and drinking at local hang outs. She even thought about getting her GED (general educational development) and taking singing lessons before the rape last year.

When asked how she tends to cope with problems, Joan laughed and said, "I drink myself into a stupor and have sex 'til I drop!"

Case Study 3: Paul, ACL 4.6

Paul, a 43-year-old, single male; diagnosed mild mental retardation and seizure disorder; lives with his mother, a college professor.

Chief Complaint

Aggressive and hostile behavior at home makes it impossible for his mother to continue to care for him.

History of Present Illness

Paul had been working in the University dining hall, mostly simple cleaning tasks. His mother transported him to and from work, and he was independent in self-care at home. However, his aggressive outbursts, presumably seizure related, had lately gotten more out of control. Paul was unable to predict when these episodes were coming, and in the latest one, he had taken a meat hammer, smashed the glass in the oven door, and made several holes in the kitchen wall. He was brought to the hospital to treat his bruises, but his mother was afraid to take him back home, insisting that he must now live elsewhere.

Medical/Psychiatric History

Paul has been mentally retarded since childhood. He has poor hearing and wears two hearing aids. He graduated from vocational school at 18, and has worked in a sheltered environment since then, mostly maintenance work for minimum wage. He has mild apraxia and a seizure disorder for which he takes medication. Because of the seizures, he is unable to drive. Periodically, he has needed hospitalization for generally accident-prone behavior (i.e., sprained ankle, broken elbow, etc.).

Occupational History

Mother has provided structure for Paul all his life. She has taught him to dress himself, make a sandwich, wash the dishes, and use the telephone. He has trouble using the washing machine and cannot handle more than a few dollars without losing it. He continually burns items when using the oven. He has been taught not to use the burners on the stove. He is easily lost when going to a new location. Paul is interested in woodwork and leather work and has been active in a group that is making craft items for sale at his church. He has never learned to be responsible for his own medication.

Case Study 4: Linda, ACL 5.2

Linda is a 67-year-old, retired, Christian, widowed mother of two grown children with a diagnosis of major depression, living alone in a condominium.

Chief Complaint

I cannot do things like I used to; nothing means much anymore.

History of Present Illness

Linda retired 2 years ago from a long career as an administrative assistant in a large corporation. Unable to afford the large suburban house she and her husband had lived in for many years, Linda moved into a condominium near her married son, David, in the city. David had to finally dispose of the many belongings his parents had collected over the years when the big house sold 6 months ago. Linda was becoming more withdrawn and irritable and, at times, refused to eat. She wanted no part of selecting what to bring with her to her new home and no longer socialized with her many friends from work. It was David's wife, Morgan, who visited her unexpectedly one day and found her on the bedroom floor with a broken hip, where she had been for almost 3 days without food or water. She endured surgery for a hip replacement and responded poorly to physical therapy treatments. After 3 weeks of physical rehabilitation, Linda was started on Prozac when a hospital psychiatrist diagnosed her with depression. An occupational therapist was called in to evaluate her and prepare her for discharge after a total of 6 weeks in a convalescent home.

Medical/Psychiatric History

Linda had enjoyed good physical health most of her life. She had an episode of postpartum depression when her daughter was born, but she recovered slowly without treatment. Her son, being younger, did not remember this episode.

Past History

Linda married at 19 to a man 15 years older. Her husband, an executive in a large automobile corporation, had provided well for his growing family. Linda, who did not like cleaning or cooking, was happy to hire others to do those things, while she spent her time organizing the PTA, volunteering at her children's school, taking the children to their lessons, and helping them with homework. At 35, Linda enrolled in a local community college where she studied economics and political science. She graduated about the same time her children did and went to work at her husband's company. Her husband died suddenly of a heart attack when Linda was 45. Since then, Linda threw herself into her job, where she was promoted and continued to work to pay the bills for her children's education. She has maintained good relations with David and her daughter Sandra, who lives in London and is not married. So far, there are no prospects of grandchildren.

Since the move, Linda has not adjusted well. She still needs to unpack boxes and organize her kitchen. She still has not met her neighbors. She feels better in the hospital than she has since the move. Prior interests are fashion, interior decorating, social gatherings, and shopping for artistic items for her home. She tells the therapist she can no longer afford to pursue any of her interests. She still uses a quad cane to walk and does not like "looking like a cripple." Her ACL is steadily rising; she currently tests at ACL 5.2.

Allen Assignment: Theory Application

Cognitive Disabilities Frame of Reference

The reference for this assignment is Allen, Earhart, and Blue (1999). The assignment has four parts, each worth 25 percent: 1) ACLS and RTI analysis, 2) treatment goals/activity analysis, 3) home adaptation, and 4) caregiver education plan.

Cases may be either selected or assigned. Please use the headings given when preparing the paper. Limit: 10 pages, 1-inch margins, 10 to 12 point font.

ACLS and RTI Analysis

You will need your ACL leather lacing kit, including instructions. Please bring the kit to class with you, as you will be role playing your case in class. You will hand in the ACL lacing test, completed as you determine your case would have done it. Use your current scoring guidelines, and Allen as a reference. (Kits are available from S & S Worldwide [1-800-243-9232]; instructional videotape for administering the ACL is available from Allen Conferences [1-800-853-2472] or Association of Allen Authorized Instructors International Web site [http://www.allen-cognitive-levels.com]).

Write a brief interpretation of the ACL test results. What generalizations can you make about your case's problem-solving ability? What aspects of your case are consistent with the test results, and which are not? Explain your reasoning.

Using Allen, predict 10 areas of difficulty in doing routine daily activities. Explain how you would evaluate these areas in OT.

Treatment Goals/Activity Analysis

Use a client-centered approach to determine your case's interests and preferences. What are some questions you would ask the client and/or caregiver during an initial interview? Explain briefly what important roles the client might set as priorities based on the case description. What precautions and/or conditions should be considered when performing the tasks that make up these life roles?

Using Allen, choose five (please number these in bold) realistic goals to be worked on in OT. These goals should be paraphrased directly from Allen, and the page number should be given as a reference. Do the following for each goal: briefly explain your reasons for choosing this as a goal using your case's specific characteristics as well as cognitive abilities and disabilities. Then, choose an intervention activity, and explain how you would adapt it to be a "just-right challenge" for your case. Consider contextual factors.

Explain how you would measure the progress of your case toward your selected goals. What improvements would you expect to see with treatment? Be specific.

Home Adaptation

How would you adapt this client's home to support his or her best ability to function? Write one paragraph about the following four areas: bathroom, bedroom (dressing area), recreational/leisure area, and kitchen. What specific tasks does the client intend to do in each of these areas? If he or she needs assistance, reminders, or changes in how the environment is set up, who will provide this for the client? Consider all environmental factors, such as lighting, placement of furniture, timing, and storage/availability of supplies for identified tasks to be accomplished in each area. How could the environment help this client to function independently and safely at home?

Caregiver Education

What can you predict about this client's need for assistance upon discharge? Use the chart in Cole (2005, p. 156) as your guide. Consider both physical and cognitive assistance. Mention the specific tasks for which your case will need the assistance you describe.

Name three activities (number these in bold, separate paragraph for each) to be used when teaching a caregiver how to assist the client. At least one of these activities should be performed in the community (e.g., fixing lunch, morning grooming/bathing, or going grocery shopping). For each activity, explain how the task environment should be set up and why. Then break the activity down into steps, and describe each in detail. Give guidelines to the caregiver for assisting the client as necessary, and explain why.

What are your recommendations to the caregiver regarding everyday management of the client at home? What are some general safety suggestions you would offer? Use everyday language when communicating with caregivers; try to avoid Allen/OT jargon.

Summary

Finally, write a summary of this client's cognitive level as you would explain it to another professional (e.g., a nurse). What are the upper limits of this client's ability? Can he or she live alone? Take medication on his or her own? Handle finances himself or herself? Plan for the future? Be left alone for all or part of the day? With what conditions? What safety precautions? What adaptations? Are home health aids necessary, and what would they need to do for the client? What level of supervision is advisable? Consider the client's financial status when making your recommendations. How will you determine when OT can be discontinued?

Case Studies

Case Study 1: Brandy, ACL 4.2

Brandy, a 23-year-old single female, appears moderately overweight, baby-faced, dressed in black, and with make up slightly overdone. She is diagnosed with schizophrenia and admitted for bizarre behavior.

Chief Complaint

"Mother threw me out, again."

History of present illness: For the past 3 weeks, Brandy has missed work several days each week. She has stayed up all night or gotten up in the middle of the night, watching the television until morning. She believes the cable television is sending her messages or showing her coded visions of the future. She has spoken to friends at work about great danger and about the coming end of the world. She gives examples from the news about chaos in the streets, random killings, and spies in our midst.

Two days ago, her mother found Brandy wandering outside behind their house wearing only black leggings and a bra (it was winter) and playing loud music on her portable radio. The neighbors called to complain. The next morning, her mother brought her to the psychiatric ward.

Medical/Psychiatric History

Brandy was first diagnosed schizophrenic, disorganized type, when she was 19. She had been put on medication, which kept the illness under control for the most part. However, she had been hospitalized four times since then. She has a habit of stopping her medication each time she has a new boyfriend. She has been followed up with monthly appointments at a local clinic after the fifth hospitalization but had missed the last appointment.

Past History

Brandy dropped out of high school at 17 because she was failing. She was involved with a fast group of teens who were suspected of drug use, and several of the group were arrested for breaking and entering. She was at constant odds with her mother and step-father and, at one point, moved out. However, after her first hospitalization, she seemed to settle down and was tutored in English and Math to prepare her for the GED, which she passed at age 21. She had many jobs but kept none until she began working for a social agency doing word processing. She had a job coach who was able to keep her out of trouble most of the time and who intervened with her boss on her behalf. Her mother was anxious for her to become independent because she was the subject of many fights between she and her husband over her continued support.

Occupational History

Brandy was independent in most self-care activities but needed help selecting and caring for clothing and preparing meals. She had a bad habit of leaving messes everywhere she went. When on medication, she was usually willing to help with housework but needed structure and supervision. Her ACL is 4.2 during the second week.

Case Study 2: John, ACL 3.8

John is a 45-year-old, unemployed male who was recently laid off as a hospital administrator. He appears disheveled and much older than his stated age. He has been married to his high school sweetheart, Liz, for 25 years and they have three children. The 21- and 18-year-old daughters are both attending college while living at home. The 12-year-old son is entering the 7th grade. John and Liz live in an upper-class neighborhood, drive expensive cars, and enjoy the high life. John never expected to be out of a job or low on cash. There is little savings because John and Liz tend to spend money easily. Since John's lay off 4 months ago, he has been noticeably more depressed and stressed out. Two days ago, he told his wife that he was thinking of driving his red sports car off a cliff. Liz became frightened and contacted their doctor. John has been admitted to the psychiatric unit for suicidal tendencies and treatment of a major depressive episode.

John is lethargic and barely audible upon an OT interview. He tends to look down at the floor and not make any eye contact. Upon review of the chart, the therapist learns that John has a Master's degree in Business Administration and has worked for the same employer for 15 years. History also reveals that John enjoyed socializing with his employees and spent many weekends playing golf and eating and drinking at a nearby sports bar. He loved his job and loved being the "boss." He took great care with his appearance and loved to wear designer clothes. He felt good about providing financial support for his family and had a strong work ethic.

John's family relationships are fairly superficial because he seemed to always be working. Liz was busy with her job as an interior decorator. John often appeased her demands for more intimacy by letting her redecorate the house as often as she liked.

Liz described recent changes in John's personality. John lost interest in sex since he got laid off and had become more introverted over the past several months. He had been hanging around in his pajamas all day, refusing to shave or get his hair cut, and often forgetting to bathe. John refused to go out of the house for any activity. His work buddies stopped calling because he never returned their calls. He had no daily routine, slept most of the day, and ate only food placed in front of him. Liz caught him eating an entire bowl of Halloween candy that happened to be within his reach. He paced the floor at night, looking pensive and worried. "I don't see any way out of this black hole," he states to the therapist.

Their youngest son is showing problems at school; he is much more interested in socializing than studying. John avoids dealing with this and calls it a passing phase. The girls are doing well at college and love being free to come and go with few limits. All three children are worried that their lifestyle and spending habits are going to change real soon if their father does not get another job.

John cannot state the correct day or date. He cannot seem to concentrate on reading and does not keep track of his belongings. He wanders around the ward, picking up objects and rearranging them. He has lost his sense of purpose since he was laid off. "I can't support my family anymore. Maybe they'd be better off without me," he laments.

Case Study 3: Raquel, ACL 5.2

Raquel is a 28-year-old, divorced, white female with a history of borderline personality and substance abuse. She lives alone in a two-room apartment and works as a receptionist/office administrator for a small law firm owned by her brother-in-law. She was admitted to an acute substance abuse program following an apparent suicide attempt.

Raquel's ex-boyfriend Lenny brought her to the emergency room after finding her semiconscious on the fire escape outside his second floor apartment. She admitted to using crack in combination with sleeping medication and heavy drinking in an attempt to end her life. Lenny had broken off the relationship a week prior to the attempt and was entertaining another woman on the night of the incident. Raquel and he had dated for 4 or 5 months, ate out together nearly every night, and Raquel had slept over at Lenny's apartment most weekends. Although Lenny rejected her repeated requests to move in with him, he was alarmed at how dependent and possessive Raquel had become.

Past history

Prior to graduation from high school, Raquel lived with her divorced mother. After high school, she worked as a waitress for low wages and depended on her good looks for tips. Forced to move when her mother remarried, and unable to afford her own apartment, she moved in with her married sister Stella. Nine years older, Stella had no children of her own. Her job and marriage suffered from staying up nights making her sister coffee when she came home drunk and talking her through troubled relationships.

Six months ago, after a family argument over Raquel bringing her boyfriend home to share the pull out sofa, Stella's husband Richard insisted that she move out. To appease his wife, he hired Raquel part-time and paid for her computer training. Surprisingly, Raquel learned the skills quickly and seemed to enjoy the social aspects of her job. (It was there she met Lenny, a client of Richard's firm.) Richard found her a small furnished studio (one large room with alcoves for bed, kitchenette, sitting area with a television, and bathroom) and paid the rent out of her wages. Still she spent most of her money on clothes and makeup and always seemed to be in debt.

Raquel struggled constantly with an intense fear of being alone, which added to her devastation when each relationship ended. To avoid loneliness, she went shopping for clothes. When they got dirty, she just bought new ones. While she loved gourmet food, she never cooked and rarely ate at home. Eating out was beginning to add unwanted pounds to her youthful, slim figure. This threatened her highly fashionable self-image.

During the 8 days of inpatient substance abuse rehabilitation, Raquel's sister was her only visitor. At a family therapy session, Stella agreed to spend an hour or two each evening assisting her sister; Richard agreed to give her another chance at work. Raquel was advised not to return to waitressing because of the temptation of alcohol. She has been referred to a Narcotics Anonymous program that meets three evenings each week, including Saturdays. At discharge, Raquel's ACL is 5.2.

Case Study 4: Morrison, ACL 4.6

Morrison is a 33-year-old, single Irish Catholic male, 15 years posthead injury, working as a medical lab assistant at hospital. Two months ago, his mother died suddenly, leaving Morrison and his elderly father to grieve in their big house. His depression worsened so that he would just sit on the lab stool, staring our the window, leaving his work undone. His boss granted him a medical leave, and a hospital psychiatrist started him on antidepressants. He was not hospitalized but referred to a home care agency for follow up.

Past history

At age 18, Morrison had won a scholarship to play football in college when a vehicle struck his bicycle from behind, throwing his body forward and then running him over. His heart stopped several times in those initial hours. He sustained massive internal injuries and stayed in a coma for 3 months. Lost forever was the athletic scholar who was destined to go to medical school. Against the odds, Morrison did recover the ability to walk with the aid of a quad cane for balance. After 2 years of rehabilitation, he could read and understand language. Still, Morrison rarely initiated conversation; his answers to questions were monosyllabic. He was unable to maintain relationships with his classmates and spent most of his time reading and watching sports on television. Morrison continued to live in his parents home, while his younger brother and sister went on to college, married and had families of their own. His interest in science and sheer perseverance allowed him to attend a community college, where it took him 10 years to earn a degree in medical technology. A meticulous worker, Morrison had no trouble finding a job. He was independent in self-care but rarely socialized except on Sundays when he attended church.

His father, a diabetic for many years, was severely overweight and visually impaired at age 70. A retired accountant, his father maintained a good income and continued to manage the finances. However, both men had relied heavily on their wife and mother for meals as well as general home management and maintenance. They were lost without her.

Current Situation

On your initial visit as Morrison's home-care therapist, you find the house in vast disarray. Church ladies had provided them with daily hot meals, but Morrison was too depressed to clean up the kitchen. In the study, a computer was set up on the desk, along with piles of unopened mail. In the downstairs bathroom, soiled clothes and bedding were stacked on top of the washer and dryer. The father reported that since his wife died, he relied on his son to help him compensate for his poor vision. He needed Morrison to read him the mail, write out the checks, and balance the checkbook on the computer. Morrison was also needed to drive the family car to buy groceries and do their errands. Even after his mother died, Morrison had no trouble doing these things. Now, he would get lost driving two blocks from home. His father was clearly willing and able to assist his son with these and other everyday activities. Morrison wanted to help, but the depression was temporarily interfering with his attention and short-term memory, problems he had fought hard to overcome after his initial injury.

REFERENCES

Allen, C. K. (1982). Independence through activity: The practice of occupational therapy (psychiatry). *American Journal of Occupational Therapy, 36,* 731–739.

Allen, C. K. (1985). *Occupational therapy for psychiatric diseases: Measurement and management of cognitive disabilities.* Boston, MA: Little, Brown & Co.; 1985.

Allen, C. K. (1987). Activity: Occupational therapy's treatment method. *American Journal of Occupational Therapy, 41,* 563–575.

Allen, C. K. (1994). Creating a need-satisfying, safe environment: Management and maintenance approaches. In C. B. Royeen (Ed.), *AOTA self-study series: Cognitive rehabilitation.* Rockville, MD: American Occupational Therapy Association.

Allen, C. K. (1998). Cognitive disabilities: How to make clinical judgments. In N. Katz (Ed.), *Cognitive rehabilitation: Models for intervention in occupational therapy.* Rockville, MD: American Occupational Therapy Association.

Allen, C. K. (1999). *Structures of the cognitive performance modes.* Ormond Beach, FL: Allen Conferences, Inc.

Allen, C. K. (2002). The official web site of Allen Cognitive Levels. Retrieved July 15, 2005, from http://www.allen-cognitive-levels.com/levels.htm.

Allen, C. K., & Allen, R. (1987). Cognitive disabilities: Measuring the social consequences of mental disorders. *Journal of Clinical Psychiatry, 48,* 185–190.

Allen, C. K., Blue, T., & Earhart, C. A. (1995). *Understanding cognitive performance modes.* Ormond Beach, FL: Allen Conferences, Inc.

Allen, C. K., Earhart, K., & Blue, T. (1992). *Occupational therapy treatment goals for the physically and cognitively disabled.* Bethesda, MD: American Occupational Therapy Association.

American Occupational Therapy Association. (2002). Occupational therapy practice framework: Domain and process. *American Journal of Occupational Therapy, 56,* 609–639.

American Psychiatric Association. (1980). *Diagnostic and statistical manual of mental disorders* (3rd ed.). Washington, DC: Author.

American Psychiatric Association. (1994). *Diagnostic and statistical manual of mental disorders* (4th ed.). Washington, DC: Author.

Austin, S. (2006, July). Cognitive disabilities model references. Poster presented at the WFOT 14th Congress, Sydney, AU.

Bar-Yosef, C., Weinblatt, N., & Katz, N. (1999). Reliability and validity of the cognitive performance test (CPT) in an elderly population in Israel. *Physical and Occupational Therapy in Geriatrics, 17*(3), 65–79.

Bayley, N. (1993). *Bayley scales of infant development (BSID-II).* San Antonio, TX: Psychological Corp.

Black, P., & Glickman, N. S. (2006). Demographics: Psychiatric diagnoses and other characteristics of North American deaf and hard of hearing inpatients. *Journal of Deaf Studies and Deaf Education, 15*(3), 303–321.

Brown, C. (2000). Clinical interpretation of "A comparison of the Allen Cognitive Level Test and the Wisconsin Card Sorting Test in adults with schizophrenia." *American Journal of Occupational Therapy, 54*(2), 134–136.

Burke, M. S., Josephson, A., & Sebastian, C. S. (1995). Clozapine for the treatment of adolescents with schizophrenia. *Journal of the American Academy of Child & Adolescent Psychiatry, 34*(2), 127–128.

Burns, T., & Levy, L. L. (2006). Neurocognitive practice essentials in dementia: Cognitive disabilities-reconsidered model. *Occupational Therapy Practice, 11*(3), CE-1–CE-8.

Burns, T., Mortimer, J. A., & Merchak, P. (1994). Cognitive performance test: A new approach to functional assessment in Alzheimer's disease. *Journal of Geriatric Psychiatry Neurology, 7,* 46–54.

Carmel, R., Katz, N., & Modai, I. (1996). Construct validity of the Allen Cognitive Level (ACL) test: Relationship of cognitive level to hand dexterity in a group of adult inpatients suffering from major depression. *The Israel Journal of Occupational Therapy, 5*(4), E230–E231.

Cole, M. (2005). *Group dynamics in occupational therapy* (3rd ed.). Thorofare, NJ: SLACK Incorporated.

David, S. (1988). Allen cognitive level and sensorimotor treatment in acute care. *AOTA Sensory Integration SIS Newsletter, 11*(1), 1–3.

Duchek, J. M., Cheney, M., Ferraro, F. R., & Storandt, M. (1991). Paired associate learning in senile dementia of the Alzheimer type. *Archives of Neurology, 48,* 1038–1040.

Earhart, C. A., Allen, C. K., & Blue, T. (1993). *Allen diagnostic module instruction manual.* Colchester, CT: S & S Worldwide.

Evans, J. D., Heaton, R. K., Paulsen, J. S., Palmer, B. W., Patterson, T., & Jeste, D. V. (2003). The relationship of neuropsychological abilities to specific domains of functional capacity in older schizophrenia patients. *Biological Psychiatry, 53,* 422.

Hagan, C. (1982). Language-cognition disorganization following closed head trauma: A conceptualization. In I. E. Yexler. *Cognitive rehabilitation: Conceptualization and intervention.* New York: Plenum.

Hagan, C., & Malkmus, D. (1979). Intervention strategies for language disorders secondary to head trauma. Atlanta, GA: American Speech Language Hearing Association Convention. Short Course.

Hamilton, B. B., Granger, C. V., Sherwin, F. S., et al. (1987). A uniform national data system for medical rehabilitation. In M. J. Fuhrer (Ed.), *Rehabilitation outcomes: Analysis and measurement.* Baltimore, MD: Brooks.

Hartman-Maeir, A., Soroker, N., & Katz, N. (2001). Anosognosia for hemiplegia in stroke rehabilitation. *Neurorehabilitation and Neural Repair, 15*(3), 213–222.

Heimann, N.E., Allen, C. K., & Yerxa, E. J. (1989). The routine task inventory: A tool for describing the functional behavior of the cognitively disabled. *Occupational Therapy Practice, 1*(1), 67–74.

Josman, N., & Katz, N. (1991). Problem-solving version of the Allen Cognitive Level (ACL) test. *American Journal of Occupational Therapy, 45,* 331–338.

Katz, N., & Heimann, N. (1990). Review of research conducted in Israel in cognitive disability instrumentation. *Occupational Therapy in Mental Health, 10,* 1–15.

Leiter, F., & Cummings, J. (1999). Pharmacological interventions in Alzheimer's disease. In D. Stuss, G. Winicur, & I. Robertson (Eds.), *Cognitive neurorehabilitation* (pp. 153–173). New York, NY: Cambridge University Press.

Levy, L. L., & Burns, T. (2005). Cognitive disabilities reconsidered: Rehabilitation of older adults with dementia. In N. Katz (Ed.), *Cognition & occupation across the life span: Models for intervention in occupational therapy* (pp. 347–388). Bethesda, MD: American Occupational Therapy Association.

Levy, L. L., & Burns, T. (2006). Neurocognitive practice essentials in dementia: Cognitive disabilities-reconsidered model. *Occupational Therapy Practice, 11*(3), CE-1–CE-8.

Luria, A. R. (1966). *Higher cortical functions in man.* London, UK: Tavistock.

Mayer, M. A. (1988). Analysis of information processing and cognitive disability theory. *American Journal of Occupational Therapy, 42,* 176–183.

Piaget, J. (1972). *The psychology of the child.* New York: Basic Books

Reisberg, B. (1986). Functional assessment staging with annotations. *Geriatrics, 41,* 30–46.

Reisberg, B., Franssen, E., Souren, L., Auer, S., Akram, I., & Kenowsky, S. (2002). Evidence and mechanisms of retro genesis in Alzheimer's and other dementias: Management and treatment import. *American Journal of Alzheimer's and Other Dementias, 17,* 160–174.

Secrest, L., Wood, A. E., & Tapp, A. (2000). A comparison of the Allen Cognitive Level Test and the Wisconsin Card Sorting Test in adults with schizophrenia. *American Journal of Occupational Therapy, 54,* 129–133.

Sevier, S., & Gorek, B. (2000). Cognitive evaluation in care planning for people with Alzheimer disease and related dementias. *Geriatric Nursing, 21,* 92–97.

Shapiro, M. E. (1992). Application of the Allen cognitive level in assessing cognitive level functioning in emotionally disturbed boys. *American Journal of Occupational Therapy, 46,* 541–520.

Chapter 17

LIFESPAN DEVELOPMENT FRAMES

"Everyone needs a fresh map of life."

– PETER LASLETT (1991)

Many current textbooks have looked at developmental theory as a common resource for occupational therapy (OT), but not a specific frame of reference. The reasons have to do with the paradigm shift in the profession, taking us away from the ages and stages concept of development, which are labeled as linear (having an inflexible order or sequence) and hierarchical (needing one foundational skill level in order to progress to the next level). Furthermore, current research has challenged the validity of stage theories, and their application in rehabilitative settings has been questioned.

Despite this new insight, developmental theories continue to influence our practice. Developmental theorists often cited in OT include Piaget (intellectual development), Erikson (psychosocial development), and Kohlberg (moral development). Physical growth and development have been outlined by many theorists through medical research and practice, including Gesell and others (Gesell & Armatruda, 1967; Yale, 2005). Dunn (2000) discusses developmental theory as a universal language through which different disciplines can effectively communicate. However, she cautions that occupational therapists cannot assume that all children with disabilities can achieve age-appropriate skills. While knowledge of normal development is necessary, flexibility is needed when applying these theories to OT practice.

In this chapter, we will review some of the more common developmental theories that impact OT. Some developmental theories begin with childhood (Piaget, 1972; Kohlberg, 1973; Wilcox, 1979; Yale, 2005; Zemke & Gratz, 1982), while other focus on adulthood (Gilligan, 1982; Levinson, 1978) and aging (Atchley, 1975, 1976, 1989; Baltes, 1997; Laslett, 1991, 1997; Havighurst, 1961). Some OT theories based on neuromaturation will be discussed in other chapters (including those by Ayres, King, and Bobaths) while others (Llorens, 1970; Mosey, 1986) will be briefly presented here.

FOCUS

In OT, developmental theories seem most relevant for treating children and older adults. However, our awareness of the typical stages of adulthood and the stressful life tasks implied (the turmoil of a midlife crisis, the pain of empty nest syndrome) can guide the questions we ask, the goals we consider, and the meaning of occupations that we choose as intervention. The American Occupational Therapy Association's (AOTA's) OT Practice Framework (2002) includes age and "life stage" as an aspect of personal context. The main focus of lifespan development as an OT approach will be assisting clients with transitional tasks (e.g., identity issues in adolescence or retirement in later life). This includes establishing or restoring client-chosen, age-appropriate occupations within continued life roles and in helping clients to adapt to the changes brought on by health conditions within and across the lifespan developmental continuum.

THEORETICAL BASE

Jean Piaget

Jean Piaget, a biologist, studied how children adapt to their environment (Huitt & Hummel, 2003). He hypothesized that human behavior is organized through schemes that represent the world and define one's actions. At birth, infants operate through schemes called reflexes. Through the processes of assimilation and accommodation in response to environmental interactions, infants soon replace reflexes with constructed schemes. Assimilation is the process of incorporating new experiences with existing schemes. Accommodation involves changing the internal structures in order to accept new environmental input.

Mental structures are more complex schemes. Piaget identified four stages of cognitive or intellectual development:

1. *Sensorimotor stage (infancy):* knowledge of the world is based on physical experiences (sensory input). Object constancy, or remembering specific individuals, occurs around 7 months. Increased mobility promotes new intellectual abilities, and the beginning of symbolic (language) abilities mark the end of this stage.

2. *Preoperational stage (toddler):* contains two substages through which intelligence is demonstrated through the use of symbols, language use matures, and memory and imagination are developed. Yet thinking is egocentric and illogical (magical) and irreversible (one right answer).

3. *Concrete operational stage (elementary and early adolescence):* intelligence is acquired through systematic manipulation of concrete objects, resulting in seven types of conservation (knowledge): number, length, liquid, mass, weight, area, and volume. Egocentric thought diminishes by the end of this stage.

4. *Formal operational stage (adolescence and adulthood):* intelligence is demonstrated through logical use of symbols related to abstract concepts.

A cross-sectional study with adult populations (Kuhn, Langer, Kohlberg, & Haan, 1977) found that only 30% to 35% of adults attain the formal operations stage. This suggests that maturation alone does not guarantee the ability to think abstractly and that special environmental experiences (such as higher education) are needed to develop higher level reasoning ability.

Piaget's theory has been widely used in many disciplines. Current educational programs based on Piaget offer discovery learning using a wide variety of concrete experiences to help children learn. Therapists may design different approaches for working with children based on their current Piaget developmental stage.

Sigmund Freud's Psychosexual Stages

Freud's stages provide a backdrop for many future theories of development. Llorens (1970), an occupational therapist, presented the psychosexual stages as one of psychodynamic growth. She specifies that "for emotional growth to proceed … it must be nurtured with affection, understanding, security, and discipline, and be stimulated by achievement and social acceptance... Children gain satisfaction in their relationships with others so that they may develop the feeling that they are loveable..." (p. 95). We will use Llorens' age groups for Freudian developmental stages. Freud believed that the personality or character of an individual developed before the age of 5. While his six psychosexual stages span only childhood and adolescence, ending in maturity by the age of 18, the frustrations, fixations, and conflicts that have occurred during these stages can persist or resurface, causing or impacting a variety of mental health conditions

in adulthood. Freud's stages are defined by the predominant source of gratification of instinctual needs.

1. *Oral stage (birth to 4 years):* needs are gratified by sucking a bottle or mother's breast. The most basic nurturing relationship with mother has implications for developing attachments and intimate or trusting relationships with others throughout life.

2. *Anal stage (1 to 4 years):* needs are gratified by control—more specifically, toilet training. In the anal stage, the child attempts to separate from parental control, while still retaining needed protection and safety. Unresolved anal issues have been blamed for adult characteristics such as messiness (stemming from lack of control and smearing or messing oneself or surroundings) or, at the other extreme, an obsession with order and cleanliness. This is the Freudian origin of obsessive compulsive behaviors or characteristics. The person who saves or collects things or continually cleans and organizes may be labeled "analretentive."

3. *Phallic or early genital stage (3 to 6 years):* child fantasizes about a sexual relationship with the parent of the opposite sex. This has also been called the Oedipal complex for little boys (age 4 to 5) or the Electra complex for girls. Libido (love) is directed toward the opposite-sex parent, and the aggressive drive is directed toward the same-sex parent. Resolution of this stage requires an emotional acceptance that such a sexual relationship is not possible, and instead, children begin to imitate the same-sex parent in order to learn gender roles appropriate for their cultural group.

4. *Latency stage (6 to 11 years):* gratification through mastery of skills. Children enter school, compete with others in sports and academic learning, and may form or strengthen defense mechanisms as necessary for acceptance and interaction with peers.

5. *Genital stage (adolescence):* begins at puberty and involves role experimentation leading to future vocation, sexual identity, independence from parents, and a re-examination of values. Llorens calls this adolescence beginning at age 11.

6. *Maturity stage (by 18 years):* maturity is achieved.

The psychosexual stages serve as a baseline for Erikson's psychosocial stages, which downplay the sexual qualities and focus on social aspects.

Erik Erikson

Erik Erikson, a German psychoanalyst, came to the United States in the 1930s (Huitt, 1997). He disagreed with Freud, his former teacher, about the role of social interaction in human development. Unlike Freud, who believed biological instincts to be the major force that completed psychosexual development by the age of 18, Erikson studied social interactions in devising his eight stages of human development, covering the entire lifespan from birth to death (Huitt, 1997). Basing his ideas on clinical observations in his practice, Erikson combined biological and social factors in identifying "sensitive periods" within which a set of crises must be resolved (Huitt, 1997). The stages are as follows:

1. *Trust versus mistrust (infancy):* child relies on the environment to meet basic psychological and social needs; inconsistency leads to mistrust. This corresponds to Freud's oral stage, in which sucking is the principal source of pleasure.

2. *Autonomy versus shame and doubt (toddler):* child develops free will, discovers the limits of control, and experiences the consequences of misuse of control. This stage corresponds with Freud's anal (toilet training) stage.

3. *Initiative versus guilt (early childhood):* child explores the fine line between independent actions (doing things for self) and the need for guidance. This stage corresponds with Freud's oedipal, or early genital stage (sexual feelings for the opposite-sex parent). The inclusion of "guilt" may be a carry over from the child competing with the same-sex parent to gain the attention of opposite-sex parent.

4. *Industry (accomplishment) versus inferiority (middle childhood):* a relatively stable stage in which the child focuses on academic learning and mastery of skills. Unlike Freud's corresponding latency stage, Erikson finds comparison of self with peers and competition for achievement and recognition to be social realities.

5. *Identity versus role confusion (adolescence):* includes two substages: 1) social identity refers to peer group membership and roles within this group, and 2) personal sense of self focusing on abilities, goals, and possibilities for the future. Two Freudian stages occur during this period: late genital stage (forming sexual relationships) and maturity. Here is an area where Erikson and Freud diverge.

6. *Intimacy versus isolation (young adulthood):* ability to give and receive love, forming long-term relationships, and forming close friendships.

7. *Generativity versus stagnation (middle adulthood):* takes an active role in guiding the next generation, either by raising one's own children, contributing to the community, or teaching and mentoring others.

8. *Ego integrity versus despair (older adulthood):* acceptance of a life well lived and appreciation for relationships one has developed over a lifetime. Despair occurs with the realization that one made mistakes that cannot be undone.

Erikson has enjoyed continued popularity as researchers in a broad range of disciplines have built upon his theory. Bingham and Stryker (1995) compared the psychosocial development of men and women and proposed the following five alternative stages for women:

1. *Developing the hardy personality (through 8 years):* feel in control, committed to specific activities, and challenged to grow.

2. *Forming an identity as an achiever (9 to 12 years):* sense of self as capable of achievement in a variety of areas.

3. *Skill building for self-esteem (13 to 16 years):* feeling worthy, deserving, and confident in the ability to cope with life.

4. *Strategies for self-sufficiency (17 to 22 years):* includes emotional and financial autonomy, sense of responsibility for taking care of self and sometimes others.

5. *Satisfaction in work and love (adulthood):* contentedness in personal accomplishments and social/personal relationships.

Erikson's childhood stages remain in the forefront of pediatric OT, where concepts of mastery and achievement continue through childhood and adolescence (Law, Missiuna, Pollock, & Stewart, 2005). These authors believe that OT interventions can facilitate the successful resolution of each age-related crisis and can assist in achieving outcomes described by Hall and Lindzey (1978). Resolution of the following occurs:

- Basic trust versus mistrust results in hope.
- Autonomy versus shame and doubt results in will.
- Initiative versus guilt results in a sense of purpose.
- Industry versus inferiority results in a sense of competence.
- Self-identity versus role diffusion results in the clarification of one's roles in society, a sense of self that continues into the future, and a sense of loyalty.

According to Law et al. (2005), Erikson's theories are "applicable across cultures, making them especially useful for occupational therapists" (p. 60).

Additionally, specific Erikson stages have been validated by researchers. Generativity in particular was validated in a longitudinal study, defining this stage as both parenthood and active mentoring, teaching, coaching, and caring for the next generation (Vaillant, 1993; Vaillant & Milofsky, 1980). Reporting on a more recent longitudinal study, Westermeyer (2004) expanded Erikson's generativity stage as significantly associated with a successful marriage, work achievements, close friendships, altruistic behaviors, and overall mental health.

Robert Peck (Bornstein, 1992) expanded Erikson's final stage, integrity versus despair, by creating three substages: 1) ego-differentiation versus work role preoccupation, focusing on the transition to retirement; 2) body transcendence versus body preoccupation, requiring adaptation to physical decline; and 3) ego transcendence versus ego preoccupation, developing an awareness of one's life achievements as a contribution to the collective wisdom of future generations.

Lawrence Kohlberg

Lawrence Kohlberg (1973) developed his theory of moral development by studying how children used concepts to make decisions about right and wrong. The theory is based on the philosophical concept of justice. His seven stages of development are as follows:

1. *Punishment and obedience:* actions are determined by physical consequences. "If I say a swear, Daddy will wash my mouth with soap."

2. *Instrumental relativism:* consists of reciprocity, like an exchange of favors. "I won't tell if you won't tell."

3. *Interpersonal concordance:* behavior is judged by intent. "I was just kidding; I didn't mean any harm."

4. *Law and order:* follows the rules and fulfills obligations out of respect for authority. "Rules are rules."

5. *Social contract:* legalistic approach based on individual rights as agreed upon by society. "I have a right to express my opinion" or "to defend myself."

6. *Universal ethical principle:* based on one's moral principles or conscience, such as the greatest good for the greatest number, sometimes in spite of or contrary to the rules or laws. "Doing the right thing" or "the Golden Rule."

7. *Ontological religious approach:* involves the cosmic and contemplative experience (Adapted from Lewis, 2003, p. 12).

Kohlberg's stages are loosely tied to age, but more so with cognitive development, which may explain why the later stages (i.e., 6 and 7) may not be achieved by many adults (Kuhn et al., 1977).

Mary Wilcox

Wilcox (1979) generally concurs with Kohlberg, but adds to it the dimension of a social and spiritual perspective. She considers the following social factors in her determination of a person's level of moral reasoning: law, value of human life, view of society and community, view of authority, empathetic role-taking, and personal meaning. As the OT profession reconsiders the spiritual context as part of its domain (AOTA, 2002), Wilcox's theory may be worth another look.

Lela Llorens

Lela Llorens (1970) provided occupational therapists with an interpretation of prevailing developmental theories, which she called facilitating growth and development. In her 1969 Slagle lecture, she defined OT's role as "a facilitation process which assists the individual in achieving mastery of life tasks and the ability to cope as efficiently as possible with the expectations made of him (or her) through the mechanisms of selected input stimuli, and availability of practice in suitable environments" (p. 93). Llorens viewed development as both a horizontal and a longitudinal process. Persons develop longitudinally by advancing through life from earlier to later stages in a stepwise sequence, while horizontal development occurs through the integration of physical, neurophysiological, psychosocial, psychodynamic, and social-cultural aspects of the self during each cycle of development. She used a chart format to illustrate relevant theories of development (horizontal), while facilitating growth from birth to maturity and throughout the lifespan. Please refer to Tables 17-1A and 17-1B for Llorens' schematic representation of facilitating growth and development.

Daniel Levinson

Daniel Levinson (1978) studied middle-aged men in developing his life transitions theory. Levinson's work, the most detailed lifespan theory addressing young and middle adulthood, inspired the familiar term "midlife crisis." Levinson identified three transitions of adult life (young, middle, and old). Each transition lasts approximately 5 years, separated by periods of relative stability (young, middle, and late adulthood). Levinson views the process of separation and individuation as continuing with each successive transition.

1. *Young adult transition (17 to 22 years):* includes four life tasks:

   a. *Forming the dream:* a young adult visualizes what he or she wishes to be in the adult world, a process that may actually begin in early childhood through creative play. The task involves finding ways to pursue the dream and make it real.

   b. *The mentor relationship:* a mentor serves to assist a young adult in making the transition into adult life. Teachers, coworkers, and supervisors can be mentors. The most important function of the mentor is to support and facilitate a realization of the dream. For many young adults, mentors are the key to becoming successful in their careers.

   c. *Forming an occupation:* making choices about one's occupation can be painfully difficult without trusted advisors (mentors). Many young adults do not have the self-knowledge or information about what different jobs entail. This is a wide open area for occupational therapists who work with young adults with disabilities.

   d. *Marriage and family:* this task entails making an emotional and financial break from one's family of origin and moving toward the monumental decision about one's life partner. Finding that special someone may not happen during the years specified, and this part of the young adult transition may continue into young adulthood. Even when

Table 17-1A

Llorens' Schematic Representation of Facilitating Growth & Development

SECTION I: Developmental Expectations, Behaviors, and Needs (selected to illustrate)

Neuro-physio-logical–Sensori-Motor Ayres	Physical–Motor Gesell	Psychosocial Erikson	Psychodynamic Grant/Freud	Socio-Cultural Gesell	Social-Language Gesell	Activity of Daily Living Gesell
0 to 2: **Sensorimotor** Tactile functions Vestibular functions Visual, auditory, Olfactory, Gustatory	0 to 2 Head sags Fisting Gross Motion Walking Climbing	**Basic Trust vs. Mistrust Oral Sensory** Ease of feeding Depth of sleep Relax. of bowels	1 to 4: **Oral** Dependency Initial aggressive Oral erotic activity	Individual mothering person most important Immediate family group important	Small Sounds Coos Vocalizes Listens, Speaks	Recognizes bottle Holds spoon Holds glass Controls bowel
1 to 4: Integration of Body Sides Gross motor plan Form & space perc. Equil. resp. Post. flex. Body scheme dev.	2 to 3: Runs Balances Hand pref. established Coordination	**Autonomy vs. Shame & Doubt** Muscular-Anal Conflict between holding on and letting go	1 to 4: **Anal** Independence Resistiveness Self-assertiveness Narcissism Ambivalence	Parallel play Often alone Recognizes extended family	Identifies objects verb. Asks "Why?" Short sentences	Feeds self Helps undress Recog. simp. tunes No longer wets at night
3 to 7: **Discrimination** Refined tactile Kinesthetic, Visual, Auditory, Olfactory, Gustatory functions	3 to 6: Coordination more graceful Muscles devel. Skills devel.	**Initiative vs. Guilt/ Locomotor-Genital** Aggressiveness Manipulation Coercion	3 to 6: **Genital-Oedipal** Genital interest Possessive of opposite sex parent Antagonism toward same sex parent Castration fears	Seeks companionship, Makes decisions Plays with other children, Takes turns	Combines talk. & eat Complete sentences Imagines Dramatic	Laces shoes Cuts with scissors Toilets indep. Helps set table
3 to Maturity: **Abstract Thinking** Conceptualization Complex relationships Read, write, numbers	6 to 11: Energy devel. Skill practice to attain proficiency	**Industry vs. Inferiority/Latency** Wins recognition thru productivity Learns skills & tools	6 to 11 **Latency** Prim. struggles quiescent Init. in mastery of skills Strong defenses	Group play & team activities Independence of adults Gang interests		Enjoys dressing up Learns value of money Resp. for grooming
	11 to 13: Rapid growth Poor posture Awkwardness	**Identity vs. Role Confusion/Puberty & Adolescence** Identification, Social roles	11 to **Adolescence** Emancipation from parents Occup. decisions Role experiment, Re-exam. values	Team games, Organizations important, Interest in opposite sex		Interest in earning money
		Intimacy vs. isolation/ Young Adulthood Commitments Body & Ego mastery				
		Generativity vs. Stagnation/ Adulthood Guiding next generation, Creativity, Productiveness				
		Ego Integrity vs. Despair/Maturity Acceptance of own life cycle				

Reprinted with permission from Llorens, L. A. (1970). Facilitating growth and development: The promise of occupational therapy. American Journal of Occupational Therapy, 24, *93–101.*

Table 17-1B

Llorens' Schematic Representation of Facilitating Growth & Development

SECTION II: Facilitating Activities and Relationships (Selected)

SECTION III: Behavior Expectations and Adaptive Skills

	Sensori-Motor Activity	Dev. Play Activity	Symbolic Activity	Interpers. Rel.	Developmental Tasks Havighurst	Ego-Adaptive Skills, Mosey, Pierce, & Newton
	Tactile stim. Identify body parts Sounds Objects	Dolls Animals Sand Water Excursions	Biting Chewing Eating Blowing Cuddling	Individual Interactions	Learning to Walk Talk Take solids Elimination	Ability to respond to mothering Mastery of gross motor responses
	Phys. exercise Balancing Motor planning	Pull toys Play grounds Clay Crayons Chalk	Throwing Dropping Messing Collecting Destroying	Individual Interactions Parallel play	Sex difference Forms concepts of social & phys. reality Relates emotionally to others Right & wrong Forms a conscience	Ability to respond to routines of daily living Mastery of 3 dimensional space Sense of body image
	Listening Learning Skilled tasks & games	Being read to Coloring Drawing Painting	Destroying Exhibiting	Individual Interactions Play small groups		Ability to follow directions Tolerate frustrations Sit still Delay gratification
	Reading Writing Numbers	Scooters Wagons Collections Puppets Bldg.	Controlling Mastery	Indiv. Interactions Groups Teams Clubs	Learn phys. skills Getting along Reading, writing, Values Soc. attitudes	Ability to perceive, sort, organize, & utilize stimuli Work in groups Master inanimate obj.
		Weaving Machinery tasks Carving Modeling		Individual Interaction Groups Teams	More mature rel. Social roles Selecting occupation Achieving emotional independence	Ability to accept & discharge responsibility Capacity for love
		Arts, crafts Sports Club & int. groups Work		Individual Interaction Groups	Selecting a mate Starting a family Marriage, home Congenial social group	Ability to function independently Control drives Plan & execute
					Civic & social respons. Econ. Standard of living Dev. adult leisure act. Adj. to aging parents	Purposeful motion Obtain/org. & use knowledge Part. in primary group Part. in variety of relationships
					Adj. to decr. phys. health, retire, death Age group affil. Meeting social obligat.	Exp. self as accept. Part. in mutually satisfying heterosexual relations

Reprinted with permission from Llorens, L. A. (1970). Facilitating growth and development: The promise of occupational therapy. American Journal of Occupational Therapy, 24, 93–101.

marriage occurs early in young adulthood, this age group rarely feels prepared for parenthood.

2. *Young adulthood (22 to 40 years):* Once the tasks of young adulthood have been resolved, one's life structure remains stable for the next 18 years. There may

be changes in one's employment or living quarters, but not in one's lifestyle or goals. For most, the 20s and 30s are spent climbing the ladder of success in one's chosen career with family life taking a back seat.

3. *Midlife transition (40 to 45 years)*: Levinson (1978) studied males at midlife, and the characteristics identified reflect this. This period represents a great deal of turmoil beginning with the realization that the adult cannot go on as before, and an internal searching and self-examination of great magnitude ensues. Three life tasks are identified for this stage:

    a. *Reappraising the past*: recognition of one's own mortality (i.e., realizing that one's time left to live is limited) gives men a sense of urgency in pursuing what they think they may have missed. This transition becomes a crisis when men resist the idea that they are getting older and try to remain in the young adult phase. The images of bald men cruising around in sports cars and pursuing women half their age are stereotypes of the "midlife crisis" for men.

    b. *Modifying the life structure*: reviewing one's life so far, and finding its shortfalls, leads to defining the changes that need to occur. Some possible changes might be changing careers, spending more time with one's family, considering aging parents, changing one's spouse, changing to a healthier lifestyle, or getting more fun out of life. Sometimes nothing changes except one's attitude and point of view. Pressures from society also need to be factored in, such as financial realities or expected family roles. The stress created by this transition can lead to physical illness, and occupational therapists need to recognize when clients are struggling so that they can assist them in adapting to some of these major life changes.

    c. *Individuation*: at midlife, individuation takes the form of resolving four polarities, which can bring about substantial changes in one's self-identity. According to Levinson, at midlife previously neglected parts of the self urgently seek expression. These polarities and examples include the following:

        • *Young/old*: "I've never thought of myself as getting old."

        • *Destruction/creation*: "Time to leave the rat race and start my own business" or "It's time to build that dream house we've always wanted."

        • *Masculine/feminine*: "I want to work closer to home so I can spend more time in the evening with my kids."

        • *Attachment/separateness*: "My wife and I have become ships passing in the night. I'll plan a second honeymoon so we can get reacquainted."

4. *Middle adulthood (45 to 60 years)*: Whatever new life structure is built after midlife tends to last for the next 15 years. Modified goals will be pursued, as middle-agers perform new roles in their lives, their families, and their communities. Again, changes may occur but not goals or basic lifestyle. This period of stability may have implications with regard to adaptation to illness or disability in the form of resistance to change. Or perhaps, the onset of chronic illness might bring on changes attributed to the next stage. For example, early retirement may catapult a 50-year-old male into the late life transition.

5. *Late life transition (60 to 65 years)*: This transition repeats the three life tasks in the midlife transition, reappraising the past, changing one's life structure, and individuation. However, in the late life transition, the tasks of individuation are different. The following tasks are extrapolated for older adults:

    a. *Physical decline*: accepting and adapting one's lifestyle to the realities of normal aging as well as possible chronic health conditions are considered when restructuring one's lifestyle.

    b. *Loss of productive role*: retirement can bring on unwanted changes, such as limiting one's income and creating a social and occupational void. This is a key area for occupational therapists to create programs for older adults as their numbers increase over the next few decades.

    c. *Coming to terms with death*: loss is a predominant theme in the lives of older adults. Coping with loss becomes a challenge that can overwhelm some people. Life review is a necessary step in reappraising one's past, a task that will determine how older persons feel about dying. Here again is a worthy goal for occupational therapists working with the elderly.

Levinson's biggest contribution to developmental theory is in defining the young and middle adult transitions. The extent of detail he offers regarding life tasks can guide occupational therapists in their understanding of the different stages of life, and what they mean for our clients' personal contexts. Additionally, the life tasks offer guidelines for what kinds of activities might be meaningful to adults at different stages of life.

Theories of Aging

In treating older adults, therapists often look to theories of aging. Developmental theorists often cited include Erikson (Huitt, 1997), Jung (1933), Atchley (1989), Cumming and Henry (1961), and Havighurst (1961). Theoretical debates about what constitutes normal aging (i.e., activity versus disengagement, and age and stage versus continuity) continue to be researched. A contemporary theory, Laslett's theory of the third age (1991) represents a possible resolution to these debates. Laslett redefines lifespan theory by bringing it into compliance with current population studies, recognizing the rapid growth and longer life expectancy of the aging population.

Age and Stage Versus Continuity

According to Daniel Levinson's (1978) adult transition theory, retirement is a part of the late life transition into older adulthood. A transition begins with a re-evaluation of one's life with regard to life satisfaction and meaning and often entails the reformulation of goals and priorities. A transition ends when the necessary changes in the structure of one's life are created to allow for continued growth and exploration of new life priorities. This transition normally occurs between the ages of 60 and 65 (Levinson, 1978). Continuity theory (Atchley, 1989) suggests that as adults age, they make adaptive choices that tend to preserve existing internal and external structures and strive to maintain their self identity and existing perceptions of self and the world. One OT application of continuity theory is Velde and Fidler's Lifestyle Performance Model (2002). In looking at the intrinsic gratification component of a person's lifestyle, notably some activities continue across the individual's lifetime. However, with advancing age, interest in a specific activity such as baseball remained while a person's level of participation changed. A longitudinal study of the retirement process as an occupational transition (Jonsson, Josephsson, & Kielhofner, 2001) attempts to support continuity theory in its use of narratives to link past, present, and future for a group of older workers interviewed before, during, and after retirement. However, an important result of this study, that despite the anticipations of the ongoing narrative, "retirement was often full of surprises and temporary periods of turbulence" (p. 44), resonates more closely with Levinson's transitions theory.

Disengagement Versus Activity Theory

Traditionally, two opposing theories have been used to explain retirement and its consequences for occupational health and well being: disengagement theory and activity theory. Disengagement theory, originally introduced by Cumming and Henry (1961), involves an older adult's inevitable mutual withdrawal from one's major life roles and responsibilities, which results in decreasing interaction between the aging person and others in the social systems to which he or she belongs. Some specific findings of these researchers follow:

- Older adults become increasingly preoccupied with the self.
- Certain institutions in society promote disengagement.
- Aggressiveness decreases and passivity increases with age.
- Decreased concern for social norms is evident.
- Withdrawal is voluntary as older adults have a greater desire for solitude.

- For many older adults, disengaging means a lower level of life satisfaction.

Disengagement theory has undergone severe criticism for several decades because it reflects the biomedical model, which equates aging with sickness and declined function. The notion that all elders are incompetent and on the verge of dying is politically unacceptable in today's culture. Our society makes every attempt to discourage social policy that ignores the elderly (Adams, 2004). Furthermore, the disengagement theory threatens the basic premise behind most publicly funded social programs, which assume that staying active means staying healthy.

Accordingly, OT has largely dismissed disengagement theory during the last half century. According to Bonder (2001), a wide variety of recent studies report that little change occurs (after retirement) in the number of activities or the intensity of participation. This suggests that while some roles such as paid work may be lost, other roles such as volunteering quickly replace them.

Activity theory (Havighurst, 1961) has contradicted disengagement theory almost from the beginning. This theory proposes that greater continued engagement in activities leads to greater life satisfaction in the later years. Occupational therapists have embraced this theory, as have most senior social programs over the last half-century. Many research studies have confirmed the positive effect that activity participation has on the health and well-being of older adults. Much medically oriented research has demonstrated the continued competence of older adults, as well as both their inclination and suitability for continued employment or a vocational involvement. Elders themselves resist the notion of retirement, as evidenced by a recent article on the Retirement Living Web site titled "Aging Baby Boomers Shun the 'R' word" (Retirement, 2004). The well-elderly study, a well known randomized controlled trial (Clark, Azen, Zemke, et al., 1997; Jackson, Carlson, Mandel, Zemke, & Clark, 1998), supports OT interventions that help community-living older adults to stay active and involved.

Third Age and Other Contemporary Theories of Aging

More recent theorists have attempted to create a compromise between the disengagement and activity theories. Atchley (1975, 1976) defined retirement as a four stage process: honeymoon, disenchantment, reorientation, and termination.

1. *Honeymoon phase:* new retirees actively pursue projects previously precluded by employment, such as traveling or remodeling their homes.

2. *Disenchantment phase:* realization that retirement has not worked out as they had hoped, requiring retirees to cope with the negative realities of retirement such as loss of income.

3. *Reorientation phase:* re-evaluation of life leads to restructuring of one's lifestyle, including a search for meaningful occupations and establishing a new daily routine.

4. *Termination:* advanced aging and the onset of disability necessitate dependence on others.

Atchley's theory, which has been validated in more recent studies (Reitzes & Mutran, 2004), paved the way for the current separation of young–old from old–old.

Peter Laslett

Peter Laslett's (1991) idea of separating young retirees from the older ones has growing credibility in light of recent research. Laslett divided life into four stages:

1. *Stage 1:* childhood and preparation for work

2. *Stage 2:* employment and raising one's family

3. *Stage 3:* third age beginning with retirement and ending with the onset of disability

4. *Stage 4:* old age and dependence

The term third age represents a change in the culture of aging based upon the reality of an extended life expectancy and a delayed onset of age-related functional decline. The third age concept has spawned a worldwide plan of action on aging: to provide for continued growth and education for successful aging to the "young old" and to better prepare them for the "fourth age" of dependency and physical decline (Baltes & Smith, 2001). Several thousands of Universities of the Third Age (U3A) have opened across the globe, beginning with the University of Toulouse in 1973, the two major archetypes being French and British U3A models (Formosa, 2000). Most offer educational programs based on the preference of members, including instruction in crochet, dressmaking, bridge, and wine appreciation as well as the study of a broad range of age-related topics dubbed "Educational Gerontology" (Withnall, 2002). Predictably, typical elderly participants (students) tend to fall within the 60 to 70 age cohort (Formosa, University of Malta, retrieved 4/22/05).

The four-age structure, which Laslett calls "a fresh map of life," gives greater importance to the third age, potentially 25 plus years, in which fully functional older adults freed from gainful employment can pursue self-fulfillment. Recent research supports the separation of the third and fourth ages, noting changes in interest in daily activities (Adams, 2004) and in social relationships (Baltes & Carstensen, 1999; Potts, 1997).

Fourth Age and Other Contemporary Theories

While Laslett's theory represents a continued hierarchy of developmental stages, it acknowledges the relative health and vitality of the 60 to 80 age group as compared with octogenarians (over 80) who may indeed exhibit the characteristics of disengagement found by Cumming and Henry (1961) so long ago. In fact, several studies over the last decade have confirmed some aspects of disengagement for this older age group. Johnson and Barer (1992) found that 50% of those over 85 years could be considered disengaged. Signs of this were 1) redefinition of social boundaries, 2) change in time orientation, and 3) decrease in emotional intensity. For the fourth-age elders, a voluntary narrowing of one's social circle has been recognized as socioemotional selectivity theory (SST) (Carstensen, 1992). Long-time friendships and family relationships take on a deeper meaning, while more superficial relationships are dropped. This voluntary disengagement allows older adults to conserve emotional energy, pace themselves, and reduce worry about others (Adams, 2004). Another study supporting SST suggests that social supports provided by new acquaintances within retirement communities are not as meaningful and do not replace the support of long-time friendships (Potts, 1997).

The fourth-age adult's time orientation changes to focus on the present, while future and past diminish. Future becomes less relevant as death approaches, while the past fades away along with the loss of contemporaries who remember them when they were younger. Emotional intensity appears to diminish in elders who have come to terms with mortality, perhaps because they have noting left to fear. Those over 85 spend more time sleeping and feel fairly comfortable with spending time alone (Larson, Csikszentmihalyi, & Graef, 1982).

Gerotranscendence, another contemporary outgrowth of disengagement theory, focuses on the positive potential of cognitive changes that occur as the aging individual constructs a new reality, one that shifts from pragmatic and materialistic to a more cosmic and transcendent world view. This internal, contemplative way of life, which trades in meaningless socialization for solitude, appears to be accompanied by an increase in life satisfaction (Tornstam, 1989, 1997, 2000). The cosmic dimension, which conceptually unites the past and present, may symbolize true wisdom for the older individual. In this state, the individual feels free to select only activities that are meaningful and to ignore the necessity for social reciprocation or convention.

Joan Erikson, Erikson's wife and frequent collaborator, wrote at age 93 about the need for solitude as a possible Erikson's ninth stage, a "deliberate retreat from the usual engagements of daily activity ... a paradoxical state that does seem to exhibit a transcendent quality" (Erikson & Erikson, 1997, p. 25).

Baltes' Theory of Selection, Optimization, and Compensation

Baltes' holistic theory builds on the work of Laslett and applies both biological and psychosocial theories of aging across the life span (Baltes, 1997). His biopsychosocial stance makes this theory especially compatible with OT.

- *Selection* refers to both biological and cultural factors. Biological selection focuses on maximizing sexual maturation in youth and shifts to the functions of cell repair and maintenance in later life. Cultural influences may promote engagement in specific occupations, such as education, sports, and vocational training during adolescence, which shifts to other occupations at each subsequent life stage. Prioritizing occupational goals becomes more significant in advanced aging as energy resources decrease.

- *Optimization* refers to the goal-directed allocation of resources, which shifts over the lifespan as the priorities of the person change. For example, home management occupations may be neglected or delegated when a career takes top priority for men and women in young adulthood.

- *Compensation* refers to the use of adaptations and/ or environmental factors to support the functions for which people choose not to expend energy at any stage of life. For example, older adults may focus on the accomplishment of personal projects (Christiansen, 2000) as preferred occupations and use a cleaning service to compensate for their lack of time spent in home maintenance.

Baltes and others focus on the balance of positive and negative factors throughout the lifespan, noting that the scale tips toward the negative as the end of life approaches (Baltes & Smith, 2001). In late life, people compensate for lost capacities through the use of adaptive devices, community resources, or the assistance of caregivers. An important point is that this theory contends that older adults continue to exert control over aging by making individual choices (selection) about their goals and how they allocate limited resources (optimization) to reach them. Baltes' selection, optimization, and compensation (SOC) theory provides a sense of continuity over the life course and illustrates how everyone, in one way or another, uses adaptation and compensation in different life stages. As such, it implies possible roles for OT across the age span and the health–disability continuum.

FUNCTION AND DISABILITY

In considering age, occupational therapists use caution and flexibility in determining the client's developmental level with respect to the different developmental theories and theorists. Historically, function has been defined as the approximate match between clients' chronological age and their mastery of the typical skills (or resolution of typical conflicts) within the applicable stage or stages of development. However, most of the traditional developmental theorists based their stages on what could be considered average for a normal population. Individuals vary widely in the way that they grow and develop, and therapists also

need to consider differences in cultural and social contexts when using a developmental yardstick with clients.

Traditionally speaking, disability is a failure to develop age-appropriate skills or to resolve the dilemmas, conflicts, or polarities appropriate for one's stage of life. Researchers in many disciplines, including education, sociology, psychology, and medicine, have raised doubts about the use of developmental ages to define abnormality. Educational psychologists have questioned the methods for testing intelligence in school-age children, claiming that they are culturally biased (Satler, 1982). Gilligan (1982), a psychological theorist who studied the adult development of women, cautions us that earlier theorists such as Erikson, Kohlberg, and Levinson based their conclusions on the observation of exclusively male subjects and that their models do not apply to women.

Illness or injury almost always impacts normal development. As clients are referred to OT, the assessment process will uncover missing skills that clients failed to learn in earlier stages of development. Furthermore, as illness interferes with normal development, the discrepancy between age and developmental level may be so great that the term age-appropriate becomes meaningless. It is the developmental stage that we as occupational therapists are concerned with since that is what determines the level of function and adaptation to the environment.

Disability can be seen as a lack of adaptive skills necessary for effective and satisfying interaction with one's environment. It can be caused by a failure to develop these skills (developmental delay), a loss of these skills (e.g., due to brain trauma), or a regression to an earlier stage of development (such as that caused by depression or schizophrenia).

CHANGE AND MOTIVATION

An individual's need for mastery motivates skill learning. What an individual seeks to master at a given age is, at least in part, determined by an internal biological clock.

However, as a person matures, the environment plays a greater part in motivation. If a person's attempts to progress developmentally are met with success, motivation will likely remain intact. Repeated failures to keep up with peers, on the other hand, may discourage a person from continuing to try. OT may encourage the rediscovery of the drive toward mastery by creating a "just right challenge." This is a task or situation that encourages the client to use higher level skills, but ones that are not beyond his or her reach.

Llorens (1970) defined a growth and development frame of reference for OT treatment of children and adults. She states that "occupational therapy is a facilitation process which assists the individual in achieving mastery of life tasks" (p. 93). In Llorens' view, occupational therapists use the "skilled application of activities and relationships" to provide growth experiences for clients, and to create growth-facilitating environments. Llorens' work with disturbed children and adolescents illustrates her focus on creating an "ego adaptive milieu" or an atmosphere within the hospital that includes aspects of physical comfort, social/cultural expectation, and support for the development of ego adaptive skills. The OT milieu facilitated children and adolescents to engage in occupations and participate with others in ways that were mutually satisfying to themselves and socially acceptable to others (Llorens & Rubin, 1967).

Mosey (1986) envisioned a recapitulation (repeat or recreation) of the ontogenesis (neurological development of an organism) frame of reference, which provides the basis for her six adaptive skills. The adaptive skills reflect the sequence of normal development, are useful for interpreting other developmental theories in the context of occupational behaviors, and can guide therapists in designing programs for clients with disabilities in order to re-establish these skills.

Mosey's six adaptive skills may be helpful in approximating a client's developmental level, as well as determining which skills need work. These skills are perceptual motor, cognitive, dyadic interaction, group interaction, self identity, and sexual identity skills. Each adaptive skill has several subskills whose typical ages of development are identified. These are described fully in her text, *Psychosocial Components of Occupational Therapy* (1986).

When there is a developmental lag or loss of skills, it was once assumed that they must be learned or relearned in the correct developmental sequence. In current practice, occupational therapists use developmental theory more as a general guideline, placing less emphasis on stages and components and more on how the client is functioning within his or her environment (Law et al., 2005). Children want to participate with others their own age, even if that means skipping a few steps along the way. Adults at various ages seek fulfillment and self-actualization in ways that do not follow the stages identified by developmental theorists.

Change occurs through the learning of new skills. This can be encouraged by setting up a growth facilitating environment. The occupational therapist looks carefully at the physical environment in terms of safety. The emotional environment may best be set through the client–therapist relationship; working with caregivers and families; and through the use of group interventions in schools, clinics, and other community settings.

EVALUATION

Interviews and collaboration with caregivers and others form the basis of collaboratively set goals. While tests of adaptive skills for each sequential stage of development may be used to supplement the interview, occupational therapists are cautioned not to use evaluations of age-specific skills in comparison with normal development when dealing with disabled populations.

Using Tests of Normal Development

Some standardized tests based on normal development have been widely used in pediatric OT practice. The Denver Developmental Screening (Frankenburg & Dodds, 1992) screens children 1 to 6 years of age for delays in personal-social, fine motor, adaptive, language, and gross motor skills. The Pediatric Evaluation of Disability Inventory (Haley, Coster, Ludlow, et al., 1992) measures functional abilities such as self-care, mobility, and social functioning from 6-month to 9-year-old children. The Vineland Adaptive Behavior Scales (Sparrow, Balla, & Cicchetti, 1984) has been a standard for the assessment of socialization, daily living, and motor skills as a determinant of developmental delay in individuals birth to 18 years. These and other standardized tests show the child's level of development compared to age-appropriate norms. As such, therapists need to use them with caution, as age appropriateness is sometimes not a reasonable goal for children with disabilities. For a more complete review of the many developmental assessment tools used in pediatric OT, the reader is referred to Mulligan's text (2003).

Understanding Client Perspective

In OT, theories of adolescent and adult development are most helpful in sorting out the difference between the issues of normal development and those that are produced by a health condition. Adults in transitional life stages (young, middle, or late life) are often full of self-doubt; may experience periods of high anxiety or depression; and may exhibit radical changes in their attitudes, activity patterns, and lifestyle. When clients experience the onset of a health condition that coincides with any of these transitions, therapists need to spend some time discussing the meaning of life stage issues with their clients. For adolescents, this might mean choosing a career, developing job skills, becoming financially independent, moving away from home, or entering an intimate relationship. Substance abuse can delay development in adolescent and adult years. Likewise, midlife has its predictable conflicts that may occur at unpredictable ages for individual clients. For example, the onset of a heart condition during midlife may symbolize the transition in attitude that normally occurs as one realizes that time is limited, death is a reality, and the person may need to change a workaholic lifestyle if that person wishes to continue with the second half of life. Older adults have many specialized issues that are better understood and clarified with developmental theories of aging.

A physical or mental health condition often cannot be separated from the other issues faced by a young, middle, or older adult, yet the health condition almost always has an impact. Both form an equally important part of the OT intervention plan.

GUIDELINES FOR INTERVENTION

Using the traditional approach in the developmental frame of reference, the occupational therapist arranges a growth-facilitating environment for the stimulation of age-appropriate behavior and skill learning. Mastery of skills and success experiences are important intervention concepts, but in client-centered practice, these need to relate to the client's desired continuing or changing life roles. This does not simply involve asking the client, "What do you enjoy doing?" or even "What are your occupational priorities?" Some important issues for client discussion from this model include continuing relationships with others, self-awareness (mood, level of stress), career or employment issues, balance or changes in activity patterns, role changes, evaluation of the past, reminiscence, values exploration, and future planning. The client's own wishes to continue his or her life structure as before, or to make some lifestyle changes, will naturally define the kinds of occupations that will have meaning. The focus of activities depends on the skills and issues clients identify as a result of the life stage discussion.

Interventions with Children or Adults with Developmental Lag

Besides the obvious physical milestones of the developmental theorists, psychosocial theories of development have long guided OT interventions with children. For example, Zemke and Gratz (1983) use Erikson's eight stages as a guideline for choices in therapeutic activities in childhood and adolescence (as well as adulthood). They suggest activities that teach independent self-care and discourage emotional dependency to help clients resolve Erikson's trust versus mistrust conflict, autonomy versus shame and doubt, and suggests activities that allow choices and self-direction within the boundaries of safety. These authors support the value of OT group interventions to encourage the development of cooperation, sharing, and self-control while adhering to social norms. This idea also supports Mosey's theory of group interaction skill development at the "project"/associative and cooperative levels, which provide a growth facilitating environment for practicing initiating ideas, cooperation, compromise, and shared leadership within the context of a group task (1986).

Transitions in Young Adulthood

Young adult issues focus on self-identity (Erikson) and establishing new adult roles such as work, home maintenance, social, community, and family (Levinson, Mosey). Persons with or without health conditions find these things difficult.

Intimate Relationships

Health conditions complicate the picture, but do not override a young adult's desire to have social (and sexual) relationships, get married, and establish his or her own home and family. For example, therapists cannot ignore the reality of a person with mental retardation or another developmental disability who seeks to develop intimate relationships and to move away from his or her parents. While other developmental milestones (cognitive, sensory, motor) may not have been reached, the client's social and emotional maturity may be very much in keeping with that of his or her peers. Occupational therapists must consider all the pieces of the puzzle when designing appropriate interventions and find ways to help clients develop the skills they are truly motivated to learn.

Employment

Young adults with health conditions may find many barriers to competitive employment, and their choices may be limited by societal attitudes as well. Using Levinson's perspective, forming the dream of what they will become needs to be considered when collaboratively setting goals because for these clients, occupational therapists may replace the mentors they would otherwise find in a vocational or work setting. Therapists will need to help clients to find the resources they will need to establish meaningful productive roles that match their physical and mental capacities. In using the developmental frame of reference, young adults with disabilities still need to have a work role, even if turns out to be voluntary or for a limited number of hours, because it is their way of connecting with the world and participating in life.

Establishing a Home

Many young adults today cannot afford their own homes. Even apartments are expensive and may need to be shared in order to meet expenses. Yet, achieving some level of independence is an important task of young adulthood; therapists should be prepared to discuss the possibilities with parents or caregivers of disabled young adults. Nancy's son has a difficult time making ends meet. He came back home after graduating from college at age 28 and has not yet left. He is having a difficult time with the life task of becoming independent and does little to help with household chores.

Transitions at Midlife

Tasks relating to middle adult transitions involve a good deal of introspection, but do not always involve major changes. Furthermore, they seem to happen at unpredictable times and to increase levels of stress that have a tendency to lead to the onset of health conditions. Clients in middle adulthood have many pressures and obligations that form a part of their identities. Advancing careers often bring increased expenses, including mortgages or high rental living quarters; memberships in clubs or community groups that enhance their networking opportunities; costs of commuting to work; and paying for services that support their jobs, such as housecleaning, parking, or child care. Parenthood has many obligations that may or may not be fully understood or fulfilled, as more young families have two parents working. The wide variety of ages at which couples have children makes a midlife transition all the more unpredictable. However, there is no doubt that many middle-aged adults feel trapped by their responsibilities and obligations, and this, coupled with lack of time to attend to their own health and well being, predisposes them to a plethora of stress-related health conditions.

Young–Old Polarity

Middle adults need to stop and think about how far they have come and where they wish to go in the second half of life. They will revisit the dream they aspired to in young adulthood and adjust their goals and life structure as a result of the conclusions they form. Resolving conflicts such as these requires a fairly high level of cognitive ability, and yet failing to do it renders the feeling of being on a treadmill, going faster and faster but getting nowhere.

Attachment–Separateness

Attachment–separateness (Levinson, 1978) will take the form of re-examining one's long-term relationships (marriage, parenthood, son or daughter to aging parents) to assess the emotional as well as physical costs and benefits. The high divorce rate during middle adulthood demonstrates the result of this life reappraisal. The marriages that survive, as well as relationships with maturing children and aging parents, often change substantially. How will such drastic life changes affect our client's occupational choices and priorities? What impact will changes in one's relationships have on family caregiving when the client experiences a physical or mental illness?

Masculine–Feminine

Masculine–feminine polarities refer to personal qualities of the individual more than gender. Both men and women can emphasize their aggressive or competitive natures (masculine) at work while taking on more supportive and nurturing roles (feminine) with family and friends. According to Levinson (1978), whichever was neglected in the first half of life will probably be emphasized in the second half. In other words, women who stayed home with their children will probably re-enter the work force, while men who climbed the corporate ladder as young adults will want to reconnect with their wives and children and spend more time in leisure pursuits. These changes in focus will affect the meaning clients attribute to occupations and may explain the changes in their motivation to pursue productive and leisure occupations.

Destruction–Creation

Destruction–creation, the last of Levinson's middle adult conflicts, parallels the masculine–feminine in turning toward whatever was neglected earlier. Destruction is not literal but refers to time wasted working long hours and the use of energy in meaningless, repetitive tasks. People who work only for income but have no personal satisfaction (such as factory workers, or other minimum wage jobs) might be viewed this way at midlife. Changing jobs or going back to school may be an outcome of this reappraisal. Creativity may be either enhanced or suffer as a result. Occupational therapists should not attempt to impose or even encourage creativity without knowing where clients fall in this continuum. Clients will find the most meaning in activities or tasks that fit their newly established goals and priorities.

Transitions at Retirement

Considering recent theoretical developments and research with regard to retirement, clients in the third age must be treated differently from those of the 80-plus age group. The preponderance of evidence points toward a continuation of active involvement in occupations and interactions with others as the key to successful retirement for the 60 to 80 age group. Therapists need to recognize that the transition to retirement is a process that many retirees handle poorly without professional help. Several adult developmental theories can guide OT interventions for this age group. These tasks include reappraising the past, re-examining one's values and goals, evaluating and nurturing selected social connections, rebalancing one's time, recognizing age- and health-related adaptations, and redesigning one's lifestyle.

Reappraising the Past

In individual work, the occupational therapist may facilitate this process by asking thoughtful questions or through evaluation activities. One useful tool in looking back over one's life is to create a time line (Figure 17-1). The client identifies significant life events along a continuum from birth to the present. Extending the time line 10 years into the future will give the therapist an indication of the client's future time perspective.

Reminiscence is another way therapists may facilitate life reappraisal (Parker, 1995). The OT perspective in planning reminiscence groups (unlike recreational groups) should focus specifically on the client's perceptions of life's accomplishments and disappointments and on identifying client-coping strategies that have failed or succeeded in the past. The outcome of this group activity may assist clients in identifying the unmet goals and meaningful occupations that will be continued into retirement.

Re-Examining Values and Goals

A natural outgrowth of the re-evaluation process may be to affirm or change one's values. The value of building wealth leads young adults to spend most of their time and energy advancing their career. In retirement, clients will need to redirect their energy toward other values such as deepening their relationships with others or contributing to their communities. Identifying enduring values

Figure 17-1. Time line evaluation at retirement with future perspective. (Created by M. Cole)

The following is a time line beginning the year you were born and continuing to 10 years from today. Place an X along this line to record each major event of your life, including year.
- Birth
- Graduations
- Marriage
- Moving to new location
- Birth of children
- Employment changes
- Retirement
- Personal injury or illness
- Specific leisure pursuits begun
- Important volunteer positions initiated or ended
- Any other important life events

X _____ X

builds a foundation for setting occupational priorities after retirement such as joining community organizations (socialization), volunteering for social causes (altruism), engaging in health-promoting or creative activities (physical and mental health), or becoming more active grandparents (meaningful family relationships). Awareness of values increases the likelihood that clients will set occupational priorities that are meaningful and satisfying in their retirement years. Occupational therapists may examine values as a part of the evaluation process or create individual or group interventions that focus on awareness of one's values.

Evaluating and Nurturing Selected Social Connections

Continued socialization has been recognized by researchers as one of the most important factors for successful aging. At retirement, daily interactions with coworkers is lost, putting new retirees at risk for social isolation. Family connections, which may not have been nurtured while working, often cause stress rather than satisfaction according to some studies. Some married retirees find that their new found togetherness 24/7 to be more intrusive than satisfying (Szinovacz & Davey, 2004). An important intervention for OT may involve identifying occupations that retired couples enjoy doing together, as well as a rebalancing of home maintenance, financial management, and social planning activities.

Retirees with grandchildren may want to change their grandparenting style with retirement. Neugarten and Weinstein (1964) identified five patterns of grand parenting:

1. *Formal:* limited contact with grandchildren with no parental responsibilities.
2. *Fun-seeking:* frequent informal contact focused on sharing leisure activities.

3. *Surrogate:* assuming parental responsibilities in the absence of parents who may be working or otherwise unavailable (usually grandmothers).
4. *Conveyer of family wisdom:* special role of transmitting family history, culture, or traditions, and of giving advice (usually grandfathers).
5. *Distant figures:* contact limited to ritualistic events, such as birthdays and holidays.

Researchers have found that the fun-seeking and distant styles are more common for grandparents under 65 years and both frequency of contact and role may change with retirement. In an unpublished study of meaningful activities for older adults in the United States and Costa Rica, family relationships and interactions with adult children and grandchildren was the primary priority for both cultures (Cole, 2001).

Rebalancing One's Time

Some developmental theories identify a change in time perspective in older adulthood to "time left to live," incorporating a recognition of the approaching end of life. Awareness of death gives a new importance to making each day count. With that in mind, occupational therapists can take a closer look at the way clients spend their time, with the following goals:
- Eliminate occupations that have little meaning such as watching television
- Identify gaps in time that can be available for meaningful occupations such as volunteering, socializing, exercising, or creative pursuits
- Recognizing or establishing routines for obligatory activities such as self-care, home maintenance, grocery shopping, and paying bills

- Balancing occupational areas of avocation, leisure, self-care, and sleep to meet the older adult's changing physical and psychological needs

A good OT evaluation for this area is the Activity Configuration, which asks clients to keep track of what they are doing each hour of the day for 1 week. For some clients, filling this out with their family members may assist elderly clients who have memory difficulties.

The outcome of an activity configuration is a discussion of one's temporal organization. The OT Practice Framework defines temporal organization as a performance process skill that involves the "beginning, logical ordering, continuation, and completion of steps and action sequences of a task" (AOTA, 2002, p. 622). Occupational therapists need to help older adults to perform occupations more efficiently in order to pace themselves and conserve energy for their most meaningful tasks. Often this means the intentional learning and practice of routines until they become automatic, requiring less physical and mental energy. For example, forming the habit of assembling all ingredients and equipment for a specific meal before beginning the preparation saves one the time and energy of making multiple trips to the refrigerator or pantry. Using routines for taking care of basic needs enables the client to spend more time and energy on enjoyment and socialization.

Recognizing Age- and Health-Related Adaptations

As noted by Velde and Fidler (2002), while one's interest in specific activities may endure over one's lifetime, the individual's level of participation may change. Occupational therapists assist clients who have health conditions that prevent them from engaging in the occupations that create meaning for them. For example, an older client who once enjoyed mountain climbing might need to adapt hiking plans for more level terrain, wear supportive foot gear, and limit the length and pace of exploratory walking.

Another OT approach that sheds light on the role of occupation in well-being is the concept of personal projects (Christiansen, Backman, Little, & Nguyen, 1999). In their study of 120 adults, perceived progress in completing personal projects that represented meaningful occupations for individuals was highly correlated with well-being. Engaging occupations, a related concept, were identified by Jonsson et al. (2001) as those that evoked a depth of passion or feeling, with a specific meaning for the retiree. The presence or absence of engaging occupations "appeared to be the main determinant of whether participants were able to achieve positive life experiences as retirees" (p. 428).

Redesigning Lifestyle

The well elderly study (Clark et al., 1997) mentioned earlier gives a good example of an OT intervention program with third-age older adults. These researchers point out that older adults often have "neither the knowledge nor the ability to determine health-relevant consequences of their occupations" (1998, p. 329). Eight modules are identified that guide small groups (8 to 10) of community-living older adults through an "occupational self-analysis" (p. 330). Each module forms a structure for several group meetings, which includes some form of didactic presentation, peer exchange, direct experience, and personal exploration. The format allows members to learn, discuss, problem solve, and make choices according to their own interests and needs. The module content areas are as follows:

1. *Introduction to the power of occupation:* discussion of how occupational choices affect well-being and create daily structure and meaning

2. *Aging, health, and occupation:* building healthy occupational habits and activities

3. *Transportation:* alternative ways to access and participate in the community

4. *Safety:* in the home and neighborhood, crime prevention strategies, body mechanics

5. *Social relationships:* dealing with loss, maintaining friendships, and finding new friends

6. *Cultural awareness:* learning and sharing diverse aspects of group members and appreciating how culture shapes daily occupations and social expectations

7. *Finances:* learning skills of budgeting, managing money, and engaging in affordable occupations

8. *Integrative summary:* lifestyle redesign journal. Reviewing the collected occupational knowledge and experience of the group using writing and photographs to construct individual road maps for the road ahead

Lifestyle means many things, but it always means change for the older adult transitioning to retirement. Occupational therapists have the skills to assist older adults in thinking about what needs changing; restructuring one's time to accommodate the changes; and balancing occupations to maintain or restore health, socialization, and personal fulfillment.

Fourth-Age Transitions

Adams (2004) compared the changes in investment in activities and interests between the young–old (65 to 74 years) and the old–old (75 to 94 years). Her findings support specific aspects of disengagement, socioemotional selectivity, and gerotranscendence theories and can guide occupational therapists in determining appropriate interventions for this population. Adams (2004) found that interest in the same activities diminished significantly from the third to the fourth age, while other interests remain keen. In summary, this study found that after age 85, interests shift away from active instrumental pursuits requiring physical or social effort, and toward more social intellectual and spiritual pursuits (p. 103). See Table 17-2 for a summary.

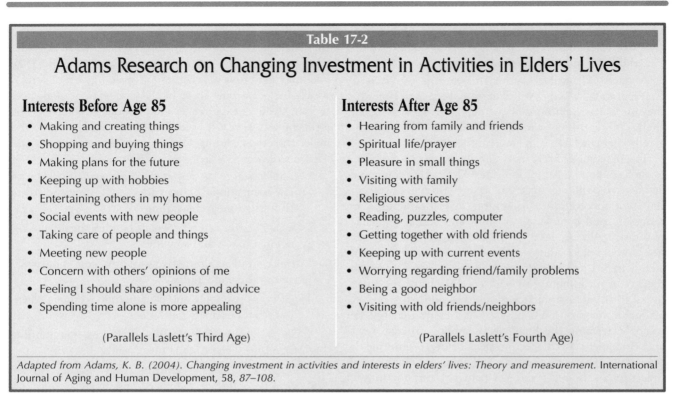

Table 17-2
Adams Research on Changing Investment in Activities in Elders' Lives

Interests Before Age 85	Interests After Age 85
• Making and creating things	• Hearing from family and friends
• Shopping and buying things	• Spiritual life/prayer
• Making plans for the future	• Pleasure in small things
• Keeping up with hobbies	• Visiting with family
• Entertaining others in my home	• Religious services
• Social events with new people	• Reading, puzzles, computer
• Taking care of people and things	• Getting together with old friends
• Meeting new people	• Keeping up with current events
• Concern with others' opinions of me	• Worrying regarding friend/family problems
• Feeling I should share opinions and advice	• Being a good neighbor
• Spending time alone is more appealing	• Visiting with old friends/neighbors
(Parallels Laslett's Third Age)	(Parallels Laslett's Fourth Age)

Adapted from Adams, K. B. (2004). *Changing investment in activities and interests in elders' lives: Theory and measurement.* International Journal of Aging and Human Development, 58, 87–108.

Occupational therapists need to be aware of the signs of gerotranscendence and to avoid forcing unwelcome socialization upon fourth-age older adults. Those activities in Table 17-2 (column 2) can serve as a guide in planning meaningful activities for this age group.

Preparing for Long-Term Care

Many older adults do not plan ahead for the time when they will be dependent on others for their care, probably for the same reasons that they do not plan for retirement; they are unable or unwilling to visualize their future. With baby boomers reaching retirement age soon, many marketing efforts focus on planning for long-term care, but these efforts focus mostly on investment in retirement communities and purchasing long-term care insurance.

Moving to a Different Location

By definition, fourth-age clients have at least one disability that causes them to be dependent on others. Choices need to be made about who will provide needed services. Cultural beliefs vary widely concerning family caregiving, and it cannot be assumed that Grandma will move in with one of her adult children. Alternative choices are staying in one's home with adaptations for safety and function and daily visits by health care professionals, moving into specialized housing such as an assisted-living facility, or entering a nursing home. Crist (1999) compared the quality of life among these choices for older adults with an average age of 87. She found that specialized housing offered the highest quality of life related to socialization, while nursing homes offered the lowest quality of life. In each of

these choices, therapists adapt the home environment to maximize occupational performance in independent activities of daily living (IADL) and self-care, recognizing that changes in personal routines and habits are difficult for the older age group. Elders who choose to live alone may need assistance in finding resources to take care of basic necessities. Occupational therapists must be knowledgeable about community services, including housekeeping, transportation, and socialization opportunities, that are not beyond the abilities of the elder client.

Changes in residence and living conditions cause stress at any age, but they may be more stressful for the older adult who simultaneously faces a decline in health status. An older adult who has well learned routines for self-care may be able to function fairly independently in a familiar environment, but that same individual may be totally dependent in an unfamiliar one. Occupational therapists may need to work with the elder and caregivers to re-establish self-care routines in a new setting and to bring in familiar objects such as quilts, pictures, books, or a wall clock with a familiar look and sound. One older adult who tended to get agitated found it a great comfort to sit and rock in a familiar rocking chair that was brought in by her daughter.

Scaling Down Belongings

The transition of moving to smaller living quarters involves making decisions about what to keep and what to give away, sell, or discard. Tasks such as these require a high level of cognition. When a fourth-age client shows signs of mild dementia, the sorting of belongings may require the help of a family member. Some tasks for the therapist, family, and client in this area are determining criteria for what to keep, what to discard, and who will be the recipients of discarded items.

- What clothing items will be appropriate for the anticipated environment, and which will require the least care and effort with independent dressing?

- What kitchen or bathroom items will be needed in the new location?

- What objects will be needed for meaningful leisure pursuits?

- Gathering personally meaningful items such as photographs, letters, souvenirs, or artwork for storage in the minimal amount of space (scrapbooks, wall shelves).

- Deciding what items of value will be given to important or significant others

- Finding charities or other needy recipients for items in good condition but no longer needed

Scaling down becomes more difficult as one ages and may become overwhelming when the elder has collected many belongings over a lifetime. Organizing objects and spaces in one's task environments is a "process skill" defined by the OT Practice Framework (2002). For the elder client, removing un-needed "clutter" will increase functional performance in activities of daily living (ADL) and IADL tasks.

Safety Issues in Physical, Cognitive, and Sensory Loss

A recent conversation with older adults living in a senior housing project focused on their fear of falling. Many of these elders had health conditions that affected their mobility, including arthritis, hip or knee replacement surgery, multiple sclerosis, and low vision. Their fear of falling prevented them from performing health maintenance activities, such as walking around the block or taking public transportation to community social activities and services. This exemplifies one of the many barriers to participation that could be addressed by occupational therapists.

RESEARCH

Developmental approaches based on theories and research from other disciplines often dominated pediatric OT practice during the 1960s and 1970s. Llorens (1970) summarized these theories and suggested a structure for their application in OT, facilitating growth and development (see Tables 17-1A and 17-1B). Mosey (1986) created a sequence of adaptive skills needed for occupational performance based on recapitulation of ontogeny. Many therapists in pediatrics still use developmental theories from other disciplines as a baseline for age-appropriate skills (Law et al., 2005). Gilfoyle, Grady, and Moore (1990) proposed a model of spatiotemporal adaptation, viewing a person's development

as a continuing upward spiral of interaction with time and space. This frame of reference builds on the work of Piaget (1971) and others. It identifies four components of adaptation: assimilation, accommodation, association, and differentiation. In association, the child relates current sensory information with current motor responses and then compares them to past experience. Differentiation is the process of identifying the specific elements in a child's situation that are relevant to another situation to refine the self-system and build more skilled adaptive responses (Gilfoyle et al., 1990).

Recent models of development in OT focus on person–environment–occupation relationships and dynamic systems theory as a way of understanding occupations over the lifespan (Davis & Polatajko, 2004; Humphry, 2002). Humphry (2002) suggests that a complex interaction between a child's innate characteristics and contextual factors determines the form of engagement in occupation for young children. Davis and Polatajko (2004) propose a model of occupational development that incorporate principles of continuity, the influence of multiple determinants, and multiple variations of patterns and mastery over the lifespan.

LEARNING ACTIVITIES

Developmental Frame of Reference

Directions: Rent a movie featuring someone with a disability. Here are some suggestions:

- *Regarding Henry*
- *My Left Foot*
- *Beaches*
- *Born on the Fourth of July*
- *I Am Sam*
- *Cybil*
- *A Beautiful Mind*
- *Mr. Jones*
- *As Good As It Gets*

Write a short paper, answering the following questions:

1. Write an occupational profile on the character in the movie you have chosen.

2. Look up the character's diagnosis and write a brief summary of the symptoms, the course, and the prognosis of illness. How does the "textbook" diagnosis compare with your character?

3. Choose a point in time in this character's life. Using three different developmental theories, identify the stages of life that apply to the character at this point in time. Write one paragraph that identifies whose theory you are applying, what

stage you chose, and what behaviors or issues in the movie exemplify these stages.

4. Write a paragraph discussing the impact of illness on the development of the character you chose. For example, where did he or she get stuck or stop developing, what regression has occurred, and what opportunities do you see for future development?

Developmental Case Assignment

For this assignment you will find an older adult (50+ years) to interview. There are three parts to this assignment:

Part A: (25 points) Write one paragraph defining the life tasks of each stage of adult development according to Levinson's transitions theory. Use a minimum of three references.

1. Young adult transition
2. Midlife transition
3. Late life transition

Part B: (25 points) Interview an older adult (50+ years).

1. Create an interview based on the attributes of each Levinson adult transition. List 10 to 20 questions you will use as a guideline. Make sure you mention all of the important life tasks for each stage. Include some predictions for the late life transition for interviewees who have not reached the appropriate age. Discuss problems, issues, and decisions he or she has faced during each transition. Identify ages at transitions (approximately start and end). Discuss how transitions affected the person's important life roles.

2. Write one paragraph describing whom you selected and why, how you conducted the interview (in person, telephone, etc.), and the contexts that affected the outcome. Give identifying data for your "client," including first name, age, gender, cultural background, vocation or job, town of residence, living situation, and family information.

Part C: (50 points) Integrate transitions and occupations. Write five paragraphs as follows:

1. Summarize the interview, highlighting the main focus areas. What did you learn by doing this interview? How do you feel about the outcome?

2. Summarize the young adult transition for your client. What occupations were involved and how were they affected or changed? How did the client establish activity patterns for the stable period to follow? How does this client's experience fit the age and stage theory of Levinson?

3. Summarize the midlife transition. What occupations were involved and how were they affected or changed? How did the client's life structure change?

How does this client's experience match Levinson's predictions for separation/individuation?

4. Summarize your discussion of the late life transition. What occupations were (or will be) involved and how were they affected or changed? How is this client planning ahead for the changes of older adulthood?

5. Choose one transition in this client's life for which OT intervention may have been helpful. Describe how OT might have contributed to smoothing out the transition. Discuss three occupational domain areas you might evaluate. Use the OT Practice Framework to guide your decision (AOTA, 2002).

REFERENCES

Adams, K. B. (2004). Changing investment in activities and interests in elders' lives: Theory and measurement. *International Journal of Aging and Human Development, 58,* 87–108.

American Occupational Therapy Association. (2002). Occupational therapy practice framework: Domain and process. *American Journal of Occupational Therapy, 56,* 609–639.

Atchley, R. C. (1989). Continuity theory of normal aging. *Gerontologist, 29,* 183–191.

Atchley, R. C. (1976). *The sociology of retirement.* New York, NY: Halsted.

Atchley, R. C. (1975). Adjustment to loss of job at retirement. *International Journal of Aging and Human Development, 6,* 17–27.

Baltes, P. B. (1997). On the incomplete architecture of human ontogeny: Selection, optimization, and compensation as foundation of developmental theory. *American Psychologist, 52,* 366–380.

Baltes, P. B., & Smith, J. (2001). New frontiers in the future of aging: From successful aging of the young old to the dilemmas of the fourth age. Keynote paper. Retrieved April 22, 2005, from http://www.valenciaforum/Keynotes/pb.html.

Baltes, M. M., & Cartensen, L. L. (1999). Social-psychological theories and their applications to aging: From individual to collective. In V. L. Bengston & K. W. Schaie (Eds.), *Handbook of theories of aging.* New York, NY: Springer.

Bingham, M., & Stryker, S. (1995). *Things will be different for my daughter: A practical guide to building her self-esteem and self-reliance.* New York, NY: Penguin Books.

Bonder, B. R. (2001). The psychosocial meaning of activity. In B. R. Bonder & M. B. Wagner (Eds.), *Functional performance in older adults* (2nd ed.). Philadelphia, PA: FA Davis.

Bornstein, R. (1992). Psychosocial development of the older adult. In C. S. Schuster & S. S. Ashburn (Eds.), *The process of human development: A holistic life span approach* (pp. 831–850). Philadelphia: Lippincott.

Carstensen, L. L. (1992). Social and emotional patterns in adulthood. *Psychology and Aging, 7,* 331–338.

Christiansen, C. H., Backman, C., Little, B. R., & Nguyen, A. (1999). Occupations and well-being: A study of personal projects. *American Journal of Occupational Therapy, 53,* 91–100.

Clark, F., Azen, S., Zemke, R., Jackson, J., Carlson, M., Mandel, D., et al. (1997). Occupational therapy for independent-living older adults: A randomized controlled trial. *Journal of the American Medical Association, 278,* 1321–1326.

Cole, M. B. (2001). Meaningful occupation among older adults across cultures. Unpublished study. Stratford, CT: Author.

Crist, P. A. (1999). Does quality of life vary with different types of housing among older persons? A pilot study. In E. D. Taira & J. L. Carlson (Eds.), *Aging in place: Designing, adapting, and enhancing the home environment*. Binghamton, NY: Haworth Press.

Cumming, E., & Henry, W. (1961). *Growing old: The process of disengagement*. New York, NY: Basic Books.

Davis, J., & Polatajko, H. (2004). Occupational development. In C. H. Christiansen & E. A. Townsend (Eds.), *Introduction to occupation: The art and science of living*. Upper Saddle River, NJ: Prentice-Hall.

Dunn, W. (2000). *Best practice occupational therapy in community service with children and families*. Thorofare, NJ: SLACK Incorporated.

Erikson, E. H., & Erikson, J. M. (1997). *The life cycle completed*. New York, NY: Norton.

Formosa, M. (2000). Older adult education in a Maltese University of the Third Age: a critical perspective. *Education and Aging, 15*, 315–334.

Frankenburg, W., & Dodds, J. (1992). Denver developmental screening test (revised). Retrieved, from http://www.denverii.com.

Gesell, A., & Armatruda, C. (1967). *Developmental diagnosis*. New York: Harper & Row.

Gilfoyle, E., Grady, A., & Moore, J. (1990). *Children adapt* (2nd ed.). Thorofare, NJ: SLACK Incorporated.

Gilligan, C. (1982). *A different voice*. Cambridge, MA: Harvard University Press.

Haley, S., Coster, W., Ludlow, L., Haltiwanger, J., & Andrellos, P. J. (1992). Pediatric evaluation of disability inventory. Retrieved, from http://marketplace.psychcorp.com.

Hall, C. S., & Lindzey, G. (1978). *Theories of personality* (3rd ed.). New York, NY: John Wiley & Sons.

Havighurst, R. (1961). Successful aging. *The Gerontologist, 1*, 8–13.

Huitt, W., & Hummel, J. (2003). Piaget's theory of cognitive development. Educational Psychology Interactive. Valdosta, GA: Valdosta State University. Retrieved July 5, 2005, from http://chiron.valdosta.edu/col/cogsys/piaget.html.

Huitt, W. (1997). Socioemotional development. Educational Psychology Interactive. Valdosta, GA: Valdosta State University. Retrieved July 5, 2005, from http://chiron.valdosta.edu/col/affsys/erikson.html.

Humphry, R. (2002). Young children's occupations: Explicating the dynamics of developmental process. *American Journal of Occupational Therapy, 56*, 171–179.

Jackson, J., Carlson, M., Mandel, D., Zemke, R., & Clark, F. (1998). Occupation in lifestyle redesign: The well elderly study occupational therapy program. *American Journal of Occupational Therapy, 52*, 326–336.

Johnson, C. L., & Barer, B. M. (1992). Patterns of engagement and disengagement among the oldest old. *Journal of Aging Studies, 6*, 351–364.

Jonsson, H., Josephsson, S., & Kielhofner, G. (2001). *American Journal of Occupational Therapy, 55*, 424–432.

Jung, C. G. (1933). *Modern man in search of a soul*. New York, NY: Harcourt, Brace & World.

Kohlberg, L. (1973). Stages and aging in moral development: Some speculations. *Gerontologist, 1*(3), 497–502.

Kuhn, D., Langer, J., Kohlberg, L., & Haan, N. S. (1977). The development of formal operations in logical and moral judgment. *Genetic Psychology Monographs, 95*, 97–188.

Laslett, P. (1997). Interpreting the demographic changes. *Philosophical Transactions: Biological Sciences, 352*(1363), 1805–1809.

Laslett, P. (1991). *A fresh map of life: The emergence of the third age*. Cambridge, MA: Harvard University Press.

Law, M., Missiuna, C., Pollock, N., & Stewart, D. (2005). Foundations for occupational therapy practice with children. In J. Case-Smith (Ed.), *Occupational therapy for children*. St. Louis, MO: Mosby.

Levinson, D. (1978). *The seasons of a man's life*. New York, NY: Ballentine Books, 1978.

Lewis, S. C. (2003). *Elder care in occupational therapy* (2nd ed.). Thorofare, NJ: SLACK Incorporated.

Llorens, L. A. (1970). Facilitating growth and development: The promise of occupational therapy. *American Journal of Occupational Therapy, 24*, 93–101.

Llorens, L., & Rubin, E. (1967). *Developing ego functions in disturbed children: Occupational therapy in milieu*. Detroit, MI: Wayne State University Press.

Mosey, A. C. (1986). *Psychosocial components of occupational therapy*. New York, NY: Raven.

Mulligan, S. (2003). *Occupational therapy evaluation for children: A pocket guide*. Philadelphia, PA: Lippincott, Williams & Wilkins.

Neugarten, B. L., & Weinstein, K. (1964). The changing American grandparent. *Journal of Marriage and the Family, 26*, 199–204.

Parker, R. G. (1995). Reminiscence: A continuity theory framework. *Gerontologist, 35*, 515–525.

Piaget, J. (1972). *The psychology of the child*. New York, NY: Basic Books

Potts, M. K. (1997). Social support and depression among older adults living alone: The importance of friends within and outside of a retirement community. *Social Work, 42*, 348–362.

Reitzes, D. C., & Mutran, E. J. (2004). The transition to retirement: stages and factors that influence retirement adjustment. *International Journal of Aging and Human Development, 59*, 63-84.

Retirement Living Information Center. (2004). Aging baby boomers shun the "R" word. Retrieved November 12, 2004, from http://www.retirementliving.com/RLart229.htm.

Satler, J. M. (1982). *Assessment of children's intelligence and special abilities* (2nd ed.). Boston, MA: Allyn & Bacon.

Sparrow, S. S., Balla, D. A., & Cicchetti, D. V. (1984). Vineland adaptive behavior scales (VABS). Retrieved, from http://www.agsnet.com.

Szinovacz, M. E., & Davey, A. (2004). Honeymoons and joint lunches: effects of retirement and spouse's employment on depressive symptoms. *The Journals of Gerontology Series B: Psychological Sciences and Social Sciences, 59*, 233–245.

Tornstam, L. (1989). Gerotranscendence: A reformulation of disengagement theory. *Aging, 1*, 55–63.

Tornstam, L. (1997). Gerotranscendence: The contemplative dimension of aging. *Journal of Aging Studies, 11*, 143–154.

Tornstam, L. (2000). Transcendence in later life. *Generations, 23*(4), 10–14.

Vaillant, G. E. (1993). *Wisdom of the ego*. Cambridge, MA: Harvard University Press.

Vaillant, G. E., & Milofsky, E. (1980). Natural history of male psychological health IX: Empirical evidence for Erikson's model of the life cycle. *American Journal of Psychiatry, 137*, 1348–1359.

Velde, B., & Fidler, G. (2002). *Lifestyle performance: A model for engaging the power of occupation*. Thorofare, NJ: SLACK Incorporated.

Westermeyer, J. F. (2004). Predictors and characteristics of Erikson's life cycle model among men: A 32 year longitudinal study. *International Journal of Aging and Human Development, 58*, 29–48.

Wilcox, M. (1979). *Developmental journey*. Nashville, TN: Abbington Press.

Yale Child Study Center. (2005). Normal stages of human development (birth to 5 years). Retrieved July 5, 2005, from http://med.yale.edu/chldstdy/history.html.

Zemke, R., & Gratz, R. R. (1982). The role of theory: Erikson and occupational therapy. *Occupational Therapy in Mental Health, 2*, 45–63.

Chapter 18

Sensory Integration and Processing

"The experience of being human is embedded in sensory events of everyday life."

– WINNIE DUNN (2001, P. 608)

Sensory motor frames of reference in occupational therapy have followed the many advances in neuroscience. This chapter reviews primarily three approaches, which may be categorized as Ayres' sensory integration (Bundy, Lane, & Murray, 2002), Dunn's sensory processing (Dunn, 1999; 2001), and sensory defensiveness (Wilbarger & Wilbarger, 1991; 2002). Sensory techniques from this frame of reference have been applied effectively with children, adults with mental health conditions, and older adults. We will begin with the earliest to emerge, sensory integration, and then present other approaches as we work our way across the age span.

Developed in the 1970s and earlier by A. Jean Ayres, an occupational therapist, sensory integration (SI) has become a standard approach in pediatric occupational therapy. Ayres (1989a) identified four phases of sensory integrative development in children, and through extensive research, developed one of the first standardized assessments of our profession, the Southern California Sensory Integration and Praxis Tests (SIPT). The SIPT has been described as "the most comprehensive and statistically sound measure for assessing important aspects of sensory integration" (Bundy, Lane, & Murray, 2002, pp. 170–171). Ayres first used sensory integrative techniques to address children with "minimal brain dysfunction," now known as learning disability. Lorna Jean King (1974, 1990) has developed sensory integrative strategies for adults with mental illness, mental retardation, and autism. Mildred Ross has designed a group approach using sensory integrative theory with older adults and others with chronic illness.

Focus

Other theorists have researched and expanded Ayres' original concepts, and currently this approach is used across the lifespan. Disorders of attention, hypersensitivity to sensory stimuli, poor postural control and balance, apraxia, and inefficient cognitive processing are some of the many occupational difficulties that have been treated with success using sensory integrative strategies. School-based therapists often use sensory integrative techniques to enhance a child's fine motor control (handwriting), focus attention, and enhance learning ability in the classroom. Adults may retain or acquire sensory modulation difficulties that interfere with their ability to work, socialize, or participate in other occupations of daily life. Using Dunn's (1999; 2002) Sensory Profile as a yardstick, occupational therapists can gain a more precise understanding of how sensory thresholds, which vary with every individual, influence both sensory perceptions and behavioral responses within the context of everyday occupations.

Theoretical Base

Neuroscientists define sensory integration as the brain's ability to organize sensory information received from the body and environment, and to produce an adaptive response. Bundy, Lane, and Murray (2002) define five basic assumptions of sensory integrative theory.

Assumption 1: The Central Nervous System Is Plastic

Plasticity refers to the brain's ability to reorganize itself in response to intervention. Ayres (1989b) writes:

... the brain, especially the young brain, is naturally malleable: structure and function become more firm and set with age. The formative capacity allows person–environment interaction to promote and enhance neurointegrative efficiency. A deficit in the individual's ability to engage effectively in this transaction at critical periods interferes with optimal brain development and consequent overall ability. Identifying the deficient areas at a young age and addressing them therapeutically can enhance the individual's opportunity for normal development. (p. 12)

	Table 18-1			
	Ayres' Sensory Integration Phases			
The Senses	**Integration of Sensory Input**			**End Products**
	Phase 1	*Phase 2*	*Phase 3*	*Phase 4*
Auditory (hearing)			Language	
Vestibular (gravity and movement)	Eye movement	Body percept		Concentration
	Posture	Coordination of two sides of the body		Ability to organize
	Balance			Self-esteem
Proprioceptive (muscles and joints)		Motor planning	Eye-hand coordination	Self-control
	Muscle tone	Activity level		Self-confidence
	Gravitational security	Attention span	Visual perception	Academic learning ability
Tactile (touch)	Sucking	Emotional stability	Purposeful activity	Abstract thought and reasoning
	Eating			
	Mother–infant bond			
	Tactile comfort			Dominance
Visual (seeing)			Language	

Adapted with permission from Ayres, A. J. (1989). Sensory integration and the child. Los Angeles, CA: Western Psychological Services.

Subsequent brain research has indicated that neurological plasticity persists into adulthood, and possibly throughout life.

Assumption 2: Sensory Integration Develops in Stages (Phases)

Ayres (1989b) conceptualized the infant brain as immature and not yet capable of processing all sensory information. She identified four phases of subsequently more complex sensory integration as a continually flowing process. The phases are summarized in Table 18-1.

Phase 1

Tactile, vestibular, and proprioceptive senses become integrated during the first year of life, creating mother–infant bond.

Phase 2

Tactile, vestibular, and proprioceptive functions are building blocks for emotional stability and a body percept (internal map), which pave the way for increasingly skilled movement against gravity, normally occurring during the second year of life.

Phase 3

Speech and language depend upon the integration of auditory sensations with other senses, vestibular,

proprioceptive, tactile, and visual. Auditory and vestibular sensory systems are intimately related as the child attends and listens to others, and moves mouth, breath, and tongue to articulate words. Integration of vestibular and proprioceptive systems give the child control over eye movements to follow a line of print. Purposeful activity is possible when eyes are directing the hands, and the body begins to work as a whole.

Phase 4

Sensory integration should be well developed as the child enters school (typically age 4 to 5). With a foundation of brain and body working together, specialization of brain and body can develop. Hand dominance is necessary for fine motor control such as handwriting; eye dominance leads the way for reading left to right. Other areas of hemispheric specialization allow the brain to organize and function more efficiently for academic learning and other areas of continued growth and development.

Assumption 3: The Brain Works as an Integrated Whole

Ayres continually stressed this idea as she conceptualized foundation skills paving the way for higher level (cortical) brain functions. This idea has been incorrectly interpreted as hierarchical, when it just as easily lends itself to a systems view of brain functioning. Lower and higher order brain functions continue to influence each other into maturity.

Assumption 4: Adaptive Interactions Are Critical to Sensory Integration

Children learn by interaction with the environment. The child climbs up a step and falls back down. The next time he tries, he will change his approach by refining the movement to produce a more adaptive response. This example demonstrates the use of feedback from the vestibular, proprioceptive, and tactile systems, which eventually form a neuronal model of correct or successful movements (climbing steps).

Assumption 5: People Have an Inner Drive to Develop Sensory Integration Through Participation in Sensorimotor Activities

Ayres (1989b) notes that every child has a great inner drive toward higher development, moving from rolling to sitting, to crawling and climbing, to walking, without much encouragement from others. The confidence a child develops in mastering each skill has been linked to the concept of self-actualization. Even children with lags in sensory integrative development tend to seek out the sensations that they need for continued growth. A child who cannot integrate sensations on a noisy playground will seek out a quieter environment to avoid sensory overload. The child with autism may seek out vibration by leaning against an active washing machine or dryer.

King's Principle of Faulty Proprioceptive Input

Lorna Jean King (1974) studied adults with process schizophrenia (primarily negative symptoms). She identified a typical "S" shaped posture, accompanied by an under-responsiveness to environmental stimuli, which she attributed to "faulty proprioceptive feedback." More recently, the symptoms of schizophrenia have been re-categorized as either positive (meaning things that occur that are abnormal, like delusions and hallucinations) or negative (meaning things that are missing, such as lack of affect, lack of motivation, and stiff or rigid movements or catatonia). The type most responsive to SI techniques is the latter, those with negative symptoms.

Dunn's Sensory Processing Model

Dunn's model focuses on the interaction between neurological thresholds for incoming sensory input and the behavioral responses generated by them. A neurological threshold is defined as the amount of stimulation required for a neuron to respond. Thresholds may be classified along a continuum from low, or a minimal amount of stimulation, to high, or a large amount of stimulation. For example, the child or adult with a high threshold might not hear a low hum of an oncoming vehicle at a distance, and will not react until the roar of a motorcycle is a few feet away. Thresholds result in different types of reactions by individuals, as they impose self-regulation (either automatic or voluntary) upon their awareness of different sensations. Neural excitation is the person's action or reaction to sensation, while neural inhibition decreases or blocks the response. Sensory modulation refers to the balancing of neurological excitation and inhibition. Persons need to modulate incoming sensations, ignoring some and paying attention to others, in order to react appropriately to situations and environments, and to focus attention to tasks and occupations. Modulation involves habituation, a learned neurological response to the repetitive firing of neurons until the stimulus is determined to no longer need attention. For example, hearing a motor vehicle moving around outside your window may arouse you from sleep, but once you have determined that it has snowed and the street is being plowed the sound is no longer a threat. Habituation occurs when the auditory stimulus is tuned out, allowing you to go back to sleep. Sensitization is the opposite of habituation. Sensitization enhances one's attention to a potentially important stimulus, and can increase the ability to detect and discriminate incoming sensations. Waking up to the smell of smoke illustrates this phenomenon, as a person senses the danger of a potential fire and tries to determine what is burning (electrical, wood, petroleum, overcooked food) and its direction or location (inside vs. outside the house) in order to take appropriate action. Heightened sensitivity might cause disability when individuals are unable to tune out incoming sensations, even when they do not pose a threat, such as in persons with attention deficit hyperactive disorder (ADHD) (Dunn & Bennett, 2002), schizophrenia (Bunney et al., 1999; Light & Braff, 2000), and brain injury (Madigan, DeLucia, Diamond, Tramontano, & Averill, 2000; Arciniegas et al., 1999).

The assessment of neurological thresholds, modulation, and resultant behaviors may be measured with Dunn's Sensory Profile (Dunn, 1999), which uses both self report and caregiver/parent perceptions of sensory processing and behaviors. Based on this tool, Dunn has identified four processing patterns of neurological thresholds and self-regulation:

1. Sensory-seeking
2. Sensory-avoiding
3. Sensory sensitivity
4. Low registration

The patterns have been correlated with temperament and personality factors such as fatigue, agitation, anxiety, depression, and self-esteem (Dunn, 2001). Preliminary research with this relatively new sensory model suggests that sensory processing patterns may be linked with lifestyle patterns, psychosocial interactions, and cognitive performance.

Although sensory processing patterns have usefulness in designing interventions for disabled populations, Dunn does not consider the patterns themselves to indicate disability. Rather they are "reflections of who we are" (2001, p. 617), and as such, can offer insights about how people can manage their daily occupations, communicate their needs, and enhance their experiences.

Wilbarger's Approach With Sensory Defensiveness

Sensory defensiveness is a "constellation of symptoms that involve avoidance reactions to sensation from any sensory modality" (Wilbarger & Wilbarger, 1991, as cited in Bundy, Lane, & Murray, 2002, p. 335). Sensory defensiveness has been attributed to a disruption in the central nervous system's process of identifying positive or negative affective qualities of incoming stimuli (LeDoux, 1996). The rapid automatic or subconscious evaluation produces defensive responses that interact with other parts of the system, such as memory of prior encounters with the stimuli, arousal or hyper arousal, and anxiety. The Wilbargers have devised methods for reducing hypersensitivity and for facilitating modulation in persons with sensory defensiveness using somatosensory input with a goal of long-term adaptation at the biochemical, cellular, and behavioral levels (Field, 1998; Pert, 1997; Wall & Melzack, 1995). Their intervention approach has education, clinical, and home-based components:

1. Clients and caregivers participate in an evaluation of sensory experiences to promote awareness of the connection between reactions and symptoms, and the presence of specific types of sensory input.

2. During clinical visits, the occupational therapist applies specific types of deep pressure and proprioceptive input.

3. The occupational therapist guides the client to integrate a sensory diet into the client's daily routines.

A sensory diet is a treatment plan that involves the therapeutic use of sensory input within the context of daily activities (Wilbarger, 1993). The specific sensory experiences contain qualities most likely to reduce defensive behaviors, and these are identified and integrated through a collaborative process with the client. Adaptation of both tasks and environments can be made. The goal involves regulating input to maintain an optimal arousal state that allows the client to engage in daily tasks, and to develop consistent routines and predictability. See the example of Jo, later in this chapter.

FUNCTION AND DISABILITY

Much of the research by Ayres and her colleagues, including the SIPT evaluation standardization studies,

sought to identify specific types of sensory integrative dysfunction. Some of the types identified are somato-dyspraxia, poor bilateral integration and sequencing, abnormal postural ocular movements, and inadequate sensory modulation. Mulligan (1998) used factor analysis to confirm four subtypes of sensory integrative dysfunction:

- Visual-perceptual deficits
- Somatosensory deficits
- Bilateral integration and sequencing deficits
- Dyspraxia

Sensory testing using the SIPT can identify both the subtype and severity of sensory integrative dysfunction in children, based on a normal bell curve that measures deviation from the norm. Other tests of sensory systems are also available.

For adolescents and adults, sensory integration deficits may co-exist with other health conditions, such as chronic mental illness, pervasive developmental disorders, acquired brain injuries, and dementia. Persons with patterns of heavy drinking or recreational drug use also have been found to have sensory integrative deficits. Various therapeutic movement activities that focus on specific sensory input have been shown to be effective in research studies with disabled populations.

CHANGE AND MOTIVATION

Therapeutic change occurs through sensory input in the context of interaction with the environment. For children or adults, occupational therapists create interventions that offer increased amounts of sensory input according to the client's changing needs. For the child with ADHD, strong vestibular input (scooter board play, spinning on a tire swing) has a calming effect that encourages the sensory integration needed to sit still and pay attention in the classroom. The adult with Parkinson's disease may be helped to keep his or her balance with the increased proprioceptive input provided by ankle weights. Lorna Jean King (1974) found that parachute play with a group of young adults with schizophrenia produced a state of calm alertness that prepared them for verbal therapy and other cognitive tasks. Linda Levy (1974) noted that rocking in a rocking chair offered comfort to persons with dementia who became agitated due to sundowners syndrome.

In summary, change occurs through guided sensory input in the context of individual or group activities.

The inner drive of children to continue the spiral upward toward greater maturity has already been mentioned. On the flip side, lack of motivation may be seen in both children and adults who have problems with sensory integration that cause them to avoid activities involving movement or specific kinds of sensory stimulation. McLean (2003) writes of Jo, a blind and deaf client who, at age 37, had the annoying habit of continually removing her clothing, and slapping and biting herself. Sensory testing found her to be tactile defensive, a problem with sensory modulation first described by Ayres in children. Occupational therapy based on Wilbarger's "sensory diet" (Wilbarger & Wilbarger, 2002), which introduced graded tactile and proprioceptive input, must have re-activated Jo's inner drive, as she sought out sensations of deep pressure, warmth, and active rhythmic movement. These strong sensory inputs combined with careful clothing selection allowed Jo to remain comfortably dressed for most of the day.

EVALUATION*

The SIPT battery has been called the "gold standard" for evaluating sensory integration and praxis (Schaaf & Roley, 2006, p. 25). Research on this assessment is ongoing, and many relationships between test results and academic learning have been found. Parham (1998) found that praxis and visual perception at 6 to 8 years of age were significant predictors of arithmetic and reading four years later (Bodison & Mailloux, 2006). The subtests of the SIPT and what they measure are listed in Table 18-2.

Ideally, clients should be evaluated for sensory integrative dysfunction using the SIPT (available from Western Psychological Services, Los Angeles, CA). However, the test itself is only for children 4 years to 8 years and 11 months, it is costly, and specialized training and certification are needed to administer it. Even when giving this test is not practical, it is important to understand what it measures and how these sensory factors relate to a child's everyday occupations in the classroom, home, and community (Bodison & Mailloux, 2006).

Frequently, informal clinical observations have been used to supplement the SIPT, including a test of prone extension, muscle tone, joint stability, postural adjustment, and equilibrium reactions. A video and corresponding manual (Blanche, 2002) outlines and demonstrates these clinical observations. The Post Rotary Nystagmus (PRN) Test measures vestibular processing as indicated by the duration of eye movement (nystagmus) following rotation (spinning) in a standardized position on a PRN board (available from Western Psychological Services) However the test does not have norms outside of the PRN subtest of the SIPT. A depressed duration of nystagmus is considered an indication of vestibular processing dysfunction when accompanied by other deficits in postural responses.

Western Psychological Services offers an array of sensory-based assessment tools for all ages and contexts. The Test of Sensory Functions in Infants (TSFI) offers a quick method to observe objectively the sensory responses of babies 4 to 18 months. Additionally, the DeGangi-Berk Test of Sensory Integration (TSI), a tool for 3- to 5-year old-children, has clear scoring and cut-offs, which allow the therapist to determine the extent of sensory processing difficulties. Most exciting is the recent publication of the Sensory Processing Measure (SPM) by Parham, Ecker, Miller-Kuhaneck, Henry, and Glennon (2007), which was standardized on over 1,000 children and provides scores of normal range, some symptoms, and definite problem range on several scales: praxis, processing of individual systems (tactile, proprioceptive, vestibular, visual, and auditory), and social participation. The SPM is actually two tools that can be used together or individually. The Home Form (Parham & Ecker, 2007) is completed by the parent/caregiver, and the School Form (Miller-Kuhaneck, Henry, & Glennon, 2007) is completed by several educational personnel, as it includes items from the main classroom, art, music, physical education, playground, cafeteria, and bus. Both tools offer the entire team the opportunity to identify when a behavior is, or is not, sensory based.

Many signs of sensory processing dysfunction may be reported by clients or their caregivers, or easily observed within the context of normal daily activities. Dunn's (1999) Sensory Profile (available from PsychCorp, [Harcourt Assessment, San Antonio, TX]) measures neurological thresholds of auditory, visual, vestibular, touch, multisensory, and oral sensory processing and identifies patterns related to modulation and behavioral and emotional responses. For children, the instrument includes parent and/or caregiver questionnaires and rating scales categorized by sensory system. Likewise, a Sensory Profile for adolescents and adults uses a questionnaire format, this time self-report, to identify typical sensory experiences and responses to different sensory input (Brown & Dunn, 2002). Some assessments for use with adults include the Schroeder, Block, Campbell (SBC) Test of adult sensory integration (Schroeder, Block, Campbell, & Savage Stowell, 1978) and the Smaga and Ross Integrated Battery (SARIB), which measures both sensory processing and cognition in adults (Ross, 1987).

GUIDELINES FOR INTERVENTION

When introducing sensory input, occupational therapists need to take their cues from the clients themselves. Clients know, more than we do, what kind of sensory stimulation they need and how much they are able to tolerate. The occupational therapist's role in this frame of reference is finding available and socially acceptable activities that involve the type and intensity of sensation clients need to normalize their sensory processing and produce adaptive responses.

Some training in sensory integration techniques is included at the advanced level of most occupational therapy educational programs. Occupational therapists who want to work with children are usually advised to seek certification from Sensory Integration International (St. Petersburg, FL, http://www.aota.org/news/announcements/40347.aspx), an organization dedicated to continued research and training of therapists in the administration and interpretation of the SIPT. Currently this organization is experiencing some legal difficulties that may temporarily affect the availability of continuing education offerings. Separately, Pat and Julie Wilbarger conduct continuing education courses in the

---

The authors would like to acknowledge Dr. Tara Glennon for her contribution to this section on sensory integration evaluation.

Table 18-2

Subtests of the Sensory Integration and Praxis Test Battery and Examples

Subtest	Brief Description	What is Measured/Home Example
Space visualization	Child must choose which of two shapes fits into a form board.	Visual manipulation: Doing a puzzle, packing a backpack.
Figure–ground	Child identifies figures hidden in a line drawing.	Visual scanning and discrimination. Finding items in a closet or drawer.
Standing and walking balance	Child holds positions on one foot or two with eyes open or closed.	Vestibular sensory functioning and motor planning. Maintaining upright posture, using a scooter or skateboard.
Design copying	Child looks a drawings of shape and copies the shape with a pencil on a test form (booklet).	Eye hand coordination, fine motor coordination, spatial perception. Related to drawing and handwriting.
Postural praxis	Child imitates positions demonstrated by the therapist.	Vestibular and proprioceptive sensory processes, awareness of body position needed to avoid bumping into things.
Bilateral motor coordination	Child imitates reciprocal movements of the therapist, using both sides of the body.	Both sides of the body work together in performing dressing, bathing, and grooming tasks.
Praxis on verbal command	Therapist verbally directs the child to take on unusual postures, both sitting and standing.	Understanding and following verbal directions is necessary for leaning how to do things or following the "rules."
Constructional praxis	Child builds a tower identical to the therapist with blocks, then replicates a more complex model.	Spatial awareness, eye–hand coordination and understanding three dimensions relates to problem-solving: pour milk, dip cookie.
Postrotary nystagmus	Therapist spins child on a board, stops abruptly, and records the number of seconds subsequent eye movement (nystagmus) continues.	Relates to vestibular system functioning, which affects muscle tone and postural stability that is necessary for the development of skilled fine motor control.
Motor accuracy	Child traces a large butterfly shape placed at midline, with a pencil and tries to stay on thick black line. Right and left hands tested separately.	Eye–hand coordination, fine motor control, hand dominance, and crossing midline. Relates to handwriting, coloring; visual tracking for reading and computer games.
Sequencing praxis	Therapist demonstrates movements for child to imitate.	Learning multi step tasks that require skilled movements, like tying shoes, braiding hair.
Oral praxis	Imitates movements of tongue, lips, cheek, teeth, jaw.	Speech and recognizing facial expressions.
Manual form perception	Child matches plastic shapes by touch with vision occluded.	Finding coins or keys in pockets, hidden areas, inside bags or drawers.
Kinesthesia	Move child's finger to specific spots, vision occluded, "go back to friend's house."	Accurate movement memory is needed for using a computer mouse, keyboarding, using a key in a lock, using an ipod.
Finger identification	Vision occluded, touch child's finger in 1 to 2 places. Child points.	Tactile discrimination and possibly defensiveness or hypersensitivity is noted.
Graphesthesia	Write on back of child's hand with finger; child imitates.	Note accuracy and behavior: defensiveness prevents wearing certain clothing/textures.
Localization of tactile stimuli	Measures location of light touch without vision.	Tactile discrimination needed for perception of qualities of objects, last tactile test likely to elicit hypersensitivity issues.

Adapted from Bodison, S., & Mailloux, Z. (2006). The Sensory Integration and Praxis Tests: Illuminating struggles and strengths in participation at school. OT Practice, Sept. 25th, CE 1–8..

treatment of sensory modulation disorders, including the sensory diet mentioned earlier. For example, with tactile defensiveness, they suggest a graded "diet" of brushing the skin with different size brushes and progressively lighter strokes to "desensitize" the skin and prevent the irritation that produces problem behaviors.

Equipment

For children, supply catalogs offer a myriad of specialized equipment for sensory integrative therapy. Most are designed to position clients and pinpoint the specific type of sensory input required to meet client goals. Bolster swings suspended from the ceiling, rocker or tilt boards, cylinders for climbing or rolling, nets filled with colored plastic balls, and boards or swings which rotate or spin

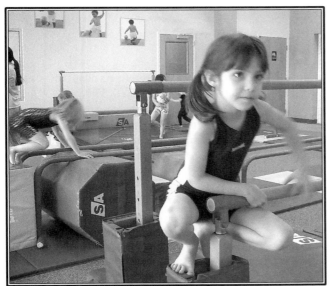

Figure 18-1. Sensory Integration programs use specialized equipment. Photo courtesy of M. Cole.

often resemble playground or gym equipment. Do not be fooled—designing effective SI interventions for clients with health conditions using any type of equipment requires a thorough understanding of sensory integrative theory and its foundations in neuroscience. In Figure 18-1, Hannah uses parallel bars to work on balance and motor planning. The vestibular and proprioceptive input also heightens her ability to pay attention and learn in school. Large mats and protective padding help to safeguard children while using the equipment.

Group Interventions

According to Koomar and Bundy (2002), groups have their place in interventions with children who need to work on cooperative play, social skills, or specific functional skills such as handwriting (p. 297). Sensory diets may be taught more practically in groups where strategies for application in daily life can be demonstrated and discussed by client members.

Groups of older adults with late stage dementia in adult day care or skilled nursing home settings can benefit from sensory stimulation. Novel stimuli such as lights, colors, calming and rhythmic sounds, and objects of varying textures, as well as striking aromas and tastes, should be offered in ways that maximize arousal and response without overwhelming or causing anxiety.

Interventions for Adults With Mental Illness

While most of the research of Ayres and her associates applies to children, several occupational therapists have written about the treatment of mentally ill adults using neurodevelopmental and sensory integrative techniques. Lorna Jean King created group interventions for clients

Table 18-3
Lorna Jean King, Principles of Sensory Integration for Group Activities

King's Principles	Goal	Examples
Choose activities that provide strong vestibular and proprioceptive input.	Arouse and normalize movement.	Pushing a heavy chair across the room.
Elicit spontaneous responses that occur below the level of awareness.	Stimulate subcortical areas (brainstem).	Reach out to "catch" a bubble.
Encourage pleasurable activities that motivate participation.	Establish limbic system connections.	Bat a beach ball over a net.
Minimize cognitive requirements.	Focus on pleasure of movement and sensation.	Spin a streamer on a stick to music.
Enable adaptive interaction with others and with the environment.	Reconnect with clients' inner drive.	Pass an egg around the circle using only elbows.

Adapted from King, L. J. (1988). Occupational therapy and neuropsychiatry. In S. Robertson (Ed.), Mental health focus. *Rockville, MD: American Occupational Therapy Association.*

with mental illness, using specific techniques and principles (Table 18-3).

King has noted the lack of sensory integration in both schizophrenic and autistic clients by observing the kinds of sensory stimulation they seek from the environment. For example, she evaluates a retarded and autistic adolescent by observing his preference for vibratory input (plays with a hand-held vibrator), proprioceptive input (constant self-hugging), and calming vestibular input (distractible and disruptive behavior is reduced by slow swinging and rocking) (Larrington, 1987).

Paul Schilder noted as early as the 1930s that schizophrenic patients are markedly under-reactive to vestibular stimulation as measured by post rotary nystagmus (rapid eye movements) (King, 1974). King linked the vestibular system abnormalities with the postural and movement limitations (pacing, adduction, and internal rotation) observed in the chronic process schizophrenic patient, more currently called the negative symptom schizophrenic. Process schizophrenia is a subtype of schizophrenia, a mental disorder that develops insidiously from childhood and is not the result of a severe or recognizable stress. Process schizophrenics do not respond readily to medical or behavioral treatment, and so tend to be chronically institutionalized.

King refers to numerous studies of the neurological deficits in schizophrenia (and also autism) that link faulty vestibular and proprioceptive processing to schizophrenic symptoms. Some of these symptoms include perceptual deficits, feelings of fatigue and slow movement, postural insecurity (fear of falling), concrete thinking, and lack of emotional response. King's hypothesis is that some schizophrenic patients have "defective proprioceptive feed back mechanisms, the vestibular component in particular being under-reactive in its role in the sensorimotor integration" (King, 1974, p. 534).

Considering today's emphasis on the biochemical etiology of all mental illness (including schizophrenia), King's postulations of the circular role of movement in altering biochemical states as well as biochemistry affecting movement remain timely. Movement and sensation are known to produce chemical changes, just as taking medication produces changes, in brain chemistry. Furthermore, King states that "this model ... applies not only to etiology but also to treatment. Although we cannot be sure which chemicals to alter, or in what direction, we can intervene in the motor behavior of the individual with the knowledge that there will be effects upon the thought processes and upon biochemistry" (King, 1974, p. 534). In later publications, King notes the role of activities in coping with stress. A strenuous action, or "fight or flight" response to stress (Gal & Lazarus, 1975), was found to be responsible for the rapid metabolism of stress hormones, thus preventing secondary damage to the system. This suggests that strenuous or heavy work activity can serve to normalize the neurotransmitter balance that has been deranged by stress (King, 1978, 1988).

The treatment techniques King utilizes in treating groups of chronic schizophrenic clients are adaptations of the techniques Ayres used with children. They are gross motor movement activities aimed at normalizing patterns of excessive flexion, adduction, and internal rotation and increasing range of motion. Vestibular and tactile stimulation are provided through the use of the standard props—hammocks, scooter boards, balls, and blankets. Heavy work patterns suggested by Rood (1954) resisted use of tonic muscle groups, and co-contraction patterns are also incorporated. Other types of equipment King has added include parachutes, balloons, and beanbag chairs.

King (1990) suggests two criteria for the selection of activities: 1) attention must not be centered on the motor process, but rather on the object or outcome, and 2) the activity must be pleasurable, evoking smiles, laughter, and a feeling of fun. Patients should not have to think about what they are doing or how they move; the goal is to elicit spontaneous movement and effect. Vestibular and proprioceptive processing occur at the brain stem level and produce automatic responses, not cortical (voluntary) responses. Therefore, if a ball is thrown to a patient and his or her hands extend spontaneously to catch it, we can assume that this automatic action reflects adaptive vestibular processing at the brain stem level. The goal of group activities using this frame of reference is to stimulate the sensory processing systems so that they will function more adaptively. As occupational therapists, we see spontaneous and purposeful motor responses as evidence that we are reaching that goal.

Approaches With Older Adults

Mildred Ross, best known for her work with the Five Stage Group, uses theories of sensory integration and motor control in creating an organized approach to the nervous systems of clients with chronic illness (Ross & Bachner, 2004). Inspired by King, Ross begins with novel sensory stimuli in orienting small groups of clients, and follows up with a movement activity intended to bring about spontaneous adaptive responses on mostly subcortical levels. In the third of her five stages, Ross departs from King in requiring that movement be refined with a perceptual-motor activity. This stage encourages clients to integrate sensory feedback from the group activity, paving the way for higher level sensory processing. In the fourth stage, Ross tests Ayres' hypothesis that controlled sensory input can produce higher cognitive functioning. A cognitive group task is presented, often requiring verbal interaction (discussing the meaning of a poem) and/or fine motor skills (drawing a picture or writing a letter). She is constantly surprised by the adaptive responses from even the most withdrawn or lowest functioning group members. For example, in stage four of Ross's group, an elderly gentleman from a nursing home, who made no eye contact and rarely spoke, noticed that a fellow group member in a wheelchair had dropped her pencil and couldn't retrieve it. To everyone's amazement, he spontaneously crossed the room to pick up the pencil and hand it to her. For those nursing home

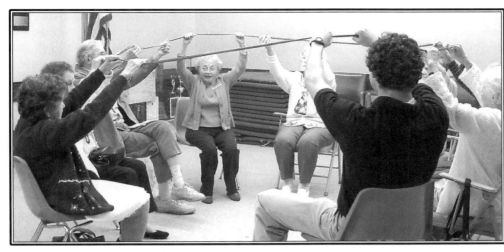

Figure 18-2. Mildred Ross demonstrating Stage II movement activity.

Table 18-4		
Mildred Ross, Sensations that Alert and Calm for the Five-Stage Group		
Senses	**Alerting**	**Calming**
Touch	Rubbing, patting, cold Example: clapping hands	Hugging, holding Example: self-massaging
Vestibular	Rotation, rapid forward movement Example: running	Slow, rhythmic movement Example: rocking chair
Proprioceptive	Light pressure Example: brushing with a feather	Moderate pressure Example: wrapping in a blanket
Visual	Bright colors, bright light Example: high contrast figures	Pastels, low intensity Example: candlelight
Hearing	Irregular, loud and contrasting Example: banging on a piano	Melodious, rhythmic, slow Example: strumming a harp
Smell	Pungent smells Examples: onions, vinegar	Sweet, faint smells Examples: vanilla, lavender
Taste	Strong flavors, crunchy Examples: hot peppers, pretzels	Smooth texture, warm Example: hot cocoa

residents deemed unfit for other activities, social awareness, emotional expression, and non-verbal interaction often emerge from the controlled sensory experiences of the Ross Five Stage Group (2005, personal communication).

Figure 18-2 shows Mildred Ross leading a Stage II movement activity in a Ross Five Stage Group of older adults in an adult daycare program.

The Ross Five-Stage Group follows:

- *Stage I:* Orientation, such as shaking hands or sharing a novel object
- *Stage II:* Movement, a gross motor activity that matches client abilities
- *Stage III:* Perceptual Motor, requiring more refined motor control
- *Stage IV:* Cognitive, making use of calm alertness that results from sensory input

- *Stage V:* Closure, such as sharing what each member liked best

Throughout the Five Stage Group, the occupational therapist continually monitors client responses to sensory input and adapts the group activity accordingly. Table 18-4 may be used as a guideline for grading activities and environmental conditions for the group.

Adapting Sensory Environments

As an OT consultant to Fairfield Hills Hospital, I (M. Cole) was asked to investigate a feeding problem for an elderly gentleman on the geropsychiatry unit. During lunch time, I went to observe the gentleman, who had good dexterity in both hands as he applied butter to a slice of bread with a plastic knife. He next removed the paper cover from a bowl of soup, and spooned it to his mouth with no apparent difficulty. "What is the problem?" I wondered. I turned my attention to the environment. Lunch was served to 25 to 30 clients (residents), in a large day room. Some clients sat at tables in the center of the room, but the majority had their lunch served on trays attached to their wheelchairs. My client's wheelchair was positioned near the corner of the room, facing the center, and as he continued to feed himself, music began to play over the speakers in the ceiling. A nurses aide told me one of the medical interns has read that playing classical music during mealtimes would create a more normal and relaxed atmosphere within the hospital setting. Soon after the music began, my client stopped eating; became increasingly agitated as time went on. I asked him if he was still hungry, noting that he hadn't touched the main course. Initially he complied and began eating some mashed potatoes. Then, suddenly and without warning, the gave the entire tray a shove, sending it crashing to the floor.

"He does this every day," the nurses aide told me. "Now I'll have to come back later and feed him. He used to be a good eater, too."

I cautiously approached him and asked him what happened. His whole demeanor had changed. It took several tries just to get his attention. His hands trembled as he finally answered with only grunt and a blank stare. It was then I noticed that the music sounded louder from where he sat. No wonder! It blared from the speaker in the ceiling directly above his head.

Another day we removed him from the day room and served him lunch in a quiet area. The gentleman's "feeding problem" disappeared. What are the lessons here?

- All individuals perceive sensory input differently. What is stimulating for one might be overwhelming to another.

- Occupational therapists can use sensory integrative concepts and techniques to test clients who appear abnormally sensitive to certain types of sensory input.

- When problem solving client occupational performance issues, occupational therapists need to look beyond the "obvious" environmental influences, and to consider all types of sensory input, including not only visual and auditory, but the other senses as well.

- When we observe occupational performance problems, we need to consider the effects of the sensory environment.

- Environmental adaptations need to include adjusting sensory input to optimize occupational performance.

CASE STUDY: BRAD

In 1976, I (M. Cole) had the opportunity to meet Lorna Jean King, when she conducted a workshop for the staff of Connecticut Valley Hospital, a state facility for mental illness. At a celebratory dinner after the workshop, quite by accident I found myself sitting next to her. At the time I worked part time in a psychiatric unit of a nearby community hospital, concurrently raising two preschoolers. Ms. King politely asked me about my family, and I proceeded to tell her about my son Brad, age 5, who spent the day in constant motion and almost never slept. She hinted that Brad might have ADHD, which could benefit from sensory integration therapy. For the sleeping problem, she suggested that I have Brad sleep in a hammock, using slow rocking motion to calm him down at night.

Eager to end the nightly bedtime struggle with my son, I immediately purchased a hammock. My husband hung it over Brad's bed (in case he fell out) and close enough to the wall for him to push against it to rock himself. We dressed Brad in a blanket sleeper, placed him in the hammock, turned out the light, and waited. Giggles soon gave way to humming, and then silence. Not every night was that easy, but we persisted until the time Brad took to fall asleep decreased from over an hour to just a few minutes. Sensory integration worked!

At the time I searched for a pediatric OT who was certified in sensory integration therapy, and found none close enough to test and treat Brad. I read all I could about the approach, and later enrolled in SI training myself. As I learned to administer the SIPT, Brad was my first subject. I tested him on the PRN board, and found he had no nystagmus. None! He wanted to keep spinning on the PRN board, and I let him. Other clinical signs of an under-reactive vestibular system included poor left-right discrimination (–2.5), poor imitation of postures (–1.4), poor motor accuracy (–1.3 both sides), poor figure-ground perception (–1.3), mixed dominance, low muscle tone, and jerky eye tracking. Granted I was still in training, and did not actually become SI certified until 1980. However, I was now convinced that Brad had what was then identified by Ayres as vestibular bilateral integration (VBI) disorder. He had been held back from first grade because of his hyperactivity, and would soon complete a "transition" year in public school. Behavior issues constantly surfaced, much to my dismay.

That summer I decided to take matters into my own hands. I hung a tire swing from a tree in the back yard, and he spent at least 30 minutes a day spinning and swinging (Figure 18-3). We built a scooter board from wood and desk chair wheels and covered it with carpeting. Our driveway ran downhill from the street, and soon Brad and the neighborhood kids took turns racing down it on the scooter board. One day I came home from work to find that Brad had built a "ski jump" out of scrap wood so he could race down the driveway on the scooter board and fly off the ramp into the backyard. Brad's inner drive was hard at work and he was having the time of his life. In August, he attended horseback riding camp. No handwriting practice or any other academic study occurred that summer (Figure 18-4).

In September, Brad began first grade as a special education student. His handwriting had significantly improved

Figure 18-3. Brad's backyard tree house with tire swing for spinning tire.

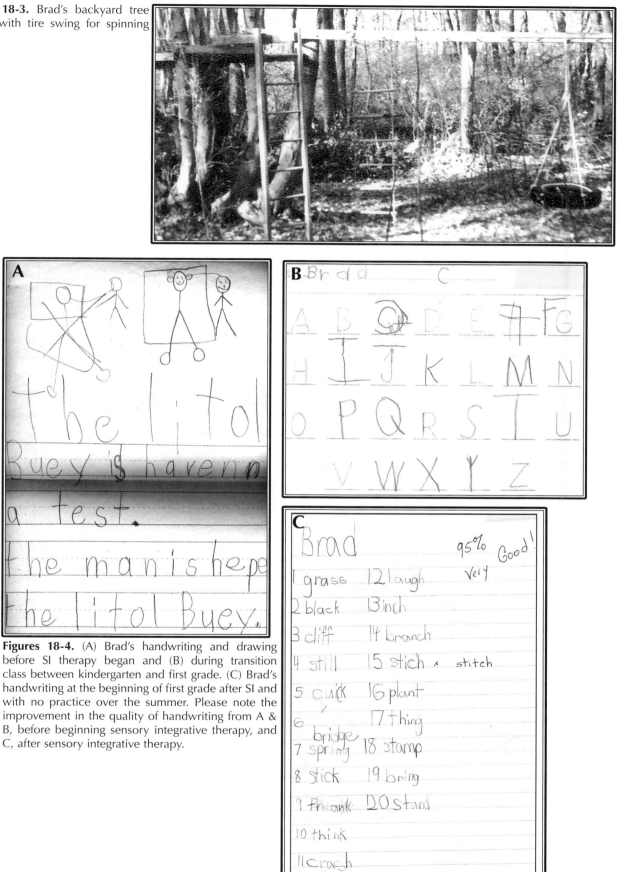

Figures 18-4. (A) Brad's handwriting and drawing before SI therapy began and (B) during transition class between kindergarten and first grade. (C) Brad's handwriting at the beginning of first grade after SI and with no practice over the summer. Please note the improvement in the quality of handwriting from A & B, before beginning sensory integrative therapy, and C, after sensory integrative therapy.

(see Figure 18-4C). Out of curiosity, I repeated the Motor Accuracy Test, and found that Brad's score had improved nearly 2 standard deviations, placing him within normal limits. Brad's IQ test (WPPSI) was 141, so with academic performance lagging one to two grade levels, he was clearly learning disabled. As his mother, I could not submit my SI testing, but I brought samples of his handwriting to an Individualized Educational Planning meeting, showing before and after summer vacation as evidence that he should be given occupational therapy in school. This was 1978, and the principal had never heard of occupational therapy, never mind sensory integration. After more than a year of "advocacy," the school board finally gave in and hired an occupational therapist. Brad was treated 3 times a week for 2 years.

RESEARCH

In a study of school-based therapists in the United States, sensory integration and neurodevelopmental were the predominant theories used (Storch & Eskow, 1996). Schaaf and Miller (2005) suggest a sensory approach for children with developmental disabilities, and suggest the development of a fidelity measure for use in intervention studies. Early efforts to do so include the identification of structural (room set-up, therapist training) and process elements. The room should be arranged to engage the child; provide physical safety; offer sensory opportunities; support optimal arousal; provide just-right challenge; ensure success; support self-organization; and create play context, collaborative activity choice, and therapeutic alliance (Parham, Cohn, Spitzer, et al., 2007). This represents a coordinated effort on the part of occupational therapy researchers to produce viable evidence of the effectiveness of interventions based on sensory integration theory.

Much of Ayres' research was devoted to the development and validation of assessment tools. The Southern California Sensory Integration Tests (Ayres, 1972, 1980) and more recently, the Sensory Integration and Praxis Tests (SIPT) (Ayres, 1989a), serve as a basis for measuring a broad range of outcomes as well as the identification of patterns of sensory integrative dysfunction (Ayres 1989b; Ayres, Mailloux, & Wendler, 1987; Bundy, Lane, & Murray, 2002). However, studies in recent years have questioned the earlier positive outcomes of sensory integrative interventions with learning-disabled children (Varga & Camilli, 1999; Hoehn & Baumeister, 1994). Despite the negative findings, sensory integrative therapy continues to be widely practiced by occupational therapists (Law, Missiuna, Pollock, & Stewart, 2005; Watling, Deitz, Kanny, & McLaughlin, 1999). A study of parents' perceptions of positive change in their children after SIT treatment include an increase in social participation, perceived competence, and self-regulation (Cohn, Tickle-Degnen & Miller, 2000).

Research efforts supporting the validation of Dunn's Sensory Profile (Dunn, 1999) include studies of reliability and confidence interval, and content, construct, convergent, and discriminant validity. Dunn's Profile has positively identified patterns of sensory processing and their relationships to patterns of temperament and relationships (Dunn, 2001). A study of children with ADHD revealed significantly different sensory processing patterns when compared with a normal sample (Dunn & Bennett, 2002). With adults, the sensory profile revealed age-related differences in processing patterns and related behaviors: Younger adults engaged in more sensory seeking behaviors, with those 80 years and older the least likely to seek out sensory experiences (Pohl, Dunn, & Brown, 2003).

According to Mulligan (2002), sensory integration has been the subject of more research than any other approach or frame of reference within the field of occupational therapy (Miller & Kinnealey, 1993; Parham & Mailloux, 2001). The consultant role, which addresses the reframing of parent and educator understanding of children's behaviors using sensory integration theory, has produced the most promising results (Case-Smith, 1997; Kemmis & Dunn, 1996; Kimball, 1999). Future researchers are advised to consider the interactions of sensory integration with sensory processing and information processing, and to reframe research questions in the context of occupation-based models.

LEARNING ACTIVITY

Grading Sensory Input

Directions: Groups of 8 to 10 students. Each student chooses one item from the following (or each student can bring their own object from home):

- Red balloon
- Bowling ball
- Jar of bubbles
- Clown hand puppet
- Five-pound weight
- Bottle of floral scented lotion
- Long scarf tied to end of stick
- Pinwheel
- Flashlight
- Bongo drum
- Music box
- Shaker of garlic powder

Students create a group activity using the object chosen. Grade the activities you do so that some would be calming and others would be alerting. Use Table 18-4 as a guide. Students then take turns teaching their activities to the rest of the group.

In discussion, group members answer the following questions after each activity:

- What sensory systems are being stimulated?
- How strong or intense is the sensory input?
- What qualities of the object or activity make it alerting or calming?

Analysis

After activities are finished, discuss the following:

- Which activities seemed most interesting or stimulating? Why?
- Which activities gave you the most pleasure or fun? Why?
- Which activities seemed difficult or tedious? Why?

In creating sensory activities, try to keep cognitive requirements minimal, so that members are free to experience sensations and hopefully enjoy them without too much distraction.

Five-Minute Writing Exercise

Directions: Describe five activities or tasks you do that help you wake up in the morning. What sensory systems are affected for each, and why are these things alerting to you?

Then describe five things you do before bedtime to calm yourself down. What sensory systems are affected for each, and why are these things calming to you?

Theory Application for Case Study: Brad

Discuss the following as if you were hired as Brad's occupational therapist when he began first grade (see p. 238, Case Study: Brad):

- What sensory systems would you focus on in therapy?
- What three activities would you do with Brad during your three 30-minute sessions per week. What equipment would you require, and how would you structure the sessions using SI principles?
- What method would you use to measure the outcome of therapy?
- Write a home program for Brad using everyday activities that incorporate the right kinds of sensory input. Describe this program so that a parent who didn't know anything about sensory integration could understand why it is important for Brad.
- Write a report for the team meeting, where you will discuss your OT goals, Brad's progress, and the reasons he should continue to receive OT services at school.

REFERENCES

Arciniegas, D., Adler, L., Topkoff, J., Cawthra, E., Filley, C., & Reite, M. (1999). Attention and memory dysfunction after traumatic brain injury: Cholinergic mechanisms, sensory gating, and a hypothesis for further investigation. *Brain Injury, 13,* 1–13.

Ayres, A. J. (1972). Types of sensory integrative dysfunction among disabled learners. *American Journal of Occupational Therapy, 26,* 13–18.

Ayres, A. J. (1974). *The development of sensory integrative theory and practice.* Dubuque, IA: Kendall Hunt.

Ayres, A. J. (1980). *Southern California sensory integration test manual: Revised.* Los Angeles, CA: Western Psychological Services.

Ayres, A. J. (1989a). *Sensory integration and praxis tests.* Los Angeles, CA: Western Psychological Services.

Ayres, A. J. (1989b). *Sensory integration and the child.* Los Angeles, CA: Western Psychological Services.

Ayres, A. J., Mailloux, Z., & Wendler, C. (1987). Developmental dyspraxia: Is it a unitary function? *Occupational Therapy Journal of Research, 7,* 93–110.

Ayres, A. J., & Marr, D. B. (2002). Appendix B: Sensory integration and praxis tests. In A. Bundy, S. J, Lane, & E. A. Murray (Eds.), *Sensory integration: Theory and practice* (2nd ed., pp. 453–476). Philadelphia: FA Davis.

Blanche, E. I. (2002). *Observations based on sensory integration theory.* Torrance, CA: Pediatric Therapy Network.

Bodison, S., & Mailloux, Z. (2006). *The Sensory Integration and Praxis Tests: Illuminating struggles and strengths in participation at school.* OT Practice, Sept. 25th, CE 1–8.

Brown, C. E., & Dunn, W. (2002). *Adolescent/adult sensory profile: User's manual.* San Antonio, TX: The Psychological Corporation (Harcourt).

Bundy, A. C., Lane, S. J., & Murray, E. A. (2002). *Sensory integration: Theory and practice* (2nd ed.). Philadelphia, PA: FA Davis.

Bunney, W., Herrick, W., Bunney, B., Patterson, J., Jin, Y., Potkin, S., & Sandman, C. (1999). Structured interview for assessing perceptual anomalies (SIAPA). *Schizophrenia Bulletin, 25,* 577–592.

Case-Smith, J. (1997). Variables related to successful school-based practice. *Occupational Therapy Journal of Research, 17,* 133–153.

Cohn, E., Tickle-Degnen, L., & Miller, L. (2000). Parental hopes for therapy outcomes: Children with sensory modulation disorders. *American Journal of Occupational Therapy, 54,* 36–43.

Dunn, W. (1999). *Sensory profile users manual.* San Antonio, TX: Harcourt Assessment, Inc.

Dunn, W. (2001). The sensations of everyday life: Empirical, theoretical, and pragmatic considerations, 2001 Eleanor Clarke Slagle lecture. *American Journal of Occupational Therapy, 55,* 608–620.

Dunn, W., & Bennett, D. (2002). Patterns of sensory processing in children with attention deficit hyperactivity disorder. *Occupational Therapy Journal of Research, 22,* 4–15.

Field, T. M. (1998). Massage therapy effects. *American Psychologist, 53,* 1270–1281.

Gal, R., & Lazarus, R. S. (1975). The role of activity in anticipating and confronting stressful situations. *Journal of Human Stress, 4,* 4–20.

Hoehn, T., & Baumeister, A. (1994). A critique of the application of sensory integration therapy to children with learning disabilities. *Journal of Learning Disabilities, 27,* 338–350.

Kemmis, B., & Dunn, W. (1996). Collaborative consultation: The efficiency of remedial and compensatory interventions in school contexts. *American Journal of Occupational Therapy, 50,* 709–717.

Kimball, J. (1999). Sensory integration frame of reference: Postulates regarding change and application to practice. In P. Kramer, & J. Hinojosa (Eds.), *Frames of reference for pediatric occupational therapy* (pp. 169–204). Philadelphia, PA: Lippincott, Williams & Wilkins.

King, L. J. (1974). A sensory integrative approach to schizophrenia. *American Journal of Occupational Therapy, 28,* 529–536.

King, L. J. (1978). 1978 Eleanor Clarke Slagle lecture: Toward a science of adaptive responses. *American Journal of Occupational Therapy, 32,* 429–437.

King, L. J. (1988). Occupational therapy and neuropsychiatry. In S. Robertson (Ed.), *Mental health focus.* Rockville, MD: American Occupational Therapy Association.

King, L. J. (1990). Moving the body to change the mind. *Occupational Therapy Practice, 1,* 12–122.

Koomar, J. A., & Bundy, A. C. (2002). The art and science of creating direct intervention from theory. In A. C. Bundy, S. J. Lane, A. G. Fisher, & E. A. Murray (Eds.), *Sensory integration: theory and practice* (2nd ed., pp. 261–306). Philadelphia, PA: F. A. Davis.

Larrington, G. (1987). Sensory integration based program with a severely retarded autistic teenager: An occupational therapy case report. In Z. Mailloux (Ed.), *Sensory integrative approaches in occupational therapy.* New York: Haworth Press.

Levy, L. L. (1974). Movement therapy for psychiatric patients. *American Journal of Occupational Therapy, 28,* 354–357.

Law, M., Missiuna, C., Pollock, N., & Stewart, D. (2005). Foundations for occupational therapy practice with children. In J. Case-Smith (Ed.), *Occupational therapy for children* (5th ed.). St. Louis: Elsevier, Mosby.

Levy, L. L. (1974). Movement therapy for psychiatric patients. *American Journal of Occupational Therapy, 28,* 354–357.

Light, G., & Braff, D. (2000). Do self-reports of perceptual anomalies reflect gating deficits in schizophrenia patients? *Biological Psychology, 47,* 463–467.

Madigan, N. K., DeLuca, J., Diamond, B. J., Tramontang, G., & Averill, A. (2000). Speed of information processing in traumatic brain injury; Modality-specific factors. *Journal of Head Trauma Rehabilitation, 15,* 943–956.

McLean, V. (2003). A well dressed woman. In D. R. Labovitz (Ed.), *Ordinary miracles: True stories about overcoming obstacles and surviving catastrophes.* Thorofare, NJ: SLACK Incorporated.

Miller, L., & Kinnealey, M. (1993). *Researching the effectiveness of sensory integration. Sensory Integration Quarterly* (Vol. XXI [2]). Torrance, CA: Sensory Integration International.

Miller-Kuhaneck, H., Henry, D., & Glennon, T. J. (2007). *Sensory processing measure School form.* Los Angeles, CA: Western Psychological Services.

Mulligan, S. (1998). Patterns of sensory integrative dysfunction: A confirmatory factor analysis. *American Journal of Occupational Therapy, 52,* 819–828.

Mulligan, S. (2002). Advances in sensory integration research. In A. Bundy, S. Lane, & E. Murray (Eds.), *Sensory integration: Theory and practice* (2nd ed.). Philadelphia, PA: FA Davis.

Parham, D. (1998). The relationship of sensory integrative development to achievement in elementary students: Four-year longitudinal patterns. *Occupational Therapy Journal of Research, 18,* 105–127.

Parham, D., Cohn, E., Spitzer, S., Koomar, J., Miller, L., Burke, J., et al. (2007). Fidelity in sensory integration intervention research. *American Journal of Occupational Therapy, 61,* 216–227.

Parham, D., & Ecker, C. (2007). *Sensory processing measure: home form.* Los Angeles, CA: Western Psychological Services.

Parham, D., Ecker, C., Miller-Kuhaneck, H., Henry, D., & Glennon, T. J. (2007). *Sensory processing measure manual.* Los Angeles, CA: Western Psychological Services.

Parham, D., & Mailloux, Z. (2001). Sensory integration. In J. Case-Smith (Ed.). *Occupational therapy for children* (4th ed.). St. Louis: Mosby.

Pert, C. B. (1997). *Molecules of emotion.* New York: Scribner.

Pohl, P., Dunn, W., & Brown, C. (2003). The role of sensory processing in the everyday life of older adults. *Occupational Therapy Journal of Research, 23,* 99–106.

Rood, M. S. (1954). Neurophysiological reactions as a basis for physical therapy. *Physical Therapy Review, 34,* 444–449.

Ross, M. (1987). *Group process: Using therapeutic activities in chronic care.* Thorofare NJ: SLACK Incorporated.

Ross, M., & Bachner, S. (2004). *Adults with developmental disabilities: Current approaches in occupational therapy* (2nd ed.). Bethesda, MD: American Occupational Therapy Association.

Schaaf, R. C. & Miller, L. J. (2005). Occupational therapy using a sensory integrative approach for children with developmental disabilities. *Mental Retardation and Developmental Disabilities, 11,* 143–148.

Schaaf, R. C., & Roley, S. S. (2006). *Sensory integration: Applying clinical reasoning in practice with diverse populations.* San Antonio, TX: Harcourt Assessment.

Schroeder, C., Block, M., Campbell, E., & Savage Stowell, M. (1978). *Schroeder Block Campbell adult psychiatric sensory integration evaluation.* Kailua, Hawaii: Schroeder Publishing.

Storch, B. A., & Eskow, K. G. (1996). Theory application by school-based occupational therapists. *American Journal of Occupational Therapy, 50,* 662–668.

Varga, S., & Camilli, G. (1999). A meta-analysis of research on sensory integration intervention. *American Journal of Occupational Therapy, 53,* 189–198.

Wall, P. D., & Melzack, R. (1995). *Textbook of pain* (3rd ed.). New York: Churchill Livingstone.

Watling, R., Deitz, J., Kanny, E., & McLaughlin, J. (1999). Current practice of occupational therapy for children with autism. *American Journal of Occupational Therapy, 53,* 498–505.

Wilbarger, P. (1993). *Sensory defensiveness.* Videotape. Hugo, MN: PDP.

Wilbarger, P., & Wilbarger, J. (1991). *Sensory defensiveness in children aged 2–12: An intervention guide for parents and other caregivers.* Denver, CO: Avanti Educational Programs.

Wilbarger, J., & Wilbarger, P. (2002). The Wilbarger approach to treating sensory defensiveness. In A. Bundy, S. Lane, & E. Murray (Eds.), *Sensory integration: Theory and practice* (2nd ed., pp. 335–341). Philadelphia, PA: FA Davis.

Chapter 19

MOTOR CONTROL AND MOTOR LEARNING FRAMES

"Contemporary motor behavior research reflects a major shift from reflex hierarchical models to systems models of motor control."

– MATHIOWETZ & BASS HAUGEN (1994, P. 733)

This combination of titles represents the evolution of this frame of reference, having its roots in neurological development, yet changing its focus in the light of current research. For pediatric occupational therapy, Kaplan and Bedell (1999) define a similar set of concepts entitled "motor skill acquisition frame of reference" (pp. 401–429). Recent studies have questioned traditional models of motor control, and newer systems-oriented approaches to motor relearning have evolved. Theories of motor control, such as the Bobath's (1990) neurodevelopmental therapy (NDT), Rood's (1954) sensorimotor approach, Knott and Voss's (1968) proprioceptive neuromuscular facilitation (PNF), and Brunnstrom's (1970) movement therapy, use principles of normal neurological development in a reflex–hierarchical or neuromaturational sequence for establishing or restoring functional movement. In today's practice, these approaches provide a backdrop for the occupational therapy task-oriented frame of reference described by Horak (1991), Mathiowetz and Bass Haugen (1994), and Shumway-Cook and Woollacott (2001), which is equally useful across the lifespan.

In this chapter, we will begin by reviewing NDT representing the traditional motor control approaches. Although NDT has been a target of criticism, its techniques continue to be widely used throughout the world (Rast, 1999). Despite current brain research that renders many of its basic assumptions out of date, NDT was recently identified by practicing occupational therapists in the United States as the second most often used frame of reference (National Board for Certification of Occupational Therapy, 2004).

Secondly, we will review the combined theories of motor learning and the task-oriented approach. These applied theories represent the paradigm shift in health sciences from the older reflex–hierarchical and neuromaturational models of motor control to one that is holistic and systems oriented and incorporates theories of learning.

NEURODEVELOPMENTAL THERAPY

Focus

Karel (a neurologist) and Berta (a physical therapist) Bobath developed NDT in England beginning in the 1940s. The approach was originally developed for the treatment of hemiplegia caused by cerebrovascular accidents (CVA), or stroke, and later as a treatment for cerebral palsy in children. Currently occupational therapists use NDT with a broad range of health conditions affecting motor control in both children and adults. NDT is considered a preparatory treatment because it is directed toward establishing sensorimotor performance components that are prerequisites for occupational performance (Levit, 2002).

Theoretical Base

The theoretical concepts came from neurology, medicine, physical therapy, and studies of human development and brain injury.

A neuromaturational approach, NDT bases both acquisition and recovery of skilled movement on the developmental sequence of mastery over primitive reflexes. Some assumptions of this approach are as follows:

- Movement control progresses from head to foot (cephalo-caudal), from trunk to limbs (proximal to distal), and from large to small (gross to fine).

- Children gradually gain control over primitive reflexes (based on sensory input) in order to perform skilled voluntary movement.

- Children internalize the sensation of movement which creates motor sequences or patterns of movement (internalized sequences of stability and mobility). Examples of patterns are rolling, sitting, crawling, standing, and walking.

- In recovery of movement, stability precedes mobility.

o Stability is created by co-contraction of complementary (opposite) muscle groups, thereby holding the body in place and mediating the effects of gravity, making skilled movement possible.

o Mobility represents a way to engage the environment through purposeful voluntary movements.

- After brain injury, abnormal movement and tone must be inhibited before normal movement and sensation can be restored. Two types of abnormal movements are identified in hemiplegia (one-sided paralysis or weakness after a stroke): flaccidity and spasticity. Both are barriers to functional voluntary movement.

o Flaccidity is limpness or low muscle tone, generally present immediately following brain trauma (stroke).

o Spasticity is high muscle tone resulting in rigidity, stiffness, and involuntary, nonfunctional (spastic) movements.

- Splinter skills are those task skills that are learned by rote and out of normal developmental sequence. Splinter skills are not encouraged in NDT, which is considered preparatory, thereby preceding the skilled movements needed for occupational performance.

Function and Disability

Function refers to the capacity to perform voluntary skilled movements needed for everyday life.

Disabilities commonly identified in stroke survivors and treated using NDT include the following:

- Loss of postural control, including the inability to stabilize one's position either at rest or during movement. For example, clients with hemiplegia following a stroke may be unable to shift their weight when standing and may lack the equilibrium responses needed to keep their balance.

- Loss of selective movement control, typically on the side of the body that is contralateral (opposite) to the site of the CVA (brain lesion). This one-sided weakness or paralysis often leads to the use of one-handed techniques for task performance. (NDT seeks to avoid this problem.)

- Abnormal tone on the affected side, leading to flaccid (too little) or spastic (too much) tone, resulting weakness or stiffness, and difficult and inefficient movements.

- Associated reactions refer to involuntary, nonfunctional movements on the affected side when moving the unaffected side.

- Poor inhibition of primitive reflexes and/or nonfunctional movements.

- Sensory disturbances also contribute to abnormal movement patterns because clients with brain injury may have lost the sensory memory for movement.

Children, from an NDT perspective, have motor dysfunction when they are unable to control their own movements. This may be attributed to lack of neural inhibition or the persistence of primitive reflexes. Common dysfunctions seen in children with cerebral palsy include lack of postural control, abnormal tone, generalized spasticity, poor inhibition of nonfunctional movements, and sensory disturbances.

CHANGE AND MOTIVATION

Change in NDT occurs through the application of specific techniques and strategies. These include handling, use of facilitation and inhibition techniques, placing hands at key points of control, and using reflex-inhibiting patterns or postures (RIPs).

Handling uses a hands-on technique of addressing problems with tone and movement control. The occupational therapist places the client in positions that decrease spasticity and activate normal movement patterns. Initially, the therapist guides client movements to retrain specific muscle groups. The goal of handling is for the client to experience what normal movement feels like. Tactile, proprioceptive, and kinesthetic messages help organize the quality of client movements and influence the status of tone (Levit, 2002).

Placement refers to the occupational therapist placing hands on key points of control, those that have the most influence over client movements. Proximal points of control influence stability in trunk, shoulder girdle, and hips, while distal points of control guide the positions and movements of arms and legs. The goal of placement is to inhibit abnormal movement and to facilitate normal movement.

Inhibition techniques include lengthening spastic muscles, positioning to decrease excessive tone, preventing unwanted movements, and teaching client methods for preventing abnormal postures and positions.

Facilitation techniques include giving clients the sensation of normal movement, providing a system for learning normal movements of trunk, arms, and legs, and direct stimulation of muscles. Occupational therapists facilitate client practice of movement while holding or constraining specific areas to restore alignment and teach clients to incorporate these same constraints when performing normal movements during daily tasks and occupations.

RIPs refer to positioning clients in ways that reduce tone by inhibiting specific primitive reflexes. For example, the tonic neck reflex may be inhibited by turning the client's head away from an extended arm, thereby decreasing tone in that arm and allowing it to move more freely. In NDT, typically occupational therapists will use RIPs to inhibit spasticity while training normal movement patterns in specific body areas (such as the affected arm in hemiplegia). The biomechanical approach may be combined with NDT when addressing issues of range of motion, strength, and endurance.

In NDT, motivation is not addressed specifically. It is assumed that training and practice will produce spontaneous improvements without intentional effort on the part of the client. However, clients may be more motivated when functional movements relate to ordinary tasks. The concept of a client's active assistance during handling supports the concept of movements used in the context of meaningful activities.

Evaluation

NDT evaluation involves both observation and handling in order to assess and record functional movement capacities and limitations (Bobath, 1990). During initial observation, the occupational therapist notes typical postures, preferred movement patterns, spontaneous use of affected side, and compensatory strategies already in place.

Handling is typically performed on a mat, where the occupational therapist looks for the following general observations:

- Client response to being moved (assist or resist)
- Normal or abnormal tone and movement on hemi side
- Response to sensory input
- Assessment of strength and movement control

Specific handling includes postures and movement sequences that relate to occupational performance. The occupational therapist looks for trunk movement, response to weight bearing and weight shifting, spontaneous equilibrium reactions, and protective responses while sitting or standing.

Selective control of arms and legs is evaluated segment by segment, moving proximal to distal (shoulder to fingers, hip to toes). In evaluating these movements, the occupational therapist looks for the following:

- Presence of placing response (holding positions when support is removed)
- Effect of tone (flaccid—move toward gravity, spastic—move toward flexion)
- Quality and strength of movements
- Segmental movements (each joint moves separately versus whole arm together)

Although NDT treatment initially occurs in a clinical setting, evaluation involves collaborative goal setting with client and family. Examples of functional goals include increasing independence in self-care and restoring safe mobility in preparation for returning to home and community.

Guidelines for Intervention

The initial goals vary according to client condition, motivation, and occupational preferences. In stroke rehabilitation, while occupations are used as both means (to practice movement) and end (to accomplish desired tasks), intervention initially involves addressing motor problems through preparatory handling and practice.

Traditionally, NDT has discouraged compensation with one-handed strategies for task performance as counterproductive because it encourages learned neglect. Much attention is given to prevention of the consequences of abnormal tone, such as asymmetrical postures, contracture of spastic muscles, possible shoulder subluxation, and abnormal movement pattern development.

Initial movement training is practiced using occupation as means (occupations are structured to incorporate specific movement strategies). For example:

- Weight bearing on affected arm using bed mobility
- Weight shifting and trunk realignment during transfers
- Bilateral arm use in wheelchair management
- Swinging a tennis racquet while seated to practice trunk balance and stability

Later in the recovery from stroke, the occupational therapist watches for signs of spasticity, including associated reactions (tone increases in affected arm when other side moves), stiffness in affected joints, and uncoordinated or nonfunctional movements. Compensation continues to be discouraged, and use of hemi side encouraged for performing activities of daily living (ADL). Occupation as end (for the sake of task accomplishment, like dressing), has the following goals:

- Using normal movement patterns to increase independence in self-care, such as bathing, brushing teeth, styling hair, or shaving
- Increasing balance and postural control during daily occupations such as standing while washing dishes, preparing meals, or changing an infant's diaper
- Increasing bilateral coordination while lifting a laundry basket, carrying a grocery bag, or playing with a beach ball

Some precautions for occupational therapists when working with stroke survivors are to always check for shoulder subluxation (out of joint) before attempting to practice arm movement. Manually restore normal alignment and hold in position during active movement. In working with the affected arm, the most difficult movements are shoulder flexion and abduction with elbow extended. Internal rotation of the shoulder (with hemi arm resting on lap) should be repositioned in neutral (palm sideways) when preparing the client for reaching and manipulation tasks (such as grasping and drinking from a cup).

Interventions with developmental disabilities in children begin with handling using inhibition and facilitation to encourage normal movement. Guidelines for children include the following:

- Engaging the child using sensory input
- Encouraging co-contraction of postural muscle groups for stability
- Moving selected body parts as the child interacts with objects or others
- Propping or positioning to assist with weight bearing tasks
- Use of supportive devices or equipment to control alignment and facilitate functional movement
- Using sensory inputs that facilitate or inhibit muscle activity
- Teaching family caregivers strategies as needed for ADL

In working with children and families, Dunn (2000) suggests that occupational therapists use NDT with caution because evidence does not support its usefulness in everyday occupations.

RESEARCH

Sherrington (1906) first called attention to the reflex model, hypothesizing that all human movement consists of a combination of reflexes triggered by specific sensory input. Rood (1954) based many of her facilitation and inhibition techniques on this concept, and reflex testing became a standard method of assessment. This model had a major influence on NDT (Mathiowetz & Bass Haugen, 1994). Adams (1971) proposed a closed loop system of motor behavior that emphasizes peripheral control of movement, which helped to explain adjustments to movements as they occur.

Hierarchical models (Jackson & Taylor, 1932; Keele, 1968; Schmidt, 1988) suggest that movement is controlled by the central nervous system (CNS) in a top-down fashion. Schmidt hypothesized that motor programs are stored in the CNS, containing instructions for responses to specific input. This model proposes an open loop system of control that sends preprogrammed instructions without the benefit of feedback. Instead of feedback, Schmidt (1988) and others suggest that feed forward or anticipatory movements account for postural adjustments during motor performance. NDT approaches are consistent with this model, which views abnormal movement as the loss of voluntary control in the CNS (Mathiowetz & Bass Haugen, 1994).

Motor learning research in the past 25 years has questioned the validity of the reflex and hierarchical models (Marteniuk, MacKenzie, & Jeannerod, 1987; Mathiowetz, 1992) by demonstrating a larger role of the environment in controlling movement. Based on growing evidence that multiple characteristics of the person, the task, and the environment contribute to functional motor recovery, Mathiowetz and Bass Haugen (1994) have proposed a contemporary task-oriented approach for occupational therapists as a systems-based approach to the treatment of movement dysfunction. This approach will be reviewed in the following section on motor learning.

MOTOR LEARNING AND TASK-ORIENTED APPROACH

Motor learning theories are shared by occupational therapists and other health care disciplines as a general rehabilitative approach to all forms of movement abnormalities and disorders. Essentially a holistic or systems approach, it draws upon theories from psychology and the behavioral sciences as well as neurology, medicine, and allied health research. Interestingly, research from other disciplines supports the concept that motor learning directly relates to specific task performance (Shumway-Cook & Woollacott, 2001; Mathiowetz & Bass-Haugen, 1994). These OT researchers have proposed a contemporary task-oriented approach to motor relearning.

Focus

Motor learning theories currently provide guidelines for restoring functional movement with clients having a broad range of health conditions. Research has demonstrated that meaningful tasks of the client's own choosing provide the greatest motivation for repeated efforts to recover and refine skilled voluntary movements in clients with acquired motor impairments (Newell, 1991; Stein, Brailowsky, & Will, 1995). These tasks relate to all of the American Occupational Therapy Association (2002) framework domain performance areas and include the impact of contexts, activity patterns, and task demands.

Theoretical Base

Shumway-Cook and Woollacott (2001) define motor control as "the ability to regulate or direct the mechanisms essential to movement" (p. 1), a concept derived from studies of reacquisition of movement after injury. Motor learning, defined as "the study of the acquisition and/or modification of movement" (p. 26) comes from research on normal development in children. These authors suggest a broader definition incorporating both motor control and learning as follows:

- Motor learning is "a search for a task solution that emerges from an interaction of the individual with the task and the environment" (Shumway-Cook & Woollacott, 2001, p. 27). The process includes perception and cognition as well as action.

- Recovery of movement functions entails the organization of both perception and action systems in relation to specific tasks and environments. This suggests that therapists should not use approaches that separate motor learning from the performance of specific tasks in specific environments. Trunk stability, shoulder and elbow extension, and grasp strength are best learned and practiced when a thirsty client wishes to reach for a cold glass of water.

- Some types of nonassociative learning, which occurs below the level of consciousness, relate to human movement. Two types are: habituation and sensitization (Kupfermann, 1991).

  o Habituation refers to a decrease in responsiveness (or desensitization) that results from repeated exposure to a nonpainful stimulus. In therapy occupational therapists might wish to desensitize clients to stimuli that trigger abnormal or nonfunctional motor responses.

  o Sensitization is an increased responsiveness following threatening or noxious stimuli. In therapy, occupational therapists often wish to increase a client's sensitivity to environmental cues that affect safe movement, such as water on the floor or obstacles in one's path.

- Learning theories such as classical and operant learning (discussed in Chapter 12) also apply to motor learning. This type of learning is called associative learning, in which the learner associates one thing with another. These concepts contribute to occupational therapists' understanding of how environmental cues affect motor responses, as well as guidelines for reinforcing desired movement behaviors. Two types of associative learning are important for restoring movement skills: procedural and declarative (Shumway-Cook & Woollacott, 2001).

  o Procedural learning refers to learning tasks that can be performed without attention or conscious thought. Procedural learning develops slowly through many repetitions and eventually becomes habitual. Many skilled movements are thought to develop through repetition under varying conditions, which results in a set of rules of movement that is stored in long-term memory as movement schema.

  o Declarative learning, in contrast, results in knowledge that can be consciously recalled, and thus requires awareness, attention, and reflection. This type of motor learning allows individuals to mentally practice a movement sequence before performing it. For example, learning to ski requires the conscious application of strategies and techniques.

- Schmidt's (1975) schema theory hypothesizes that motor learning involves sets of general rules (as opposed to specific movement patterns) that can apply in a variety of contexts. A schema is a generalized motor program that consists of four parts: 1) the initial situation (e.g., body position and task demand), 2) the parameters used (muscle groups, weight shifts, eye–hand coordination), 3) the outcome or knowledge of result, and 4) the sensory consequence, or how the movement felt. Swinging a golf club might be an example of a schema.

- Newell's (1991) ecological theory clarifies the role of perceptions in motor learning. Practicing tasks promotes learning of an optimal motor strategy through increased coordination of perception and action in response to environmental constraints. Perception provides the following information for motor learning:

  o Recognition of the goal or task (through demonstration)

  o Recognition of regulatory cues (relevant to the task, such as size or weight of an object to be moved)

  o Knowledge of performance, or feedback during performance (how the movement felt)

  o Knowledge of result, or feedback on goal achievement, outcome, or consequence (move a full glass of water too fast and it will spill)

- All motor learning approaches acknowledge the importance of practice. Research has shown that variable practice, using movement skills with varying conditions, leads to increased ability to adapt and generalize learning.

- Contextual interference refers to practice of movement skills in random order. Research shows that random practice significantly increases motor performance during transfer (unfamiliar) tasks (Magill & Hall, 1990).

- Individual characteristics, such as level of experience or intellectual abilities, influence the effectiveness of random practice (Rose, 1997). Random practice leads to learning and application of skills under novel conditions (Schmidt, 1988).

- Transfer of learning, important for all motor relearning programs, occurs more easily when conditions are similar. The more closely the clinic conditions resemble the home environment, the more likely that motor skills will adapt.

- Recovery refers to regaining the same level of functioning as before the onset of injury or illness. Spontaneous recovery occurs without the benefit of intervention. Forced recovery refers to function gained through therapeutic intervention. Altering the methods or mechanisms through which one accomplishes a task qualifies as adapted or functional recovery.

Function and Disability

Functioning is defined within the context of specific tasks. Acquisition of skills for doing a task may be separated into early (experimental) or late (refinement) stages of learning (Gentile, 1992). Several theorists have attempted to define the progression of learning with regard to motor tasks.

A three-stage model of motor learning (Fitts & Posner, 1967) includes the following:

- *Cognitive stage:* client develops a thorough understanding of the task, its demands, and the required skills and strategies. Client experiments with a variety of strategies for dressing. Child tries out different movements for climbing stairs.

- *Associative stage:* practicing and refining selected motor strategies for doing a task.

- *Autonomous stage:* the motor skill becomes relatively automatic and no longer requires sustained attention.

In defining function, contemporary theorists (Newell & van Emmerik, 1989; Southard & Higgins, 1987) describe a gradual increase in the degrees of freedom within which skilled movements are performed. Shumway-Cook and Woollacott (2001) describe the tendency to "freeze" one's joints in the early stages of learning a new skill, so that movements are stiff and inefficient. Joint movement (degrees of freedom) gradually increases with practice (e.g., learning to use a hammer).

No specific criteria for function and dysfunction have been developed in OT for this newly defined frame of reference (Kaplan & Bedell, 1999). For children, age-appropriate tasks can be selected collaboratively with the child, family members, teachers, and/or others. For adults, client-identified roles often determine the tasks that are important within the context of cultural and social contexts.

Change and Motivation

Systems theory suggests that skill acquisition for specific task performance is highly influenced by the match between the person, the task demand, and the environment. Change consists of learning motor strategies by trial and error at first, and later by practice and refinement of skilled movements. Collaborative problem solving with clients involves adapting both task and environment to better match a client's current capacities. Occupational therapists will need considerable skill in task analysis and will focus on environmental adaptations that facilitate motor skill acquisition.

Motivation comes with the selection of tasks that are challenging and meaningful, tasks that are identified as priorities by the clients themselves. For example, a child wishes to learn to play soccer so he or she can join the team. A young adult wishes to be able to perform work tasks so that he or she can return to work.

Postulates of change apply the general principles of motor learning and research that were reviewed in the basic assumptions section.

Kaplan and Bedell (1999) have articulated four general postulates (1 through 4 below) and eight specific postulates of change (5 through 12 below) that guide interventions with children. These principles could just as easily apply to adults with motor deficits (adapted from Kaplan & Bedell, 1999, pp. 421–422). The following circumstances make motor skill acquisition more likely to improve:

1. A match among the task requirements, environmental demands, and the client's abilities.

2. The client understands what is to be achieved and is provided with clear information about the expected motor skill performance and outcome.

3. The client is encouraged to independently problem solve to find his or her own optimal movement strategies to perform tasks.

4. The client is provided with a task that is challenging (i.e., within the client's zone of proximal development) (Vygotsky, 1978).

5. In the early stages of learning, feedback is focused on movement outcome and the critical features of the task and environment (not on motor performance).

6. In the early stages of learning, feedback is summarized (rather than detailed) and provided when movement performance is above acceptable level.

7. In later stages of learning, clients are encouraged to self-evaluate their own movement performance and outcome by focusing on feedback from theri own body and the environment.

8. Client practices whole versus part of a task.

9. If the client uses randomized practice (different applications of skills), movement skills are more likely to generalize to a variety of contexts.

10. For open tasks (ones that must adapt to changing circumstances), the task demand is varied during practice.

11. The client practices and is provided feedback about motor skill performance and outcome in natural (not clinical) settings.

12. When motor skills are practiced in varied daily routines, they are more likely to be used in a wider range of circumstances (Kaplan & Bedell, 1999, pp. 421–422).

As a starting point, Vygotsky (1978) suggests that the therapist define a client-specific range of performance expectations based on the client's zone of proximal development. This begins with the tasks that currently can be performed independently and moves toward those tasks that can be performed adequately with therapist assistance. A dynamic assessment, during which the therapist can observe the client's response to different types of cues and assistance, is needed to define his or her zone of proximal development.

Evaluation

Evaluation, by definition, needs to be conducted during occupational and role performance in natural settings. Occupational therapists collaborate with clients to determine occupational problems with role and task priorities. Mathiowetz and Bass Haugen (1994) suggest that occupational therapists observe clients performing selected functional tasks in various contexts. Each part of the system—the attributes of the person, the task, and the environmental contexts—would need to be evaluated to determine appropriate OT interventions. Shumway-Cook and Woollacott (2001) suggest that self-report or proxy report (parent, caregiver) can be a valid way to determine functional capacity when client is temporarily unable to perform certain activities.

Guidelines for Intervention

With specific task accomplishment as the goal, intervention would focus on assisting clients in developing the optimal motor and cognitive strategies for achieving functional goals. Task demand and environmental context can be altered, and specific attributes of the client's body structure and function, such as muscle strengthening, stretching, supporting, or splinting, may be incorporated into the problem-solving process. Thus, remediation (establishing or restoring), adaptation, and compensation (modification) are not separated, but represent one holistic approach.

A recent variation of task-oriented motor learning for treating stroke survivors is constraint-induced movement therapy, or forced use of the affected side by constraining the unimpaired limb during waking hours. In a study comparing two groups of chronic stroke survivors (1-year post stroke), an experimental group with the unaffected arm constrained for 2 weeks in conjunction with intensive practice of functional tasks with the affected arm, exhibited significantly greater motor skills, greater carry over into life tasks, and maintenance of these gains in a 2-year follow-up (Taub, Miller, Novack, et al., 1993). Based on this and other studies, it is estimated that 20% to 25% of clients with chronic stroke symptoms may benefit from this treatment (Blanton & Wolf, 1999).

Research

The studies already cited provide strong evidence of the effectiveness of motor learning using a task-oriented approach. Mathiowetz and Bass Haugen (1994) did a comprehensive literature review comparing the neuromaturational

and motor learning approaches. These researchers refer to the paradigm shift in theoretical models of motor behavior (Abernethy & Sparrow, 1992), away from traditional (reflex, hierarchical, neuromaturational) models, and toward more systems-oriented models. In a recent study of constraint-induced treatment of adult stroke survivors, participants reported no significant improvements in average performance or satisfaction until 4 to 6 months post intervention (Flinn, Schamburg, Fetrow, & Flanigan, 2005). While the motor learning approach is relatively new, research so far is promising. The main concern for OT with both of these approaches is their use within the context of occupation-based models. This research is beginning to emerge within specific models (Flinn, 1999; Gibson & Schkade, 1997; Gray, 1998).

The Carr and Shepherd (1998) approach has many similarities with the motor learning approach described here. These Australian physical therapists use the principles of kinematics and kinetics to assist clients with CNS motor dysfunction in four categories of motor performance: standing and sitting, walking, reach and manipulation, and balance. Their guidelines are well researched and are entirely compatible with the OT task-oriented approach descried in this chapter (Sabari, 2002).

LEARNING ACTIVITIES

Neurodevelopmental Therapy

Internet Search

Directions: Type in key words related to NDT and summarize the following:

- What health conditions are considered to be the focus of this approach? List and describe.

- What disciplines are considered to be qualified to use this approach?

- What type of training is needed to become qualified to use this approach? Where is training offered and how much does it cost?

- What advice is offered to persons with health conditions and their caregivers regarding ongoing applications of NDT?

- What are the current issues and concerns according to current research?

- What new evidence has been generated by current researchers and how might each be useful in OT?

Laboratory Activity

Directions: From your textbooks on normal development, devise a list of primitive reflexes that occur in children from birth to 3 years. Look up the traditional procedures for testing the presence of each reflex. With a partner, practice eliciting these reflexes or testing to see if they are present.

Next, look on the NDT Web sites for techniques to inhibit the primitive reflexes you have identified. Practice the procedures for inhibiting reflexes with your partner.

Please refer to other textbooks on neuromaturational approaches as necessary.

Case Study: Wally

Wally, a 68-year-old, thin, black male, works as a caretaker in a church where he also lives with his wife. He was admitted to the hospital after suffering a CVA, leaving his right arm and leg flaccid, and his speech slurred and dysarthric. He is also depressed.

Present Illness: While mopping floors in the church where he works, Wally's right arm, leg, and face became numb and he fell to the floor. He was found by his wife shortly after and taken to the emergency room. He was admitted to a medical floor with a diagnosis of left CVA and basal ganglia hematoma with right hemiparesis. Since the illness, he has also stated that he is very depressed. He feels useless because of his disabilities acquired from the CVA. Wally is worried that his wife will not be able to care for him if he returns home and that he will have to go to a nursing home. He and his wife may have to go on welfare.

Profile: Wally has been married for almost 30 years. His 31-year-old stepdaughter died of cancer less than a year ago and the family is still struggling with the crisis. He has been working in the church for 17 years and lives in a small apartment in the church basement with his wife. His wife states that she will now have to find a new place to live as it is probable that her husband will have to retire. She does want him to come home, but she is unsure if she will even be able to care for him. Wally's wife loves to cook and give him treats, but feels very guilty for not forcing him to take his high blood pressure medications more consistently.

Medical/Psychiatric History: Wally has had hypertension for 9 years, has a history of ulcers, and had retinal surgery 6 years ago. He has no history of psychiatric illness.

Mental and Physical Status: Wally appears to be a very neat, clean, and well-groomed individual. His eye contact is very inconsistent, especially when approached from the right side. His motor activity is impaired and he does not ambulate at this time. He needs supervision with wheelchair mobility. His right arm and leg are flaccid and he has a right facial droop. Wally's speech is slurred and dysarthric; he confabulates and has word-finding difficulties, making him hard to understand.

His affect is depressed. He states that his right arm and leg are "useless" and he wants to "cut them off." The client does smile and laugh when progress is made or when he makes funny mistakes. His formal thought is confused much of the time, especially on Mondays when he seems to have forgotten how to transfer, bathe, and dress. His perceptual deficits include visual disturbances, crossing the midline, figure–ground difficulties, and severe right neglect.

Intellectual deficits include disorientation to place and time and impairment of short-term memory. He is impulsive and lacks safety awareness; his judgment is severely impaired. His insight includes slight understanding of his illness and its impact on his future. Cognitively, he can follow two-step commands. His motivation is erratic, depending on his mood.

Theory Application for Wally

Neurodevelopmental Therapy Approach

Directions: Use the NDT approach to complete the following:

- Write one paragraph describing your application of NDT in addressing ADL. How would you explain your OT interventions to Wally's wife using layman language?
- Summarize Wally's function and disability using an NDT perspective. Choose three goals you would work on in OT using the traditional approach.
- What three tasks might you focus on with Wally in eliciting voluntary movement on the affected side?
- How could you incorporate NDT principles into Wally's daily routines? Give three examples.
- What recommendations would you give Wally's wife in carrying over NDT training after discharge?

Motor Learning Approach

Directions: Use the motor learning approach to complete the following:

- Summarize Wally's function and disability using a contemporary task perspective.
- What three tasks might Wally choose to focus on as implied in the case? What tasks would be priorities for Wally's wife for when he returns home?
- Describe the procedure you would use to evaluate Wally's ability to perform the tasks he has chosen. Use one of these as an example and describe your approach in detail.
- How would you summarize an intervention plan for Wally using a motor learning approach?

Comparison of NDT and Motor Learning

- Describe the similarities and differences in the way you define occupational problems and set goals for Wally.
- How is your approach to evaluation similar and different?
- How could you deal with Wally's motivational issues in each of these approaches?

- What are the differences in intervention strategies and techniques?
- What changes would you make in the environment and task demand in NDT versus motor learning approaches?
- What is the role of adaptation and compensation using each of these?
- Which approach would you use with Wally, and why?

REFERENCES

Abernethy, B., & Sparrow, W. A. (1992). The rise and fall of dominant paradigms in motor behavior research. In J. J. Summers (Ed.), *Approaches to the study of motor control and learning* (pp. 3–45). Amsterdam: Elsevier.

Adams, J. A. (1971). A closed-loop theory of motor learning. *Journal of Motor Behavior, 3,* 111–150.

American Occupational Therapy Association. (2002). The occupational therapy practice framework: Domain and process. *American Journal of Occupational Therapy, 56,* 609–639.

Blanton, S., & Wolf, S. L. (1999). An application of upper-extremity constraint-induced movement therapy in a patient with sub acute stroke. *Physical Therapy, 79,* 847–853.

Bobath, B. (1990). *Adult hemiplegia: Evaluation and treatment* (3rd ed.). London, UK: Heinemann.

Brunnstrom, S. (1970). *Movement therapy in hemiplegia.* New York: Harper & Row.

Carr, J. H., & Shepherd, R. (1998). *Neurological rehabilitation: Optimizing motor performance.* Oxford, UK: Butterworth-Heinemann.

Dunn, W. (2000). *Best practice occupational therapy in community service with children and families.* Thorofare, NJ: SLACK Incorporated.

Fitts, P. M., & Posner, M. I. (1967). *Human performance.* Belmont, CA: Brooks Cole.

Flinn, N. (1999). A task-oriented approach to the treatment of a client with hemiplegia. *American Journal of Occupational Therapy, 53,* 345–347.

Flinn, N., Schamburg, S., Fetrow, J. M., & Flanigan, J. (2005). The effect of constraint-induced treatment on occupational performance and satisfaction in stroke survivors. *Occupational Therapy Journal of Research, 25,* 119–127.

Gentile, A. (1992). The nature of skill acquisition: Therapeutic implications for children with movement disorders. In H. Forssberg & H. Hirschfeld (Eds.), *Movement disorders in children* (pp. 31–40). Basil: S. Karger.

Gibson, J. W., & Schkade, J. (1997). Occupational adaptation interventions with patients with cerebrovascular accident: A clinical study. *American Journal of Occupational Therapy, 51,* 523–529.

Gray, J. M. (1998). Putting occupation into practice: Occupation as ends, occupation as means. *American Journal of Occupational Therapy, 52,* 354–364.

Horak, F. B. (1991). Assumptions underlying motor control for neurologic rehabilitation. In M. J. Lister (Ed.), *Contemporary management of motor control problems: Proceedings of the II STEP Conference* (pp. 11–27). Alexandria, VA: Foundation for Physical Therapy.

Jackson, J. H., & Taylor, J. (1932). *Selected writings of John B. Hughlings, I and II.* London, UK: Hodder & Stroughter.

Kaplan, M. T., & Bedell, G. (1999). Motor skill acquisition frame of reference. In P. Kramer & J. Hinojosa (Eds.), *Frames of reference for pediatric occupational therapy* (2nd ed.). Philadelphia, PA: Lippincott Williams & Wilkins.

Keele, S. W. (1968). Movement control in skilled motor performance. *Psychological Bulletin, 70,* 245–248.

Knott, M., & Voss, D. E. (1968). *Proprioceptive neuromuscular facilitation* (2nd ed.). New York, NY: Harper & Row.

Kupfermann, I. (1991). Learning and memory. In E. R. Kandel, J. H. Schwartz, & T. M. Jessell (Eds.), *Principles of neuroscience* (3rd ed.). New York: Elsevier.

Levit, K. (2002). Optimizing motor behavior using the Bobath approach. In C. Trombly & M. V. Radomski (Eds.), *Occupational therapy for physical dysfunction* (5th ed.). Philadelphia, PA: Lippincott Williams & Wilkins.

Magill, R. A., & Hall, K. G. (1990). A review of the contextual interference effect in motor skill acquisition. *Human Movement Science, 9,* 241–289.

Marteniuk, R. G., MacKenzie, C. L., & Jeannerod, M. (1987). Constraints on human arm movement trajectories. *Canadian Journal of Psychology, 41,* 365–368.

Mathiowetz, V. G. (1992). Informational support and functional motor performance. *Dissertation Abstracts International, 52,* 11A.

Mathiowetz, V. G., & Bass Haugen, J. (1994). Motor behavior research: Implications for therapeutic approaches to central nervous system dysfunction. *American Journal of Occupational Therapy, 48,* 733–745.

National Board for Certification of Occupational Therapy. (2004). Practice analysis study of entry-level occupational therapist registered and certified occupational therapy assistant practice. *Occupational Therapy Journal of Research, 24,* s1–s31.

Newell, K. M. (1991). Motor skill acquisition. *Annual Review of Psychology, 42,* 213–237.

Newell, K. M., & van Emmerik, R. E. A. (1989). The acquisition of coordination: Preliminary analysis of learning to write. *Human Movement Science, 8,* 17–32.

Rast, M. (1999). NDT in continuum: Micro to macro levels in therapy. *Developmental Disabilities Special Interest Section Quarterly, 2,* 1–3.

Rood, M. S. (1954). Neurophysiological reactions as a basis for physical therapy. *Physical Therapy Review, 34,* 444–449.

Rose, D. J. (1997). *A multilevel approach to the study of motor control and learning.* Boston, MA: Allyn & Bacon.

Sabari, J. S. (2002). Optimizing motor control using the Carr and Shepherd approach. In C. Trombly & M. V. Radomski (Eds.), *Occupational therapy for physical dysfunction* (5th ed.). Philadelphia, PA: Lippincott Williams & Wilkins (pp. 501–519).

Schmidt, R. A. (1975). A schema theory of discrete motor skill learning. *Psychology Review, 82,* 225–260.

Schmidt, R. A. (1988). *Motor control and learning: A behavioral emphasis* (2nd ed.). Champaign, IL: Human Kinetics.

Sherrington, C. S. (1906). *The integrative action of the nervous system.* New Haven, CT: Yale University Press.

Shumway-Cook, A., & Woollacott, M. (2001). *Motor control: Theory and practical applications* (2nd ed.). Philadelphia, PA: Lippincott Williams & Wilkins.

Southard, D., & Higgins, T. (1987). Changing movement patterns: Effects of demonstration and practice. *Research Quarterly for Exercise and Sport, 58,* 77–80.

Stein, D. G., Brailowsky, S., & Will, B. (1995). *Brain repair.* New York, NY: Oxford.

Taub, E., Miller, N. E., Novack, T. A., Cook, E. W. III, Fleming, W. C., Nepomuceno, C. S., et al. (1993). Technique to improve chronic motor deficit after stroke. *Archives of Physical Medicine and Rehabilitation, 74,* 347–354.

Vygotsky, L. S. (1978). *Mind in society: The development of higher psychological processes.* Cambridge, MA: Harvard University Press.

Chapter 20

PSYCHODYNAMIC FRAME

"Passion lives here."

– THEME OF THE 2006 WINTER OLYMPIC GAMES IN TORINO, ITALY

Psychoanalytic theory has reinvented itself many times since Freud's day. In all of its manifestations, passion, and emotion, the pleasure-seeking principles of human motivation remain central. Psychodynamic theory is one of the few occupational therapy (OT) approaches that deals effectively with emotional issues. Other theories have not offered adequate explanations for human emotions. Behaviorists try to extinguish them, cognitive therapists try to regulate them; still, emotional crises continue to create havoc in the lives of our clients and emerge as barriers to occupational performance. How do we explain the sudden eruptions of anger and frustration, the persistence of hopelessness, or the lapses into addictive behaviors to numb emotional pain? Passion, whether directed toward aggression—as in the fierce competition of Olympic sports—or toward libido—the expression of love for people or principles, often defies logic. Passion exudes from the core of the human spirit without the need for reasons or scientific evidence. Its irrational nature when applied to interpersonal relationships is undeniable. Maybe it is time to admit that there just might be something going on beneath the surface—that perhaps occupational therapists need to use psychodynamic strategies to explore the emotional turmoil of the unconscious.

One sign of renewed interest in emotion is the emergence of spirituality as a concern in OT. The person's ego, or sense of self, is conceptually similar to the human spirit in client-centered OT. Whenever we talk about the meaning of occupations, we are referring to emotions, affect, and motivation. Both Hasselkus (2002) and Fidler and Velde (1999) explore the relationship of spirituality and everyday occupation. This spirituality is not defined as religion but as the experience of meaning (Burkhardt & Nagi-Jacobson, 1994; Howard & Howard, 1997; Urbanowski, 1997; Urbanowski & Vargo, 1994). In the Canadian client-centered model, "the person is seen as possessing physical, affective, and cognitive components, central to which is the essential core of being, the spiritual element" (Law, Baptiste, Carswell, McColl, Polatajko, & Pollock, 1998, p. 2). Current definitions of the human spirit as the person's essence or soul bear a striking resemblance to the concept of the "self" in ego-psychology. Furthermore, research studies from ego-psychology and object relations can provide evidence to support the use of creative media as OT interventions. The psychodynamic frame of reference in OT encompasses concepts from object relations, ego psychology, humanism, and human spirituality (Bruce & Borg, 2002).

Historically, OT theorists have acknowledged the usefulness of psychodynamic concepts in mental health practice. Diasio (1968) explored the psychoanalytic view of motivation and the environment. The Fidlers (1963) point out the importance of the unconscious and view activities as part of a communication process with human and nonhuman objects to effectively gratify instinctual needs. Mosey (1986), in considering analytical frames of reference, emphasizes the "structure for linking psychoanalytic theories, the symbolic potential and reality aspects of activities, and the process of altering intrapsychic content in the direction of providing a more adaptive basis for interaction with the environment" (p. 385). Llorens (1966) refers to "socially acceptable, ego-adaptive functioning" (p. 178) in describing the effects of client involvement in activity groups, thus focusing on OT techniques that help develop and strengthen the functions of the ego.

FOCUS

In OT, the most useful concepts from psychodynamic theory may be clustered into five areas:

1. Social participation and relationships
2. Emotional expression and motivation for engagement in occupations

255

3. Self-awareness through reality testing and feedback from others

4. Defense mechanisms such as denial, projection, and sublimation through the symbolism of activities and occupations

5. Projective activities such as communication and clarification of occupational goals and priorities

1. Social Participation and Relationships

Attachment theory has its roots in object relations, a neo-Freudian theory. Relationships do not typically occur in a vacuum—often they revolve around shared activities, such as having dinner together, playing games, working on projects like gardening, and participating in community events or celebrations. Fonagy (1998) applies attachment theory to explain why some adults fail to integrate their experiences with the meaning of that experience or why they lack the ability to empathize or understand a situation from someone else's perspective. Attachment theory refers to the satisfaction of emotional needs through interaction with both human and nonhuman objects. For example, studies have demonstrated that pets, especially dogs and cats, supply ongoing comfort, reduce stress, and reduce feelings of loneliness during adversity or stressful transitions for older adults in nursing homes or retirement communities (Banks & Banks, 2002; Sable, 1995).

2. Emotional Expression and Motivation

Spiritual issues such as human emotions and motivation impact occupations for clients across the lifespan in every area of OT practice. It would be a mistake to limit the use of the psychodynamic approach to mental health. This frame of reference seeks to explain how emotions and drives impact all the performance areas of occupation in the American Occupational Therapy Association (AOTA) OT Practice Framework (2002). When we observe unexpected or irrational emotional behaviors, it may be time to explore what is going on beneath the surface, in the client's unconscious. Psychodynamic theory gives occupational therapists some tools for doing this through the projective arts like drawing, creative writing, movement, and story telling. In focusing on the person's "inner life," psychodynamic theory encompasses self-identity, interpersonal relationships, and the drive toward mastery, within the concepts of libido (life force) and aggression (death force). Simply put, these involve a person's motivation to love and to work.

3. Self-Awareness

One of the important roles of the ego is to integrate all the different aspects of the self. The context areas listed in the OT Practice Framework (AOTA, 2002) have a special importance as potential sources of need satisfaction, and these environmental factors continue to shape the "self."

This relates to Christiansen's (1999) concept of occupation as self-identity and a sense of coherence, which defines the meaning of daily experiences within the context of one's surroundings. Object relations and attachment theories tell us that people learn about who they are (self-concept, self-esteem, self-efficacy, self-worth) through interaction with others. An important tool for OT practice might be our therapeutic use of self and our skilled application of group process in order to help clients give and receive feedback from each other about aspects of their occupational performance and participation in life.

4. Defense Mechanisms

Most occupational therapists have worked with clients who have unusual behaviors that do not seem reasonable—self-destructive behaviors such as addictions, risk-taking sexual habits, failure to adhere to a diabetic diet, or continuing to smoke despite the onset of emphysema. Psychodynamic defenses are unconscious mechanisms that are functional for the client in helping to maintain self-control, reduce anxiety, or mediate otherwise painful realities or experiences. Sometimes these seemingly nonfunctional behaviors have a symbolic meaning for the client; for example, a self-destructive behavior may be the client's way of acting out an internalized rage that would otherwise cause the ego (self) to disintegrate. Even something as simple as the client's response to chronic pain has been explained in psychodynamic terms (Watkins & Watkins, 1990).

5. Projective Arts and Activities

Psychodynamic approaches are especially useful in dealing with emotions and exploring the symbolic meaning of occupations. Occupational interventions that use creativity as a projection of the self to promote self-awareness and insight are best understood from a psychodynamic perspective. This includes movement to music, painting, sculpting, and writing poetry—these are the same creative activities that are often used in helping clients to become more in touch with their spiritual dimensions.

THEORETICAL BASE

An understanding of the psychodynamic frame of reference would not be complete without a brief review of Freudian psychoanalytic theory. Freud's concept of the unconscious relates to aspects of the human spirit that cannot be observed or easily defined. Freud suggests three ways by which observation of unconscious content is possible: projections (drawings, music, drama, and creative writing), dreams (symbols and their meaning), and free association (spontaneous connections of objects, symbols, and emotions) (Table 20-1). Researchers have studied projections such as drawings, associations, and symbols to define the role of the unconscious in motivating both adaptive and

	Table 20-1	
	Freud's Psychosexual Stages	
Ages	**Stage (Source of Gratification)**	**Fixation Characteristics (Problems by Theme)**
Birth to 1	Oral stage (sucking, biting)	Trust, dependency (psychosis)
1 to 3	Anal stage (toilet training)	Control, autonomy (neurosis, character disorder)
3 to 5	Phallic stage (early genital)	Sex roles (oedipal/Electra complex)
5 to 12	Latency stage (sublimation)	Skill development, superego (guilt)
12 to adult	Genital stage (puberty)	Sexual identity, mature relationships

deviant behaviors (Fonagy, Gergely, Jurist, & Target, 2002). Psychodynamic theory provides an explanation for many of the irrational, even bizarre behaviors we observe in persons with a variety of illnesses, for example, suicide attempts, risk-taking behaviors, paranoia, self-starvation, or sexual deviance, that are otherwise unexplainable. Occupational therapists seeking to understand the meaning of occupations, also need to explore the emotional connections and unconscious motivations clients demonstrate through their occupational behaviors.

Included in the following overview is a discussion of ego functions and their relevance to OT. Attempts to validate the concept of the ego have led to definitions of 12 ego functions, their role in defining the self, and the process of interaction with the environment (Bellak, Huruich, & Gediman, 1973). Finally, contributions from the OT literature will be summarized. Dickerson (1992) has clarified the role of affect and emotion in human experience and decision-making, citing research findings. Fidler & Velde (1999) refer to the "dynamic of congruence, or match, of an activity with the nature and characteristics of the person" (p. xi). In recent years both Fidler and Velde (1999) and Hasselkus (2002) have looked beyond the "purposeful" nature of activities and focused on their symbolic and metaphorical meaning in the dimension of spirituality.

FREUD'S PSYCHOANALYTIC THEORY

The following is intended as a brief review of the original concepts of Freudian psychoanalytic theory. A more thorough understanding may be obtained by referring to other basic psychology texts. Psychoanalytic theory is exceedingly complex, and there are many variations currently in use.

Personality Structure

Freud (1953) organized personality into three parts: *the id*, *the ego*, and *the superego*. This structure is still accepted by many psychotherapists regardless of their discipline or theoretical preferences.

The Id

The id is defined as the unconscious. It is the part of the personality that houses primitive drives and instincts, as well as needs and conflicts, that the ego is unable to integrate. The id is the biological component of the personality, and is thought to operate through primary process thinking. *Primary process thinking* is the earliest to develop in the infant. It is illogical and undisciplined and operates on the pleasure principle, demanding immediate gratification of needs and drives. Dreams, with their illogical sequences and symbolic representations of conflicts and emotions, also reflect primary process thinking.

The Ego

The ego is the psychological component that has contact with the external world. It functions logically and works to achieve a balance between internal drives and external expectations. The ego operates through a *secondary process*, one that is learned through experience in reaching compromises and applying logic and discipline in an attempt to adapt to the environment. Ego psychologists expanded on this concept, which is equivalent to the "self."

The Superego

The superego is the social component of the personality that serves as an individual's moral code, sense of good and bad, or right and wrong. While people are usually aware of their values and beliefs, the superego is often illogical and unrealistic in its quest for idealism and perfection. These moralistic ideals are thought to be internalized from one's parents and one's culture.

Symbols, Projections, and Communication with the Unconscious

Rarely, except in episodes of psychosis, does the content of the unconscious become known. Psychoanalytic therapy's main thrust is to help an individual become aware of his unconscious conflicts and fixations so that the mature ego can deal with them effectively and resolve

Figure 20-1. Freud's Theory of Personality (1953). (Created by M. Cole.)

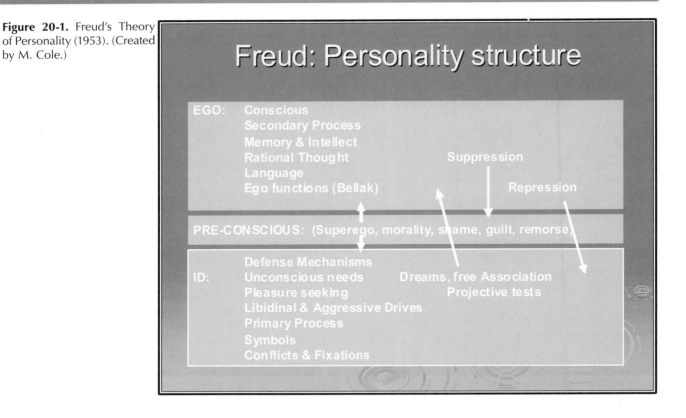

them. However, the nature of primary process makes awareness of unconscious material very complex. Primary process is not organized or logical and is not remembered in words or complete thoughts. Highly emotional material may take the form of symbols, which represent experiences that originally produced them. The memory of being locked in a closet as a childhood punishment may have been *repressed,* only to re-emerge in adulthood as an unexplained dread of small enclosed spaces. The client may turn down a high-paying job if it means taking an elevator or refuse to submit to a needed magnetic resonance imaging (MRI). It is the therapist's role to help the adult client to interpret the meaning of emotional responses that create such functional barriers and to remember and work through the original traumatic experience.

The content and lines of communication among the id, ego, and super-ego are represented in Figure 20-1. Repression and suppression are defense mechanisms. Repression locks painful memories in the unconscious, where they cannot be voluntarily retrieved. Memories of physical or sexual abuse during childhood generally fall into this category. In contrast, suppression is a conscious process of avoiding difficult or emotional issues, or putting them off until a more appropriate time. For example, a student may suppress a conflict with parents until after taking a difficult exam. Defense mechanisms are thought to operate on an unconscious level most of the time. In OT, we may view defenses as barriers to communication (e.g., displacing one's anger onto an inappropriate object) or barriers to the therapeutic process (e.g., denial of a disability). OT interventions can have the goal of breaking through client defenses (barriers) in order to facilitate therapeutic occupational goals.

Psychic Energy, Libido, Aggression, Anxiety, and Depression

In Freud's view, the amount of *psychic energy* is limited, and must be shared by all three parts of the personality (1953). This explains why people cease to function when too much energy is being used in trying to deal with unresolved conflicts from the past. A healthy individual is able to resolve conflicts as they arise and, therefore, keep psychic energy available for the ego to grow and develop and interact effectively with the environment. In mental illness, psychic energy may be trapped in the id and may produce nonadaptive behaviors that doctors call symptoms.

Two specific forms of psychic energy are described by Freud (1953): the libidinal and the aggressive drives. *Libido* is the sexual energy that represents the urge to perpetuate life, to be intimate, to love, and to reproduce. This is also called the life force, and is demonstrated by a person's tendency to form relationships with other people. The *aggressive drive* is equated with the death force, and is associated with hostility, hatred, and the urge to destroy. It is expressed in the tendency to be self-sufficient and to keep others at a distance. Both the libidinal and the aggressive drives are part of the id, and both seek expression through objects. It is a function of the ego to control these drives and to allow their expression in ways that are socially acceptable. It is a function of the superego to guide an individual's libidinal and aggressive drives toward constructive and morally acceptable expression.

Anxiety, in Freud's view, is defined in relation to both drives and the ego's control function (1953). Anxiety is an alerting response that lets us know that something is wrong and needs to be changed and that some action needs to be taken to get us out of danger. However, unlike the existentialists who view anxiety as a normal condition of life, Freud views anxiety as pathological. Freudian anxiety develops out of the conflicts over control of the available psychic energy within the personality itself. This anxiety goes beyond fear of realistic danger from the external world. It is the fear that the id may take over, forcing the individual to act irrationally or in ways that are morally wrong, or that the superego may take over, causing a pervasive sense of guilt and self-punishment. As long as the ego maintains control, anxiety can be safely held in check and dealt with realistically. High levels of neurotic anxiety, however, may necessitate the unconscious use of ego defense mechanisms to help reduce the tension and protect the survival of the ego. These mechanisms will be reviewed later in this chapter.

Depression may be conceptualized psychodynamically as anger turned inward. *The Diagnostic and Statistical Manual or Mental Disorders, Fourth Edition* (DSM IV), while defining a depressive episode in terms of specific behaviors, also characterizes depression as diminished pleasure in activities, feelings of worthlessness or excessive guilt, loss of energy, and the inability to express emotions other than sadness or hopelessness (Sadock & Sadock, 2003). These symptoms are consistent with the psychodynamic concept that the aggressive drive is being directed against the self. As an OT activity, expressive media can sometimes reveal the guilt and self-loathing that lurks in the unconscious of a depressed individual.

Occupational therapists may facilitate the expression of psychic energy through activities. This helps the client in a variety of ways. Through activities, the aggressive drive can be directed toward productive work, constructive home-making, or competition in sports. The libidinal drive can energize the client to development of social skills, nurturing skills, and cooperation with others. Various ego functions might be encouraged in OT groups, such as appropriate expression of feelings, both loving and aggressive, or the sharing of perceptions to help members develop a realistic sense of self.

Psychosexual Stages and Mental Illness

Freud (1953) believed that personality is largely determined by one's early childhood experiences. Spanning a range of 18 years, from birth to maturity, psychosexual stages of development are differentiated by changes in the objects that potentially provide needs satisfaction. An *object is someone or something that gratifies or frustrates a need*; objects can be human or nonhuman. The classic example of an object in the oral stage is mother's breast. A nonhuman substitute for mother's breast is the bottle. When children's needs are gratified, they thrive and are able to develop to the next stage. However, when children's needs are continually frustrated, they develop *fixations* that can remain in the unconscious and cause many problems in adulthood that we know as symptoms of illness. Freud's psychosexual stages of development are outlined in Table 20-1.

The psychosexual stages are critical to our understanding of mental illness. In spite of current discoveries of the genetic and biochemical origins of some illnesses, most psychopathology is still explained in terms of Freud's levels of personality organization (Sadock & Sadock, 2003). In general, the earlier the conflict occurs, the more severe the illness. While there are not rigid parallels between the stages and the development of certain illnesses, fixations in the early stages are likely to result in faulty or incomplete development in later ones. For example, dissociative identity disorder, also known as multiple personality disorder, is defined by the exaggerated use of the defense mechanism dissociation. The etiology, in almost 100 percent of the cases, includes an early traumatic event (oral stage) that causes the child to "dissociate" from overwhelming emotional pain by creating separate personalities (Sadock & Sadock, 2003). Likewise, failure to develop self-control in the anal stage may result in the overdevelopment or misuse of defense mechanisms as the ego's attempt to compensate for lack of self-control in later stages. Borderline personality disorder and obsessive-compulsive disorder (OCD) are examples (Sadock & Sadock, 2003).

CONCEPTS FROM EGO PSYCHOLOGY

Ego psychology, an outgrowth of psychoanalytic theory, focuses on the conscious rather than the unconscious aspects of the personality and is therefore, by definition, more observable and measurable. The ego is best understood as the self. A client's sense of self, or self-concept, can determine his or her degree of involvement in OT intervention. If Milton sees himself as a capable musician and a worthwhile individual, he will be motivated to overcome disability. If Rebecca defines herself as a nurse, she will make the effort to overcome her depression to return to that occupation. In this frame of reference, the ego is seen as a powerful motivating force that can either resist or facilitate therapeutic change.

Hartmann (1939, 1964) suggested that the process of psychoanalysis was not a reconstruction of what once existed buried in the unconscious (the Freudian view). He saw that psychotherapy requires that the mature ego establish correct causal relationships and judgments of the emerging memories. The significance of Hartmann's work is in establishing the autonomy of the ego as separate from the id in psychoanalytic theory. Ego psychology has been developing since 1923, and has had many spokesmen, including Adler, Sullivan, Hartmann, Erikson, Lewin and Rapaport (Fine 1979). The common element is an emphasis on the ego.

Table 20-2	

Twelve Functions of the Ego and Their Relevance to Client Occupations

Ego Functions*	Occupational Therapy Example
1) Reality testing	Client accurately interprets sensory information in the environment to identify an emergency situation and respond appropriately.
2) Judgment	Client knows how to ask for help when unable to perform a task, such as replacing a light bulb in an out of reach location, or lifting heavy items when moving.
3) Sense of self and the world	Client expresses a realistic awareness of own abilities and roles in society, and maintains stable relationships with others.
4) Control of drive, affect and impulse	Client refrains from tasting fruit in the supermarket until the selected items are paid for.
5) Object relationships	Client effectively uses objects to meet basic needs in socially acceptable guidelines
6) Thought processes	Can apply reason when solving problems in everyday living, can learn and remember how to perform occupations
7) Adaptive regression in service of the ego	Voluntarily choosing playful occupations which one enjoys, such as romping with a pet, or playing ball with a child—behaviors typical of an earlier stage of development.
8) Defensive functioning	Employing healthy defenses such as altruism—clients with arthritis helping others with similar difficulties to adapt valued occupations
9) Stimulus barrier	Ability to tune out visual and auditory distractions in order to focus on the task at hand.
10) Autonomous functioning	Clients use occupational therapist's expertise in order to make informed choices in setting occupational goals
11) Synthetic integrative functions	Clients consider all aspects of a situation when acting to meet individual needs while at the same time adhering to social and environmental expectations
12) Mastery/competence	Clients build self confidence through their ability to successfully perform occupations.

*Adapted from Bellak, L., Huruich, M., & Gediman, H. (1973). Ego functions in schizophrenics, neurotics and normals. New York, NY: Wiley & Sons.

Bellak et al. (1973) operationalized the functions of the ego, making them more amenable for research purposes (Table 20-2). Each will be discussed briefly with respect to concepts applicable to OT practice.

1. Reality Testing

Reality testing is perhaps the most important function of the ego in therapy. It is the ego's ability to use perception and judgment to differentiate between internal needs and external demands. This process involves the use of interaction with the environment and with others in shaping and reshaping one's views of self and the world. It is this process that is responsible for adaptation to the environment. The ego becomes aware of needs and drives from the id but delays their gratification until they can be satisfied in ways that are socially acceptable. Reality testing is an integral part of the therapeutic use of groups. The process of integrating one's own perceptions, views, or beliefs with those of others is called consensual validation.

OT interventions involving the use of concrete tasks provide another kind of reality testing, one on a sensory level. Manipulation of objects and materials provides

sensory input—taste, touch, smell, vision, hearing, and proprioception (position, pressure, balance, etc.)—which can lead one to challenge internal perceptions. Robert felt he had no energy and, therefore, could not complete a woodworking project. When the group members persuaded him to try it, however, the sensory stimulation provided by sawing and hammering the wood (proprioceptive and auditory) helped release the needed energy. Robert learned through experience that by engaging in appropriate motor activities, he was able to direct his energy to produce a positive effect on the environment (a completed project). If the group then also provides positive feedback on his wood project, Robert is further inclined to change his view of himself from the ineffective "I can't" to the effective "I can!" It is important here for the occupational therapist to be aware of Robert's abilities in choosing a task, thus ensuring that his experience is likely to be a successful one.

2. Judgment

Judgment is another function of the ego that is often the focus in OT. Clients need to use good judgment whether applied to motor planning (using a walker or shower grab bar) or responding to social situations (using tact when expressing negative emotions). Good judgment requires the following cognitive processes: accurate and realistic perception of the situation, identification of intended behaviors and likely consequences, prediction of the behaviors' effect on others, control of response until options are considered, and an appreciation of what it takes to accomplish something. On a well-known psychological test, the client is asked the question, "What is the thing to do if you find an envelope in the street that is sealed, addressed, and has a new stamp?" The most acceptable answer is "mail it" (Wechsler, 1981, p. 126). How one arrives at this response requires a complex process of perception, reasoning, and anticipation of consequences. Additionally, knowledge about one's culture and social norms guides decisions about what is right and wrong. Judgment is a cognitive skill of the highest order and one of the most difficult to learn or teach.

3. Sense of Self

Many aspects of sense of self appear in the literature, and their meaning can be somewhat confusing. Three discrete aspects will be defined here: *self-concept*, *body image*, and *self-esteem*.

Self-Concept

Self-concept, or self-identity, is sometimes used interchangeably with the word ego. Developmentally, the idea of self originates when the infant begins to differentiate self from mother, and then from the environment in general. Psychotic individuals are understood by ego psychologists to have regressed beyond the point where they are able to differentiate self from others. These psychotic individuals are said to have "poor" or "loose" ego boundaries. This factor makes psychotic clients particularly sensitive to their environment. When someone in the group is angry, for example, it is often the psychotic client who is first to notice it, although he may not express his awareness realistically or appropriately.

Following Freud's original formulations, the attempt was made to correlate the various clinical entities with the points of fixation in psychosexual development (1953). Primarily, the oral stage is associated with psychosis, the anal stage with neuroses, and the phallic stage with hysteria. Ego psychologists have elaborated and changed this original oversimplified concept of mental illness, but have retained the idea that the ego or self-concept is fundamentally different in these three levels of mental health conditions (Leichsenring & Hiller, 1990). Psychological testing such as word association (Jung, 1910), interpretation of inkblots (Rorschach, 1921), and association with photographs (Murray, 1951) are a few of the earliest attempts to measure ego functions with particular regard to self-concept.

The idea that concept of the self is a common problem area for mentally ill individuals has lead occupational therapists to make self-concept and its related ideas, body image, self-esteem, and self-perception, the focus of OT intervention. Fidler (1978) made the connection between doing (occupation) and becoming (self-identity) as a natural part of human development, supporting the value of occupations as a powerful force for therapeutic change (self-actualization). Drawing and word association activities, often taking their cues from the various psychological tests, have been useful in promoting knowledge of the self. Self-esteem is better approached in OT through successful experiences and feedback from others. Person drawings, in particular, are a useful therapeutic tool, for both evaluation and intervention in OT.

Body Image

Body image is the perception of one's physical self that forms the basis of self-awareness. According to theories of child development, the earliest learning involves the association and differentiation of somatosensory sensations. These provide a kind of geographical knowledge of the body, how it works, and what defines "me." Body sense, according to Allport (1958), allows a child to develop a sense of personhood. It is the sensory motor exploration of early play that helps the child define the boundaries of his or her body and distinguish "me" from "not me." In adulthood, body sense continues to provide a basic reference point from which environmental interactions take place. The sensory systems, for example, help people know how they feel. Influences from the body guide day-to-day behavior. For example, you may stay home from work because you feel fatigued, or you may go for a walk because you feel restless. The child achieves a sense of control over his body by reaching out to the environment to satisfy body needs: a bottle satisfies hunger, a toy satisfies need for pleasure, mother satisfies the need for comfort. As adults, we continue to reach out to the environment and to others, based on our perceptions of our bodies and what we need.

Illness tends to produce distortions in body image, and this may be a source of problem behaviors. As occupational therapists, one of our goals is to determine whether our client's body image is realistic. Using activities that encourage clients to become aware of their feelings and sensations can help to correct body image distortions. Movement activities and person drawings are two examples of possible activities. Movement, dance, physical sports, and exercise may be help clients to develop a realistic body image.

Self-Esteem

Self-esteem describes the subjective feelings of one's own ability. As with sensory motor, perceptual, and cognitive processes, feelings are innate and develop as the child matures. However, feelings or affects are intricately tied to objects, and their expression determines how people relate to one another and to their world. Rapaport (1953) attempted to articulate a theory of affect, suggesting that affect originates as psychic energy and is seen as a signal emitted by the ego to indicate an internal feeling state needing to be noticed. Spitz (1959) offered a theory of affect development in the infant as 1) crying, 2) smiling, and 3) stranger distress or fearfulness. Language development then allows the child to express a multiplicity of feeling states of increasing complexity.

The expression of affect or emotion is an important function of the ego. As suggested by Rapaport (1953), it is one of the ways the ego has to control and direct energy from the id. Acting out has been described earlier as a more primitive, less socialized form of expression of affect through action. Those with special talents are able to express affect through artistic media, such as painting, music or poetry, and drama. While these ways are socially acceptable, the most commonly acceptable way to express affect is by describing it verbally with words.

As occupational therapists, we often observe in our clients (and sometimes in ourselves) a lack of ability to communicate emotions to others. In the psychodynamic frame of reference, a common goal of OT is the appropriate expression of emotions.

4. Self-Control

Control was the earliest of the ego functions to be recognized, when Freud conceptualized the ego's main function to control the instinctual drives from the id. Impulse control may be seen as a derivative of this earlier conceptualization. Lack of impulse still helps to explain several current mental disorders (DSM IV [American Psychiatric Association, 2007]), such as pathological gambling, kleptomania (impulsive theft), pyromania (starting fires), and the impulsive aggressive behaviors (intermittent explosive disorder) that may be seen in juvenile delinquency and episodes of school violence or domestic violence.

Lack of self-control also helps to explain physically related disorders, such as abuse of pain or sleep medications, overeating and obesity, and the abuse of substances such as alcohol or nicotine. In psychodynamic terms, motivation operates unconsciously according to the pleasure principle. In the absence of ego control, pleasure seeking is given free rein.

Occupational therapists may wonder why clients continue to smoke, drink, gamble, or behave in self-destructive ways. This theory suggests strategies that strengthen ego functions, such as building self-esteem and using rational thought and good judgment, will help the client to maintain appropriate self-control..

5. Object Relations

Freud viewed object relations as the foundation of an individual's capacity to love and to work. The Fidlers (1963) define OT in terms of the development of relationships with human (therapist) and nonhuman (environment) objects. In human relationships, the client develops the ability to satisfy some of his or her basic needs, such as recognition, self-esteem, and belonging, through a

therapeutic relationship with the occupational therapist. In the safety of a therapeutic environment, the client uses realistic feedback from the therapist or other clients to correct his unrealistic concepts and expectations of self and others. Nonhuman objects are related to the client's ability to work. The client can learn, in OT, to use the symbolic as well as actual properties of objects to help satisfy aggressive drives and needs.

Attachment Theory

As a contemporary outgrowth of object relations, attachment theory further defines the parent–infant bond as the model for subsequent interpersonal relationships (Bowlby, 1988). Initially, infant behaviors seek to establish and maintain the proximity of caregivers through 1) signals that draw parents to them (smiling), 2) aversive behaviors (crying) for the same reason, 3) skeletal/muscle activity (locomotion) to stay close to parent/caregiver, and 4) goal-corrected partnerships. Goal-corrected partnerships, emerging around age 3, are based on internal working models, which include memories of early attachment interactions, expectations of caregiver attributes of others, autobiographical memories that form an internal image of the self, and acknowledgment of the psychological characteristics (i.e., desires, emotions, intentions, beliefs) of others as different from the self. A child's early attachments have been proposed as a basis of "social intelligence and meaning making" (Marvin & Britner, 1999). They called this an internal interpretive mechanism, which generalizes the early experiences to all subsequent attachments with significant others. This theory highlights the importance of early nurturing but also considers genetic or inherited attributes, such as a predisposition to antisocial behavior (Reiss, Neiderhiser, Hetherington, & Plomin, 2000). Attachment theory is further discussed later in this chapter.

6. Thought Processes

Thought processes are the cognitive functions of the ego having to do with *attention, memory, learning and logical thought, compromise, problem-solving,* and *judgment.*

Attention

Attention is the ability of the ego to focus on something for a period of time. It requires not only alertness of the mind but a readiness to take in new information. Information coming in through the sensory systems is screened for relevance, and the brain focuses on aspects of the environment to which a response is appropriate. Sustained attention, or concentration, is needed for the individual to participate in OT groups.

Memory

Memory is central to psychoanalytic theory, as seen in Freud's persistent efforts to recapture early childhood events. Rapaport (1942) recognized the relationship between memory and emotional factors. The ego was thought to censor memory in accordance with the intensity of associated emotional factors. In other words, events that were extremely painful are repressed; the ego pushes them below the level of consciousness, and they cannot be remembered at all. Also, the ego can alter the perception of a traumatic event so that the senses are numbed and the brain will not receive more stimuli than it can handle. In this case, the memory of the event would be inaccurate or unrealistic. The current metaphor most closely associated with memory is that of a computer, with information storage and retrieval as the primary activities. It is believed that one's memory process reflects individual styles of secondary process functioning. In other words, what someone remembers about an event is dependent upon how he perceives and understands an event in the first place.

Learning and Logical Thought

Learning and logical thought are skills of the ego that have been given little attention by followers of psychoanalysis; yet, their use is central to the notion of making therapeutic change. It has been noted by ego psychologists since the 1950s that intellectual development (learning) occurs most favorably in a warm, secure environment. This observation is helpful to OT in order to recognize the importance of creating and maintaining this kind of secure environment. Occupational therapists protect clients from physical harm by removing from the task environment potential dangers such as toxic odors and wet or slippery floors. Psychological safety is provided when the occupational therapist offers respect, empathy, and nonjudgmental acceptance in the therapeutic relationship.

The kind of thinking attributed to the ego is secondary process thinking. This is also called reasoning or logical thought. It is the ability of the ego to consider facts in the light of reality and put them to use in guiding behavior. *Problem-solving* is a cognitive skill that requires the use of logical thought. In fact, all of the functions of the ego contribute to problem-solving: accurate perception and reality testing, memory, control of impulses, and appropriate use of defenses. The process of solving problems is quite complex, but the ability to do so is often a deciding factor in whether our clients are considered to be competent in activities of daily living (ADL). Occupational therapists are often asked to evaluate a client's problem solving ability.

7. Adaptive Regression

Regression is going backward from a later to an earlier stage of development. In 1964, Arlow and Brenner defined regression as the re-emergence of modes of mental functioning characteristic of earlier phases of psychic development. They further state that regressions are usually transient and reversible. Pathology is not determined by the depth of the regression (oral, anal, etc.) but by its irreversible nature, by the conflicts that it engenders, and by its interference with the process of adaptation. As a function of the ego, we refer to the reversible type, whereby persons voluntarily revert

to "play mode" when relaxing with friends after a stressful day of work or engaging in physical competition with others within the context of a sport such as wrestling or football. A healthy individual may occasionally regress in an effort to relieve stress or just "have fun." Judgment plays a part in knowing when regression is appropriate (kidding around with friends) and when it is not (bar room brawls). In OT, we may encounter clients (such as "workaholics") who have a difficult time relaxing and just enjoying life. At the other extreme, some clients may play too much and need to exert more self-control and responsibility (such as substance abusers). This "adaptive regression in the service of the ego" differs from the regression as a defense mechanism in that it is conscious, voluntary, and reversible. As a defense mechanism, the opposite is true, as described in the next section.

8. Defense Mechanisms

Defenses are broadly understood as a way of warding off anxiety and ensuring the safety and preservation of an intact ego. Exaggerated defenses, on the other hand, often create internal barriers to occupational performance. For example, a person with OCD spends a great deal of time checking and rechecking every step of a task, making it difficult to manage time effectively. The recurrent obsession might be self-doubt, "Am I sure I packed everything I need in my tote bag?" and the resulting act or compulsion would be repeatedly taking everything out of the bag putting it back in. Early psychologists focused on this aspect when developing the techniques of psychoanalysis. The goal of psychoanalysis was to break through a person's defenses so as to uncover the memory of critical childhood events or patterns.

Sadock and Sadock (2003, pp. 208–209) have classified defense mechanisms into four categories:

1. *Narcissistic defenses:* projection, denial, and distortion
2. *Immature defenses:* acting out, blocking, hypochondriasis, introjection, passive-aggressive behavior, regression, schizoid fantasy, and somatization
3. *Neurotic defenses:* controlling, displacement, dissociation, externalization, inhibition, intellectualization, isolation, rationalization, reaction formation, repression, and sexualization
4. *Mature defenses:* altruism, anticipation, asceticism, humor, sublimation, and suppression.

The contemporary ego psychologists view mature defenses as performing a healthy adaptive function, and these will be most relevant to our work in OT. Those defenses that are dealt with most often in OT are reviewed here. The reader is referred to Sadock and Sadock (2003) for a more thorough description of the previous defenses.

Sublimation

Sublimation was identified by Anna Freud in 1936 as a healthy and acceptable rechanneling of libidinal and aggressive drives into constructive activity. While sublimation is no longer a focus in psychological literature, the concept remains central to OT because of its implications regarding activity, creativity, and tasks or work. As occupational therapists using a psychodynamic frame of reference, we continue to see clear evidence of this rechanneling of energy. The concept allows us to understand why work is such a central part of living and why the loss of the work role produces both aggressiveness and anxiety and a sharp decline in one's self-worth. Neutralization (Hartmann's updated substitute for sublimation) refers to the de-energizing of the libidinal and aggressive drives. It is the "successful defense" by which the mature ego masters reality.

Projection

Projection is another defense, originating with Freud (1936), that continues to hold value in OT. The modern day variation was described by Melanie Klein (1948) as projective identification. In this mechanism, parts of the self are split off and projected onto an external object or person. Projection provides the ego with a means of getting rid of bad parts of the self. Sam is angry with his boss, but he believes the anger is bad, so he projects the anger onto his boss. Now Sam can like himself and feel justified in believing his boss is the bad guy who gets angry. Good parts of the self may be projected also, to avoid separation or keep them safe from the bad parts. Projection at higher levels leads to misinterpreting the motives, feelings, attitudes, or intentions of others.

Projection as a concept is used extensively in OT in the form of projective techniques. Projective techniques are generally creative modalities such as drawing, sculpture, poetry, creative writing, or drama, which allow/encourage a person to express the hidden parts of the self. A client is said to project parts of himself, particularly affects such as anger or love, in the form of symbols or shapes in art or characters and situations in writing or drama. When done in adulthood, these images or fantasies are then open to interpretation by the mature ego. As therapists, we encourage our clients to apply logic and mature judgment to the products of their projective creations when we ask them to explain them. One Vietnam veteran participating in an OT projective arts group was asked to explain his elaborate drawing of the atrocities of war. The guns, the dead body parts, and the destructive remains of buildings symbolized for him the bad parts of himself that he found so hard to accept.

Regression

Regression was also an emphasis of Freud's early work as it helped to explain "fixations" as a cause of mental illness (1936). The importance of regression has recently been enhanced by its relation to borderline and psychotic conditions. Psychotic individuals are said to be regressed to the oral stage (birth to 1 year), the earliest stage in Freud's psychosexual stages of development. Borderline (character disorder) individuals are thought to be regressed to the anal stage (1 to 3 years) and fixated there. This view of regression may help to explain the behavior of our clients with these diagnoses in terms of the functioning of the ego. To do so, however, would require a thorough understanding of Freud's psychosexual stages of development.

Regression has another implication that is important for the occupational therapist in planning intervention. This is the concept of "regression in the service of the ego." Ernst Kris (1936) first used this term to imply a purposeful regression to earlier modes of functioning without the loss of overriding ego control. The artist who smears paint on a canvas to express extreme affect but retains the control to return to the normal world (while the psychotic client cannot) is a good example. The technique of "free association," or the uncensored, often illogical associations of words and images, has been cited as another example.

The therapeutic usefulness of regression to the ego lies in its contribution to a clearer self-understanding. When we ask our clients to wedge clay or use finger paints, these processes reflect the typical (sometimes forbidden) fascination of the anal stage (smearing feces). Our therapeutic purpose for doing this is not to encourage regression, but to free the individual to express affect in an uninhibited way, with the hope of recapturing the innate urge toward mastery that may be trapped there. The client, after engaging in such a creative process, returns to a more mature level of functioning, but he or she retains an awareness of the affect discovered during the regression. This affect is essential if clients are to change the way they understand and use occupations as a part of their recovery from illness and reintegration into social and community roles.

Acting Out

Acting out can best be defined as an action, usually repetitive and compulsive in nature and often self-destructive, that serves the unconscious purpose of resolving a repressed internal conflict by external means. It reflects a primitive lack of control over actions that are typical of the infant and regressively present in psychosis and character disorder. In observing the social interactions of clients with mental illness, occupational therapists often see emotions being "acted out" instead of talked about. For example, anger at someone is expressed by walking out of the room and slamming the door. An action is substituted for a mature verbal description of a feeling state. Occupational therapist group leaders should discourage acting out responses. These are inappropriate and unproductive for both the client and other group members. The more mature ego skill of verbal expression of affect should be encouraged.

Identificantion

Identification, as a defense described by Freud, was meant quite literally as the taking onto oneself the characteristics of another. The concept originated as a logical outcome of the Oedipal conflict, in which sexual desire for the opposite sex parent is replaced by identification with the parent of like sex. Anna Freud (1936) described this phenomenon as "identification with the aggressor." The child's identification with the feared "aggressor" is used, in part, to explain the repetition of behavior patterns in families. An example is when an abused child grows up to abuse his or her own children. Erikson (1950) contributed greatly to the popularity of this concept in his extensive discussion of the identity crisis occurring in late adolescence.

9. Stimulus Barrier

As a function of the ego, the brain copes with incoming sensory stimulation by screening out irrelevant stimuli and allowing the person to process only sensory information that requires a response. For example, people visiting a big city for the first time may feel bombarded my many strange sights, sounds, smells, and movements while navigating a busy street or shopping mall. Normally, the ego provides a "self-protective deafness" (Bellak et al., 1973) to fend off potential sensory overload. Failure to screen out sensory input can cause the entire nervous system to shut down, rendering the person unable to function in certain environments. Some persons with schizophrenia lose this protective function during episodes of psychosis. Other health conditions can also interfere with the stimulus barrier ego function, such as stroke, head injury, or developmental disability. Occupational therapists should be aware of this and avoid exposing such individuals to environments such as crowded busses, department stores, concerts, or sports arenas that are likely to produce such extreme sensory stimuli.

This ego function overlaps with the sensory motor frames, and can also be understood from a neurological perspective.

10. Autonomous Functioning

Ego autonomy, as recognized by Hartmann (1939), includes perception, intention, object comprehension, thinking, and language. These mental processes develop independently of the conflict resolution within Freud's psychosexual stages. Their development is more related to interaction with the environment. In OT, we often equate a client's autonomy with the ability to think and act independently. Autonomy may be understood as the opposite of dependency. For example, Amy, age 14 with cerebral palsy, may need to become less dependent on parents and helpers when entering public high school. Besides independence in physical self-care, Amy may need to gain confidence in her ability to make her own decisions, choose her own friends, and pursue her own interests. Amy's goal in OT may be to become more autonomous in her thinking as well as her behavior with peers and in social situations. In this example (and others), autonomy goes hand in hand with the ability to use rational thought, good judgment, and self-control regarding one's intentions, commitments, and responses to others.

11. Synthetic Integrative Function

This ego function involves the balancing of different parts of the personality—ostensibly Freud's id, ego, and superego—in order to satisfy physical and emotional needs in socially and culturally acceptable ways. To do this, the ego guides the person's interaction with the environment. For example, a mother might take her toddler grocery shopping and observe the child taking a candy bar off the shelf and eating it. This meets the child's need or wish to taste the sweet candy (pleasure-seeking), but mother teaches the child that such behavior is not socially acceptable. The child learns that she must delay gratification until mother pays for the candy bar before she can eat it. The child's ego learns to follow this social rule, thus integrating her internal need with outer reality. Healthy growth and development involves engaging in relationships with others in a give and take manner that is mutually satisfying. Children learn to share and take turns, and such reciprocal social relationships continue into adulthood. Thus, this ego function interacts with object relations and attachment theory, described previously. In OT, we might involve clients in building social networks or finding needed social support. Our clients may need to offer empathy and support to others in order to obtain needed support for themselves. Older adults may need help with integrating these roles when facing declining health and decreased independence.

12. Mastery/Competence

The *mastery/competence* function of the ego is defined by Bellak et al. (1973) as adaptive performance in work and relationships, and the subjective feelings of competence. White (1959) defines competence as "an organism's capacity to interact effectively with its environment..." (p. 297). OT's current concepts of personal causation (Kielhofner, 2002) and self-efficacy (Bandura, 1977, 1995; Polatajko & Davis, 2005) come from White's (1967) original observation of feelings of competence, the result of a well-developed ego, that includes a history of successful experiences in coping with the environment.

Coping

Coping is the ego's ability to rescue oneself in times of illness or crisis. In an emotional crisis, many of the ego defenses described previously may be viewed as coping mechanisms, protecting the ego from destruction by diverting psychic energy. In the case of physical trauma, the ego uses body sense and reality testing to determine what functions of the body remain intact. The ego's sense of self will often provide the motivation to find ways to compensate for lost functions. For example, a client with right-sided hemiplegia will learn to write with his or her left hand. Compensation is a coping strategy.

Another example of a coping strategy is energy conservation. When physical and mental deterioration occur, energy for use in everyday activities is severely limited. Careful planning before embarking on a task can prevent the client from wasting energy in needless movements. For example, after I (M. Cole) had an operation, I was only able to stand up or walk for 15 minutes before stopping to take a rest. When preparing a meal, I had to learn to use the 15 minutes to gather absolutely everything I needed to make meatballs, then assemble them while sitting at the kitchen table. The cooking had to be done in an electric frying pan on the table, rather than at the stove. I had to learn to be satisfied with accumulating a mess around me, rather than cleaning as I went along, and to use a wet sponge to wipe my hands, rather than washing at the sink every few minutes. For clients with chronic disability, conserving energy is a coping skill that is absolutely essential for continued functioning at a level that is consistent with the client's self-identity.

Creative Media and Spirituality from an Occupational Therapy Perspective

Why do people feel uplifted or energized by music? Why do they become engrossed in theatrical performance or enjoy a good cry at the movies? Creative arts do more than convey an intellectual message—they also touch our spirit in ways that often cannot be explained. Spirituality has been defined in OT as the experience of meaning. The "movie prescription" has been successfully used in client groups to help them find meaning in various ways. For example, the movie *The Lion King* gets people thinking about their purpose in life, and the way that cultural messages get passed on from one generation to another. Interventions that create spiritual connections sometimes relate more closely to client satisfaction than outcome measures used in mental health treatment. Babbis (2002) has described ethnography studies of three women with anorexia nervosa who have much to say about the helpfulness of expressive media interventions. These cases elucidate the need to for occupational therapists to pay special attention to individuals who have uncovered painful emotions and memories in the course of creative activities and to provide a safe structure within which to explore their significance in creating positive outcomes.

FUNCTION AND DISABILITY

A healthy ego is synonymous with a strong sense of self; body image, self-identity, and self-esteem are realistic and can serve as the basis of adaptive function. A functioning adult is free from conflicts and fixations, and is able to satisfy his or her needs and direct his or her drives in ways that fit in with the social environment and culture. A balance exists in the functioning individual that allows the psychic energy to flow freely between the id, ego, and superego. The ego is in control and defense mechanisms are not exaggerated so that the individual with a healthy ego can use most of his or her energy to grow and develop and interact effectively with others. In Fidler's model, the healthy person is able to work productively with others to accomplish a task (Fidler & Fidler, 1963). The defenses the individual uses are mature ones, like sublimation of aggression in work, identification with idealized others, and the suppression of immediate gratification.

Disability in the psychodynamic frame of reference is defined in terms of inadequate psychosexual development, the presence of conflicts and fixations, and the imbalance of psychic energy among the three parts of the personality. These abnormal states can produce symptoms of neurosis, psychosis, or character disorder, which imply a disturbance in the ability to perform occupations associated with satisfactory participation in life situations.

From Mosey's (1970a) perspective, mature ego skills are necessary in order to participate in a variety of dyadic relationships and group interactions. Dyadic interaction, or relationships between oneself and another individual, develop sequentially as follows:

- *Trusting familial relationships:* such as parents or caregivers
- *Association relationships:* such as playing with other children
- *Authority relationships:* such as accepting guidance from teachers or coaches
- *Chum relationships:* such as peer groups and friendships
- *Intimate relationships:* such as dating, marriage, close friendships
- *Nurturing relationships:* such as becoming a parent, caregiving, teaching, or mentoring others

These represent different types of attachment and suggest ways that both children and adults can meet each others' social and emotional needs. Failure to meet these needs with others in ways that are satisfying to self and others, contributes to our understanding of a client's disability in social participation.

Mosey (1970a, 1970b) also proposed five levels of group interactions:

1. *Parallel:* members work side by side while following the leader and rules.
2. *Project (or Associative):* members begin to interact around a task.
3. *Egocentric cooperative (or Basic cooperative):* members help one another with the group task.

4. *Cooperative (or Supportive cooperative)*: members socialize and express feelings.

5. *Mature*: taking on a variety of group roles, balance of productive and social goals.

Function includes the ability to interact at all of these levels when appropriate. Donohue (2005; 2007) has developed a measure of social participation that has validated Mosey's original theory. Therefore, this tool, the Social Profile, may be used in this frame of reference as a measure of function and disability in the occupational area of social participation.

The presence or absence of mature ego functions will guide our setting of goals in OT. Disability can take the form of poor reality testing, poor or unrealistic body image, poor self-identity, poor self-esteem, impulsiveness or passivity, inability to control or regulate emotions, unbalanced use of defenses, and inability to cope. In OT, problems with ego functions create barriers to occupational performance, and goals may involve overcoming these barriers.

CHANGE AND MOTIVATION

In the Freudian view, people change as a result of insight, defined as self-understanding and reflection upon their perceptions of past experience. Through the therapeutic relationship, clients work to become aware of the emotions, motivations, and conflicts that are hidden in their unconscious. This process is called *working through*.

From an ego-adaptive perspective, change occurs through the learning and performance of adequate ego functions. These skills can be learned within the therapeutic relationship or in the social context of therapeutic groups where the consequences of problem behaviors can be readily seen and discussed. Foundation skills can be worked on through simple, well-structured, reality-oriented tasks that focus on the development of sensory motor, perceptual, and cognitive skills. Motivation can be enhanced through success experiences in OT.

Explanations of motivation also represent a continuum between id and ego. In the Freudian view, the id works on the *pleasure principle*, which seeks to gratify needs and drives and to reduce tension and anxiety. Looked upon in this way, we might define life satisfaction as the absence of anxiety. However, satisfaction of needs requires interaction with the environment. The ego mediates and negotiates on behalf of the id so that needs can be met and drives satisfied through the development of mature social or person–environment relationships. Motivation comes from directing psychic energy toward the *mastery of ego skills* and the *symbolic expression of emotions* through engagement in occupations.

When energy is bound up in dealing with conflict, persons may not be motivated to develop ego skills. As the ego is available to help reduce tensions and to satisfy needs through mature relationships and meaningful work

activities, persons will be motivated to increase ego skill development. Azima (1982; Azima & Azima, 1959) explored the use of creative arts to address personality characteristics, including the clients' perceptions of self and others as well as the symbolic expression of unconscious conflicts and motivational or emotional fixations. The occupational therapist can set up therapeutic occupations that allow clients to practice adequate ego skills and experience successful and satisfying consequences. A strong self-concept and high self-esteem are also motivating; these foster a sense of control and lead people to direct their energy toward even greater skill development and self-actualization.

EVALUATION

OT has a rich history in the use of projective techniques for both assessment and intervention. Creative media, such as drawing, sculpture, and finger painting, have formed the basis of a number of test batteries. Drake (1999) summarized many of these (Table 20-3) and gives some general guidelines for their use, such as the following:

- Choosing media that relate to client goals
- Noting whether for formal or informal use
- Always generating client input about their creative efforts
- Corroborating findings with more objective assessments or observations
- Focusing on the aspects of the assessment that address client priorities

For example, drawings can measure outward qualities such as fine motor control or perceptual qualities such as spatial awareness as well as internal qualities such as self-esteem and mood. Scoring for these assessments varies widely, and some assessments are more standardized and well researched than others. Standardized assessments should follow the format described in the manuals that accompanied them.

Other projective tests worth considering follow:

- *Kinetic House–Tree–Person Drawings (KHTP), Burns (1987)*: Instruct the client to draw a house, draw a tree, and draw a whole person (not a cartoon or stick person). A pencil with eraser and 8.5- x 11-inch paper are used. Questions about the drawing and interpretations vary.

- *Forer Vocational Assessment, Forer (1983)*: Ask the client to finish incomplete sentences in 12 work-related categories such as goals, job turnover, reactions to criticism, reactions to authority, coworker relations, etc. This assessment uncovers some psychosocial issues related to the occupational performance area of work.

- *Kinetic Family Drawing and Kinetic School Drawing, Burns and Kaufman (1972)*: Ask the client to draw you his or her family or classmates doing something

	Table 20-3	
Assessments That Use Expressive Media		
Test and Date of Publication	**Whom and What It Measures**	**Media/Subtests**
Goodenough Harris Draw-a-Person Test, 1926/1960	Intelligence in children. Scoring includes many factors such as the features present, proportion, and detail.	Pencil and blank paper
Fidler Battery, 1959+	For adults with mental illness. Emotions, attitudes, interpersonal, cognitive, and sensory motor skills	Clay, drawing, finger painting, collage, movement, and group games
Azima Battery, 1959+	For adults with mental illness. Ego defenses, mood, reality awareness, perceptions of environment, and energy level.	Free pencil drawing. Draw a person of each sex. Unstructured clay project. Finger painting
Goodman Battery, 1967	For adults with mental illness. Cognition, organization, problem-solving, self-esteem, ego boundaries, emotional overlay, control issues, etc.	Tile task, spontaneous pencil drawing, figure drawing, clay task
BH Battery, Hemphill 1970+	For adults with mental illness. Client tells a story about the finger painting. Therapist rates functional and neuro-behavioral responses.	Mosaic tile task. Finger painting task
Magazine Picture Collage; Lerner, 1982+	Mental health and long-term care. Observations of process of cutting and gluing and selection of color, title, and comments about client-made collage. Therapist uses a score sheet to rate.	Cut out pictures of client's choosing from old magazines; glue them to construction paper.
Build A City; Nelson-Clark, 1975+	Groups format, instructed to "build your ideal city"—30-minute time limit. Rating scale completed by the occupational therapist includes group roles, a running record of member interactions, and positive and negative qualities.	Standard tools and materials, including scissors, construction paper, Styrofoam, blunt table knife, string, clay, and pipe cleaners

(Adapted from Drake, M. (1999). The use of expressive media as an assessment tool in mental health. In B. Hemphill-Pearson (Ed.), Assessments in occupational therapy mental health: An integrative approach. Thorofare, NJ: SLACK Incorporated.)

together. These drawing tasks are useful in working with children and for family-centered therapy.

In OT, these tests can also serve as a basis for individual or group discussions. Interpretation should also follow Drake's guidelines for eliciting client input and corroborating findings with other assessment methods.

Evaluations of personality type come from another branch of psychodynamic theory, that of Carl Jung. Jung divided personality into two basic types: introverted and extroverted (1921). The Myers-Briggs Type Indicator (MBTI) (Myers, 1944, 1956) is an example of an assessment tool based on the theories of Jung. This tool assesses personality preferences for four mental processes: directing energy, processing information, making decisions, and organizing one's life. Based on answers to a short set of dichotomies, the assessment places the participant into one of 16 categories. This assessment has been used to predict learning styles, direct career choices, and explain the dynamics of relationships with individuals or in groups (Myers & McCaulley, 1986).

As a learning experience, take the MBTI (http://www.capt.org/take-mbti-assessment/mbti.htm). Print your score and interpretation, and bring it to class to discuss.

INTERVENTIONS

Using Activities to Test Reality

Carving or stamping designs onto leather is an activity filled with symbolism. First of all, consider that leather is the skin of a dead animal. Using a knife to cut and carve cowhide can be symbolically associated with the expression of hostility, aggression, or even homicidal tendencies. Secondly, the movements of pounding a stamping tool with a hammer or wielding a carving blade across a thick leather surface have the potential to absorb huge amounts of psychic energy. Sublimation of the aggressive drive, in the psychodynamic view, underlies the natural drive to compete in the workplace, to strive for success.

Table 20-4

An Addict's Poem

Gotta tell my wife I love her
Gotta kiss my kids hello
Should invite the neighbors over
One more drink before I go

Haven't sold my monthly quota
Pour another, and don't be slow
I'll be sober by tomorrow
Give those suckers a good show

Is it really twelve, it can't be
Feel so wasted, can't drive home
Just one more so I can face her
Bartender how much do I owe?

– Anonymous

Symbolic and Transitional Objects

How often do people puzzle over the meaning of dreams, or the reasons for their attraction and attachment to physical objects? The connection of symbols with emotions can be understood using object relations theory, the idea that people seek to gratify emotional needs through objects. Fine (1999) confirms the importance of symbolism in creating meaning for life's occupations. She states, "There is an unfortunate tendency in the so-called cognitive revolution to reduce the mind to an information processing system disconnected from experience and context" (p. 13). In contrast, acknowledging the unconscious inner life opens the door to a fuller understanding of clients' current relationships with the external environment as well as their involvement in preferred activities (Vaillant, 1993; Zemke & Clark, 1996). OT interventions that apply the symbolic meaning of activities or encourage self-expression through art, poetry, drama, dance/movement, or creative writing all help clients get in touch with their emotions.

Activities to Express Emotions

Occupations are said to cross cultural boundaries easily, and this is particularly true of expressive media. Painting transcends the limitations of language, its message communicated with shape, color, and intensity directly to the intuitive human spirit within. For those clients who do not communicate easily using language, for whatever reason, drawing, painting, and sculpture represent alternative ways to connect, often without the barriers of social or political correctness. Likewise, storytelling, or narratives relating to one's occupational experiences, allows clients the freedom to express emotions as well as the facts of their individual history.

Moving to music, playing instruments, and interpretive dance represent other creative activities through which clients can express emotions. For example, older adults with dementia or aphasia resulting from acquired brain injury might choose music that reflects their mood, create a lively rhythm with drums or strings, or move in ways that convey their prevailing affect. Clients unable to communicate in more traditional ways might express feelings of connection with each other and socialize through movement or musical expression.

Closely related to music is poetry. Persons with complicated emotions, such as those with substance abuse issues, can use poetry to help them sort out the many nuances of affect that influence their addictive behaviors and their profound helplessness to control the outcome for themselves and those they love. Table 20-4 is an example. The therapeutic use of drama has been demonstrated by psychologists throughout the 20th century. In OT, play reading in groups is a nonthreatening way to get clients to express emotions. For example, the play "Twelve Angry Men" offers a variety of parts that require the appropriate verbal expression of hostility while a sequestered jury debates the merits of a criminal case. Another useful dramatic technique is the "empty chair." Clients are asked to visualize a person with whom they have a troubled relationship or unresolved issues seated in the empty chair and to speak to that individual as if he or she were present. For example, Marge never got the chance to tell her father how she felt about him before he died. Using the empty chair technique can give clients a way to work through some conflicted relationships within the safety of the therapeutic group.

Storytelling, creative writing, and journaling are often used as vehicles for self-expression. These may be structured by the occupational therapist for use with individuals or groups. For example, writing a "letter to the departed" is another creative way to deal with unresolved relationship issues.

Group Interventions

Task-oriented groups are an excellent example of OT intervention using the psychodynamic frame of reference. It is a context in which all of the ego skills discussed can be evaluated and worked on. Cole (2005) has extrapolated from Fidler's (1969) original concept three phases for conducting task-oriented OT groups. The first phase, planning, focuses on facilitation of group brainstorming, persuasion, and decision-making as members decide on a meaningful task for the group. The second phase, or actual doing of the activity or task, is then organized and carried out by group members (to the best of their ability), with selective interventions by the OT group leader. The third phase, evaluation, involves a discussion of the process, including feelings about the task and outcome, problem-solving that occurred during the first and second phases, and mutual

Figure 20-2. Pet therapy at an Adult Day Care Center—dog Griffin demonstrates attachment theory in the person–animal relationship.

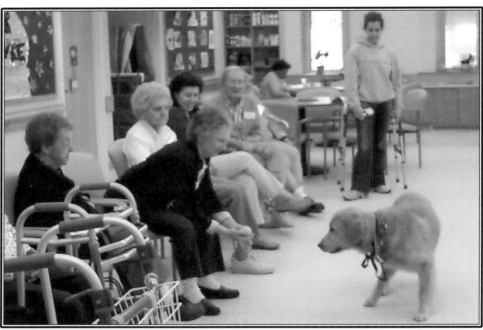

feedback regarding each members' contribution to the task and outcome.

OT interventions that encourage exploring the unconscious and uncovering painful or conflicting memories to be resolved remain a less popular, but an equally legitimate, application of psychodynamic theory.

Pet Therapy

One up-and-coming OT intervention based on object relations theory is pet therapy (Figure 20-2). Current studies use object relations and attachment theory to explain the therapeutic benefits of pets. People create relationships with animals in order to satisfy needs, use skills, socially engage, and find meaning in life. Animals provide a means by which individuals can love and be loved unconditionally. The interactive nature of caring for animals is deeply satisfying to many individuals. Pets provide affirmation of the self and an unconditional source of need gratification. Animals can provide a sense of security through their protective nature. Furthermore, service animals have been shown to improve self-esteem, internal locus of control, and psychological well-being in individuals with severe ambulatory diseases (Latella, 2003).

Symbolic Legacies in Hospice Care

A young Hospice volunteer, who held evening classes in jewelry making in her home, discovered the symbolic meaning of the jewelry quite by accident. Someone in her class, diagnosed with ovarian cancer and given less then three months to live, wanted to make a special necklace for each of her teenage daughters to wear on their wedding day. A similar type of symbolism may be found in the making of commemorative quilts from pieces of clothing or fabrics that symbolize important life events. Writing letters to loved ones; memoirs about family events, ancestors, or other significant events; or writing an ethical will offer persons facing terminal illness with opportunities to articulate the emotional connections, values, beliefs, and words of wisdom they wish to pass along to significant others in their lives. Such spiritually meaningful activities might connect with Jung's concept of transcendence in later life as a way to contribute to the "collective unconscious" (Jung, 1955). Grieving, depression, fear, anger, and pain can overwhelm a person with terminal illness. The occupational therapist's role might be to enable the creative expression of these strong emotions through a symbolically meaningful activity.

RESEARCH

Application of psychodynamic theory has a long and rich history in the OT literature. While the journalists and the general public question whether Freud is "dead" (Gray, 1993), many outgrowths of his theory continue to be researched and published (Fonagy, 1998; Fonagy et al., 2002).

Dickerson (1992) argues that occupational therapists have become too cognitively oriented, "... that the pendulum has gone too far in the other direction, away from the affective component addressed in the object relations (psychodynamic) frame of reference" (p. 48). She compares the research on affect from both cognitive and somatic perspectives, and finds considerable evidence that affect is separate from, and not dependent upon, cognition. Evidence for this includes the following:

- Affect is primary—people make decisions and judgments based on emotion, not cognition. Cognitive appraisal comes afterwards.

- Affect is basic—a universal response among cultures, and animals.

- Affective reactions are instantaneous, automatic, and often unwelcome.

- Affective reactions are difficult to verbalize, often relying on nonverbal channels of expression (visceral or somatic level).

- Affective judgments tend to be irrevocable, and therefore difficult to change with cognitive interventions such as reasoning or confrontation

Dickerson's arguments certainly have face validity. Have we not met clients who stubbornly say "I can't" and resist any efforts to demonstrate their occupational performance strengths? Persons with depression often cling to the belief that their life is worthless despite a long list of impressive achievements. Persons who experienced the Depression years continue to save things they might use some day, believing they cannot afford to spend money on themselves. Persons with anorexia nervosa believe they are "fat" despite overwhelming evidence to the contrary. In OT interventions, using projective arts that facilitate expression of affect and emotion may give therapists and clients needed insights as to why they believe as they do, and to understand what must be done to overcome this barrier to occupational performance.

An idea central to OT is the interaction of emotion and occupation. Greene and Cole (1991), compared clients' emotional investment in OT groups with that of traditional group psychotherapy. They found a significant preference for OT task groups among groups of both psychotic (schizophrenia, bipolar disorder) and character disorder (borderline) client members. This finding implies that OT interventions have a stronger impact than traditional talk therapy.

Studies of attachment theory, the modern day outgrowth of object relations, also help to validate the role of occupations in human life. In attachment theory, the self is seen from two perspectives: 1) self as the agent responsible for constructing self-concept and generating the experiences that distinguish the individual, and 2) self as the mental representation, otherwise known as identity (Fonagy et al., 2002). Occupations contribute to both perspectives, by first providing the milieu within which persons experience life, and then providing opportunities for reflection and interpretation of the meaning of past occupational experiences within the context of our social relationships. Christiansen (1999) links occupation with identity, viewing "occupation as the principal means through which people develop and express their personal identities" (p. 547). Zimmerman

& Becker-Stoll (2002) studied the role of attachment in adolescent identity formation, and found that between the ages of 16 and 18, internal working models of attachment predicted a stable (strong self) or diffuse (weak self) identity status. Bilsker and Marcia (1991) found that adaptive regression in young adulthood, such as participation in sports and playful occupations with others, serves an important function in the identity formation process. Hartmann's (1939) notion of adaptation as an autonomous ego function is applied in a study of children developing in the midst of environmental turmoil and violence (Mayes, 1994). Mayes notes that in the face of adversity, individuals adapt by reaching a relative state of autonomy that deviates from the average. In other words, occupational therapists may recognize that clients' adaptations are subjective and dependent upon their individual surroundings and circumstances.

Attachment theory also incorporates the role of social and emotional support. Kates and Rockland (1994) applied general principles of supportive psychodynamic therapy for persons with schizophrenia, which included building a therapeutic alliance, supporting adaptive defenses, providing social skills training, and vocational rehabilitation. Appelbaum (1994) stresses the role of creating environments to promote learning, optimize anxiety, encourage mature relationships, and strengthen adaptive defenses in fostering a strong sense of self.

Disability studies that provide evidence for the psychodynamic approach include anxiety disorders, depression and suicide, and chronic pain. Hoffmann and Bassler (1995) show how psychodynamic formulations of anxiety can best be addressed by active strengthening of adaptive ego functions as well as disclosure of conflicts concerning self-control. A controlled clinical trial of 99 subjects supported an object relational view of suicidal behavior, finding suicide attempters significantly more likely to report a history of childhood loss combined with recent loss in adulthood (Kaslow, Reviere, Chance, et al., 1998).

LEARNING ACTIVITIES

Case Study: Meryl

Meryl traces her obsessive compulsive behaviors to an auto accident when she was sixteen. Now in college and physically recovered with a only a scarred breast and injured collarbone remaining, "things began to fall apart." She explains this as a reaction to her expectation that she should now feel "normal," only she doesn't. In fact, she has never dealt with the psychological trauma of the accident at all. Instead, she keeps her anxiety in check by performing the ritual of sitting in coffee shops for hours watching other people, safe from behind her textbooks (which she should be studying). She has eating rituals too. Each item of food has to have its own plate, so that it is not unusual for her to have five or six plates in front of her, taking up lots of space and driving her family crazy when she's home. Because of her rituals, Meryl feels that she cannot have normal relationships with peers. She spends a great deal of time fantasizing about the relationships she'd like to have, like having candlelight dinners with men or casual conversations with girlfriends over coffee. She lives in a suite on campus, but has her own bedroom where she eats, sleeps, and basically keeps to herself. In meeting with an occupational therapist about recurring shoulder pain, she puts on a heroic front, but bursts into tears while describing her occupational difficulties with dorm and college life.

Directions and Discussion

1. Look up the definition of OCD, and briefly describe the symptoms. What is the etiology from a psychodynamic perspective?

2. What occupations present difficulty for Meryl in her current life roles? List and explain them.

3. How would you evaluate Meryl's psychological and social difficulties with occupation?

4. Using expressive media, design interventions for each of the following issues:

   a. Remembering the details of the accident to which she attributes her obsessions and compulsions.

   b. Expressing the sources of underlying anxiety which energize her need to repeat obsessive-compulsive rituals.

   c. Identifying barriers to the development of self and social identity.

5. For each issue, write the following: What media would you use (art, drama, writing, crafts, movement), and how would it be structured? Write several questions you would ask her for each. Explain the reasons for choices and expected outcomes for each intervention.

Wellness: Psychodynamic Frame

Directions: Use colored markers (8 or more colors) and a sheet of white paper to *draw your mood*. Your mood is an internal emotional state, not necessarily connected to specific events. You will be more likely to get in touch with emotions by closing your eyes and allowing your mind to wander. Don't censor yourself. There are no right or wrong emotions. If you come up blank, try one of the following as a guide:

- A place you'd rather be
- The colors you feel drawn to
- A person you wish you could talk to
- Something you want to avoid

- A feeling you wish would go away
- The weather inside your head
- The shapes and lines that define who you are on the inside

Do not wait for an "idea" to form. Just pick a color and begin drawing. Allow your instincts to guide you. Continue until the entire page is covered, or until you come to a natural end.

Reflections

1. What name would you give the mood or emotion you drew?

2. To what extent were you able to give up conscious control?

3. How did it feel to draw without a topic or subject?

4. What made this project hard or easy for you?

5. How could you use drawing to facilitate communication about emotions with clients?

Group Activity: Emotions and Symbols

Supplies: Eight small round balloons, paper, pencils, and scissors

Directions: Work in groups of 8 members. Think about a recent problem that has caused you for feel upset. How would you define the problem? Take 10 to 15 minutes to write down a brief description of the problem and your emotional reactions. What is particularly bad about it, and what might be some negative consequences for you? Write three words to further define your "upsetness" in this situation.

Discussion

Take turns sharing your emotion words with the group. You don't need to give any details you feel uncomfortable sharing. The writing you have done symbolizes the problem and your negative emotions.

Activity

Each member takes a balloon. Rip up the paper describing your problem, and put all the pieces inside the balloon. Then blow up the balloon and knot the end. It is important that the whole group do this next step together. Take the balloons to a high spot, like the roof, a tower, or a nearby bridge, and throw them over the edge. Watch them drift away, and imagine that your upset feelings are drifting away with them.

Reflection

Discuss how it felt to do this activity. How has your feeling about the problem changed? What feelings remain, and how might you otherwise express them? What is the effect of symbolic expression of emotions? How might you use symbolism to help clients in OT?

Table 20-5

Psychodynamic Toolbox

Emotional Barrier*	Activity and Symbolism	Intervention Guidelines
Depression: hostility turned inward	Kicking a beach ball, throwing darts, punching a heavy bag, hitting a pillow, hammering nails into wood	Encourage movements that allow the expression of hostility in a safe way. Ask client to give the object (ball, bag, target) a name. Discuss significance and emotional responses.
Dependency: clinging	Empowering through use of technology, learning correct and safe use of power tools, playing board games.	Increase self-confidence through the successful accomplishment of tasks that have highly visible and well-defined goals.
Uncontrolled anger: irritable and prone to outbursts of temper	Digging in a garden, planting, playing tennis or racquetball, wedging clay, making pottery, kneading dough, baking bread	Encourage sublimation of aggressive drive into creative and positive work tasks. Express hostility safely through competitive sports.
Obsessive-compulsive: need for control		Meet need for order, grade toward less structure and tolerance for ambiguity.
Overwhelmed with grief: cries easily		Encourage expression of emotion. Define/discuss lost objects (e.g., significant other, loss of roles/abilities through illness or trauma) through artistic media
Grandiose, agitated and impulsive, manic tendencies		
*		
*		

Add other emotional barriers/activities/guidelines—continue chart on another page.

Psychodynamic Toolbox

Directions: Use the symbolic properties of activities to create appropriate interventions for emotional barriers to occupational performance. Using the examples given in Table 20-5 as a guide, fill out the rest of the table. Give at least three ideas for each. Discuss.

REFERENCES

Allport, G. (1958). *Becoming: Basic considerations for a psychology of personality.* New Haven, CT: Yale University Press.

American Occupational Therapy Association (AOTA). (2002). Occupational therapy practice framework: Domain and process. *American Journal of Occupational Therapy, 56,* 609–639.

American Psychiatric Association. (2007). *Diagnostic and statistical manual of mental disorders* (4th ed.). Washington, DC: Author.

Appelbaum, A. H. (1994). Psychotherapeutic routes to structural change. *Bulletin of the Menninger Clinic, 58,* 37–54.

Arlow, J. A., & Brenner, C. (1964). *Psychoanalytic concepts and the structural theory.* New York: International University Press.

Azima, F. (1982). The Azima battery: An overview. In B. Hemphill (Ed.), *The evaluative process in psychiatric occupational therapy* (pp. 57–64). Thorofare, NJ: SLACK Incorporated.

Azima, A., & Azima, F. (1959). Outline of a dynamic theory of occupation. *American Journal of Occupational Therapy, 13,* 1–7.

Babbis, F. (2002). An ethnographic study of mental health treatment and outcomes: Doing what works. *Occupational Therapy in Mental Health, 18*(3/4), 1–137.

Bandura, A. (1977). *Social learning theory.* Englewood Cliffs, NJ: Prentice Hall.

Bandura, A. (1995). *Self-efficacy in changing societies.* Cambridge, MA: Cambridge University Press.

Banks, M. R., & Banks, W. A. (2002). The effects of animal-assisted therapy on loneliness in an elderly population in long-term care facilities. *The Journals of Gerontology Series A: Biological Sciences and Medical Sciences, 57*(7), M428–M432.

Bellak, L., Huruich, M., & Gediman, H. (1973). *Ego functions in schizophrenics, neurotics and normals.* New York: Wiley & Sons.

Bilsker, D., & Marcia, J. E., (1991). Adaptive regression and ego identity. *Journal of Adolescence, 14,* 75–84.

Bowlby, J. (1988). *A secure base: Clinical applications of attachment theory.* London, UK: Routledge.

Bruce, M., & Borg, B. (2002). *Frames of reference in psychosocial occupational therapy* (3rd ed.). Thorofare, NJ: SLACK Incorporated.

Burkhardt, M., & Nagai-Jacobson, M. (1994). Reawakening spirit in clinical practice. *Journal of Holistic Nursing, 12,* 9–21.

Burns, R. C. (1987). *Kinetic-house-tree-person drawings: An interpretive manual.* New York: Brunner-Routledge.

Burns, R. C., & Kaufman, S. F. (1972). *Actions, styles, and symbols in kinetic family drawings (KDF): Clinical interpretative manual.* New York: Brunner/Mazel.

Christiansen, C. H. (1999). Defining lives: Occupation as identity: An essay on competence, coherence, and the creation of meaning, 1999 Eleanor Clarke Slagle lecture. *American Journal of Occupational Therapy, 53,* 547–558.

Cole, M. (2005) *Group dynamics in occupational therapy* (3rd ed.). Thorofare, NJ: SLACK Incorporated.

Diasio, K. (1968). Psychiatric occupational therapy: Search for a conceptual framework in light of psychoanalytic ego psychology and learning theory. *American Journal of Occupational Therapy, 22,* 50–57.

Dickerson, A. E. (1992). The relationship between affect and cognition. *Occupational Therapy in Mental Health, 12,* 47–59.

Donohue, M. (2005). The social profile. Unpublished Assessment Tool. New York University, New York.

Donohue, M. (2007). Interrater reliability of the social profile: Assessment of community and psychiatric group participation. *Australian Journal of Occupational Therapy, 54,* 49–58.

Drake, M. (1999). The use of expressive media as an assessment tool in mental health. In B. Hemphill-Pearson (Ed.), *Assessments in occupational therapy mental health: An integrative approach.* Thorofare, NJ: SLACK Incorporated.

Erikson, E. (1950). *Childhood and society.* New York: Norton.

Fidler, G. (1969). The task oriented group as a context for treatment. *American Journal of Occupational Therapy, 23,* 43–48.

Fidler, G. (1978). Doing and becoming: Purposeful actions and self actualization. *American Journal of Occupational Therapy, 32,* 305–310.

Fidler, G., & Fidler, J. (1963). *Occupational therapy: A communication process in psychiatry.* New York: Macmillan.

Fidler, G., & Velde, B. (1999). *Activities: Reality and symbol.* Thorofare, NJ: SLACK Incorporated.

Fine, R. (1979). *A history of psychoanalysis.* New York: Columbia University Press.

Fine, S. (1999). Symbolism: Making meaning for self and society. In G. Fidler, & B. Velde (Eds.), *Activities: Reality and symbol.* Thorofare, NJ: SLACK Incorporated

Fonagy, P. (1998). Moments of change in psychoanalytic theory: Discussion of a new theory of psychic change. *Infant Mental Health Journal, 19,* 163–171.

Fonagy, P., Gergely, G., Jurist, E. L., & Target, M. (2002). *Affect regulation, mentalization, and the development of the self.* New York: Other Press.

Forer, B. (1983). *The Forer vocational survey.* Los Angeles, CA: Western Psychological Press.

Freud, A. (1936). *The ego and the mechanisms of defense.* New York: International University Press.

Freud, S. (1953). History of the psychoanalytic movement. In J. Strachey (Ed.), *The standard edition of the complete psychological works of Sigmund Freud.* London, NK: Hogarth.

Greene, L., & Cole, M. (1991). Level and form of psychopathology and the structure of group therapy. *International Journal of Group Psychotherapy, 41*(4), 499–521.

Gray, P. (1993). The assault on Freud. Time, November 29th, 47–49.

Hartmann, H. (1939). *Ego psychology and the problem of adaptation.* New York: International University Press.

Hartmann, H. (1964). *Essays on Ego psychology.* New York: International University Press.

Hasselkus, B. (2002). *The meaning of everyday occupation.* Thorofare, NJ: SLACK Incorporated.

Hoffmann, S. O., & Bassler, M. (1995). Psychodynamics and psychotherapy of anxiety disorders. *Z Arztl Fortbild* (Article in German), *89,* 127–132.

Howard, B. S., & Howard, J. R. (1997). Occupation as spiritual activity. *American Journal of Occupational Therapy, 51,* 181–185.

Jung, C. (1910). The association method. *American Journal of Psychology, 21,* 216–269.

Jung, C. (1921). Psychological types. In C. D. Green, (Ed.), *Classics in the history of psychology.* Retrieved September 25, 2007, from http://psychclassics.yorku.ca/Jung/types.htm.

Jung, C. (1955). *Modern man in search of soul.* Orlando, FL: Harcourt, Inc.

Kaslow, N. J., Reviere, S. L., Chance, S. E., Rogers, J. H., Hatcher, C. A., Wasserman, F., et al. (1998). An empirical study of the psychodynamics of suicide. *Journal of the American Psychoanalytic Association, 46,* 777–796.

Kates, J., & Rockland, L. H. (1994). Supportive psychotherapy of the schizophrenic patient. *American Journal of Psychotherapy, 48,* 543–561.

Kielhofner, G. (2002). *Model of human occupation: Theory and application* (3rd ed.). Baltimore, MD: Lippincott, Williams & Wilkins.

Klein, M. (1948). *Contributions to psychoanalysis 1921, 1945.* London, UK: Hogarth Press.

Kris, E. (1936). The psychology of caricature. *International Journal of Psychology, 17,* 285–303.

Latella, D. (2003). Animal assisted therapy: A curriculum for occupational therapy. (Dissertation.) Bridgeport, CT: University of Bridgeport Press.

Law, M., Baptiste, S., Carswell, A., McColl, M. A., Polatajko, H., & Pollock, N. (1998). *The Canadian occupational performance measure* (3rd ed.). Ottawa, CA: Canadian Occupational Therapy Association.

Leichsenring, F., & Hiller, W. (1990). Primary and secondary process thinking in normal probands, neurotic and borderline patients. *Psychosom Med Psychoanal, 36*(1) 62–78.

Llorens, L. (1966). Occupational therapy in an ego oriented milieu. *American Journal of Occupational Therapy, 20,* 178–181.

Marvin, R. S., & Britner, P. A. (1999). Normative development: The ontogeny of attachment. In J. Cassidy, & P. R. Shaver (Eds.), *Handbook of attachment: Theory, research and clinical applications* (pp. 44–67). New York: Guilford Press.

Mayes, L. C. (1994). Understanding adaptive processes in a developmental context. A reappraisal of Hartmann's problem of adaptation. *Psychoanalytic Study Child, 49,* 12–35.

Mosey, A. (1970a). *Three frames of reference for mental health.* Thorofare, NJ: SLACK Incorporated.

Mosey, A. (1970b). The concept and use of developmental groups. *American Journal of Occupational Therapy, 24,* 272–275.

Mosey, A. (1986). *Psychosocial components of occupational therapy.* New York: Raven Press.

Murray, H. A. (1951). Uses of the thematic apperception test. *American Journal of Psychiatry, 107,* 577–581.

Myers, K. (1944, 1956). Briggs Myers type indicator handbook. Retrieved February 27, 2006, from http://www.teamtechnology.co.uk.

Myers, I. B., & McCaulley, M. H. (1986). *A guide to the development and use of the Myers-Briggs type indicator.* Novato, CA: Consulting Psychologists Press.

Polatajko, H. J., & Davis, J. A. (2005). Methods of inquiry: The study of human occupation. In C. Christiansen, & C. Baum (Eds.), *Occupational therapy: Performance, participation, and well-being* (pp 189–208). Thorofare, NJ: SLACK Incorporated.

Rapaport, D. (1942). *Emotions and memory.* New York: Harper.

Rapaport, D. (1953). On the psychoanalytic theory of affects. *International Journal of Psychoanalysis, 34,* 177–198.

Reiss, D., Neiderhiser, J., Hetherington, E. M., & Plomin, R. (2000). *The relationship code: Deciphering genetic and social patterns in adolescent development.* Cambridge, MA: Harvard University Press.

Rorschach, H. (1921). *Psychodiagnostics: A diagnostic rest based on perception.* New York: Grune & Stratton.

Sable, P. (1995). Pets, attachment, and well-being across the life cycle. *Social Work, 40,* 334–341.

Sadock, B., & Sadock, V. (2003). *Kaplan & Sadock's synopsis of psychiatry* (9th ed.). Philadelphia, PA: Lippincott, Williams & Wilkins.

Spitz, R. (1959). *A genetic field theory ego formation: Its implications for pathology.* New York: International University Press.

Urbanowski, R. (1997). Spirituality in everyday practice. *Occupational Therapy Practice, 2,* 18–23.

Urbanowski, R., & Vargo, J. (1994). Spirituality, daily practice, and the occupational performance model. *Canadian Journal of Occupational Therapy, 61,* 88–94.

Vaillant, G. E. (1993). *The wisdom of the ego.* Cambridge, MA: Harvard University Press.

Watkins, J. G., & Watkins, H. H. (1990). Dissociation and displacement: where goes the "ouch?" *American Journal of Clinical Hypnosis, 33,* 1–10, discussion 11–21.

Wechsler, D. (1981). *Wechsler adult intelligence scale* (Revised ed.). New York: The Psychological Corporation.

White, R. H. (1959). Motivation reconsidered: the concept of competence. *Psychological Review, 66,* 297–333.

White, R. H. (1967). Competence and the growth of personality. In *Science and psychoanalysis, vol. XI, The ego.* New York: Grune and Stratton.

Zemke, R., & Clark, F. (1996). *Occupational Science: The evolving discipline.* Philadelphia, PA: FA Davis.

Zimmerman, P., & Becker-Stoll, F. (2002). Stability of attachment representations during adolescence: the influence of ego-identity status. *Journal of Adolescence, 25,* 107–124.

Chapter 21

FRAMES OF REFERENCE INTEGRATION

INTRODUCTION TO FRAMES OF REFERENCE

Have you ever looked through a pair of rose-colored glasses? If so, you've probably noticed how rosy everything looked. Wearing dark-colored glasses on a cloudy day may have the opposite effect. Both will affect how we interpret what we see and will, subsequently, impact our emotional responses, interactions, decisions, and behaviors. It is the same with a frame of reference but more complex because it involves all of our sensory and cognitive experiences.

Understanding Frame of Reference

To further illustrate the nature of a frame of reference, read the following example while everyone closes their eyes to better visualize the scenario:*

"Imagine yourself asleep in the upstairs bedroom with no one else in the house. You are suddenly awakened in the middle of the night by a loud noise. You are now lying alert but motionless in your bed, listening intently. What could it be? (pause)

"There are several options. Option 1) thunder. You keep listening but the sound does not repeat itself. You look out your bedroom window and the stars twinkle back at you. The moon lights up the sky, and there is no lightening or rain. Comparing your knowledge and experience regarding thunderstorms with these cues, you eliminate this explanation. Option 2) a nearby explosion or car crash. Maybe you get out of bed and scan the surroundings outside your bedroom window. You listen for sirens, signs of fire engines, flashing lights. There are none. You search your memory for more information about the sound you heard. It was blunt and muffled with a tinkling afterwards. You realize now that the sound must have been close by. How does this realization make you feel? (pause)

"Option 3) a burglar. He or she might have entered your house by breaking a window. This is the option you most fear. What thoughts run through your mind as you contemplate this possibility? (pause) Hesitantly, you get out of bed and begin to investigate. Maybe you quietly dress yourself and put on shoes or a coat. Maybe you locate a portable phone or cell phone, just in case. You now listen much more intently for sounds within the house. You quietly open the door a crack, the one that leads to the hallway and stairs, and you listen. Silence. Still thinking, you consider 'What would a burglar do if he sees me? Am I in danger?' You shut the bedroom door and lock it. Then you notice the night light is working. There is electricity working... on TV, the burglars would shut it off, so ... maybe it isn't a burglar after all. Then you hear a faint 'meow' coming from the direction of the stairs.

"Option 4) the cat. What do you know about cats? They are nocturnal, you recall. At night they are apt to prowl, to investigate their surroundings. They might even jump onto tables and counter tops that are off limits during the daytime. The meows sound louder, closer. Encouraged, you unlock and open the bedroom door. Your cat, Mittens, enters, purring and rubbing against your legs. Would a cat do this with a stranger in the house? Probably not. But then, what was that loud noise? (pause)

"Emboldened, you walk out into the hall and look around. There at the bottom of the stairs, caught in a beam of moonlight, is a broken vase surrounded by water and scattered long stem roses. Relieved that you have solved the mystery, you climb back into bed, Mittens now purring at your feet. Clean up can wait until morning. You may now open your eyes."

*Adapted from Cole, M. (1998). What, exactly, is a frame of reference? In K. Sladyk (Ed.), The occupational therapy student primer: A guide to college success. Thorofare, NJ: SLACK Incorporated.

Figure 21-1. Model and frame of reference analysis.

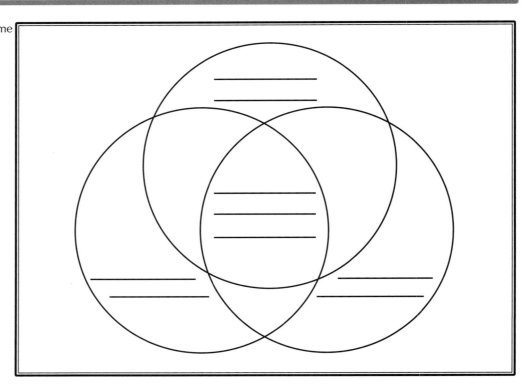

Drawing Activity

Draw a Venn diagram with three intersecting circles (see Figure 21-1 for an example). Label them person, environment, and situation/event. What variables fall within each circle that impact the outcome of this scenario? Describe how these three concepts interacted in order to produce an adaptive response. How might this part of our exercise relate to occupational therapists working with clients?

PRACTICE FRAMEWORK PROCESS: INTEGRATING MODELS AND FRAMES OF REFERENCE

The Framework Process Model uses the Venn diagram to demonstrate the interaction of three concepts of service delivery: evaluation, intervention, and outcomes. The core of the model, where all three circles overlap, represents the client–therapist relationship, which follows the client-centered approach (See Figure 2-3) (American Occupational Therapy Association [AOTA], 2002, p. 615). This "collaborative" therapeutic relationship applies the principles of Carl Rogers, and other humanistic and existential concepts that have been reviewed in earlier chapters. Each partner in the collaboration brings different knowledge, beliefs, and viewpoints to the process. The client brings subjective expertise, while the occupational therapy (OT) practitioner brings a professional body of knowledge coupled with "clinical reasoning and theoretical perspectives to critically observe, analyze, describe, and interpret human performance" (AOTA, 2002, p. 615). This description of the Framework Process allows the occupational therapist to choose from any of the occupation-based models to guide clinical reasoning for the subsequent evaluation, intervention, and outcomes. The model chosen will define the way that person–occupation–environment interactions are perceived. The use of an occupation-based model early in the Framework Process serves the vital purpose of bringing into focus a broad range of possible barriers to engagement in occupation—client factors, contexts of performance, and the demands of that task chosen.

Frames of reference are incorporated into the Framework Process at both evaluation and intervention phases of service delivery. While neither models nor frames of reference are mentioned in the outcomes phase, their use is implied in the measurement of initial goals, which were chosen within a theoretical perspective. During evaluation, the "theories and frames of reference that the occupational therapist selects to guide his or her reasoning will influence the information that is collected during the occupational profile" (AOTA, 2002, p. 616). The occupational profile subsequently influences the selection of targeted outcomes (client priorities, goals). Specific assessments used during the "Analysis" (p. 617) phase of evaluation that are derived from specific frames of reference imply that the resulting interventions will either confirm or refute the therapist's initial hypothesis, which represents the collaborative definition of the occupational problem or barrier.

The Framework further specifies that intervention planning requires the application of "approaches based on theory and evidence" (p. 618). After the intervention has been implemented, the therapist and client engage in a review process "relative to achieving targeted outcomes." At this point in the Process, if the client has not progressed as expected, the occupational therapist needs to reconsider not only the intervention methods but also the model and frame of reference that guided its choice. In order to "modify the plan as needed" (p. 618), the therapist may also need to switch to a different frame of reference.

LEARNING ACTIVITIES

The following learning activities are intended to be applied at the beginning, during, and at the end of students' study of frames of reference. It is also suggested that students use the Reed's Venn Diagram method (see Chapters 4 and 11) for analyzing frames of reference, including those discussed here and those referenced elsewhere in their curriculum.

Discussion

During this visualization experience, you imagined one sensory event (a loud noise) and formulated four different theories (or hypotheses) as possible explanations. These might represent four different frames of reference, or different ways of interpreting the same event.

- What other explanations came to mind?
- What experiences have you had that might have required a similar reasoning process?
- How did your prior experiences affect the process?
- How did you conduct "research" to substantiate or refute each option?
- How did your emotions affect your thinking? How did emotions affect your behavior?
- What other actions or decisions did you contemplate during the scenarios?
- How do you think this exercise relates to occupational therapists working with clients?

Case Study 1: Craig

Craig is a 39-year-old married male with two children admitted to the neuropsychiatry unit for alcohol abuse, depression, and suicidal ideation. He states, "Alice and the kids would be better off without me."

In the recent past, his wife went away for the weekend with friends. Craig refused to go but felt abandoned and unable to care for the children. He began drinking Friday night and Saturday morning took his 5-year-old son to a friend's house. On the way home he drove his car into a ditch on the side of the road, was taken by ambulance to the emergency room (ER), and treated for a contusion on the left side of his head and a broken left elbow and collar bone. In addition, his blood alcohol was high, and he was arrested for drunk driving.

The son of an alcoholic father of Irish decent, Craig was often the target of his father's anger because he could not learn how to read and found it difficult to sit still in school. He quit after the 8th grade and learned to do body work on cars from one of his two older brothers. He is still enraged at his parents for labeling him the "family dummy," causing him to feel inadequate and helpless.

Craig did a stint in the United States Army, where he was sent to the Middle East on a peace-keeping mission. He learned to operate a radio and to shoot with a rifle and a semiautomatic. Once, while there, he was stabbed in the back by a fellow United States serviceman in a bar. He did not remember the incident but did recall spending most of his off-duty time drinking.

Back home, he made good money as an auto body repairman working with his two older brothers. His first marriage failed after a few years, and he has been taking antidepressants on and off since then. He met his current wife at an Alcoholics Anonymous (AA) meeting. The 10-year-old daughter is hers from a prior marriage.

Now detoxified and back on antidepressants, he comes to OT dressed in black boots, jeans, and a black leather jacket. He asks you to read him the questionnaire and fill in the blanks for him. You ask him to draw a person doing something and he does so willingly, using the cast on his left arm to hold the paper while he uses a right, back-handed grip to draw in great detail (Figure 21-2). When he's finished, he tosses it back at you saying, "Analyze that!"

Craig participates in other program activities. He makes the coffee, enjoys playing horseshoes, walks the grounds and smokes, and often wins at poker.

Occupational priorities are to return to work, spend more time with his son, catch up on his yard work, and win the lottery so he can get out of debt. His wife wants him to stop drinking and to interact more with her. She also would not mind if he sold his motorcycle "before he kills himself or someone else."

Theory Application

Choose three different frames of reference that might provide guidelines for evaluation and intervention for Craig. Then do the following for each:

1. Write a summary of the case from that frame's perspective. What three performance areas would you expect Craig to choose as priorities and why?

Figure 21-2. Craig's "Person taking a walk." (Reprinted with permission.)

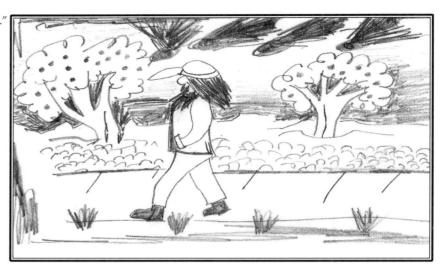

Use the OT Practice Framework as a guide to performance areas.

2. List and explain five problems with occupational performance from this frame's view. How would you assess each of these problems' occupational areas? Choose some specific tasks from Craig's priority areas as a focus for problem descriptions.

3. What might be some ways Craig would be motivated from this frame?

4. What contextual factors might present barriers to functioning, and how might they be modified?

5. What intervention plans would you suggest for Craig over the next 4 to 6 weeks? Design one individual session (1 hour) and one group session (1 hour) as examples.

Frames of Reference Review and Panel Discussion: Class Exercise Sign-Up

In preparation for the final exam, organize a panel discussion. For the purposes of review, please select one of the following categories (work in pairs):

1. History of theory (theorists, years developed, when/ how used in OT—for each frame listed following)

2. Allen cognitive disabilities

3. Toglia Dynamic Interactional

4. Behavioral theories (behavior modification and self-management)

5. Psychodynamic

6. Developmental theories

7. Sensory integration

8. Motor control

9. Motor learning

10. Biomechanical and rehabilitative frames

11. Cognitive behavioral

Each group will do the following:

1. Review all notes, quizzes, and readings on your topic using these basic headings: Focus, Basic Assumptions, Function/Dysfunction, Postulates of Change, Motivation, Assessment, and Intervention Strategies. Do this on the computer and e-mail it to each other. Use the Table 21-1, and summarize the content to no more than 10 words in each box. This will not be all you need to know about the theory, but it will make the similarities and differences more apparent. Fill in only your column in preparation for the Panel Discussion, but in class, fill in the rest as a study guide.

2. Be prepared to answer the following questions in class:

   a. How does your frame of reference differ from each of the others? What are the similarities? What are the essential differences?

   b. What specific theorists have contributed to this OT frame, and how do they differ from each other (if applicable)?

   c. Give a case example of how this frame of reference might be used.

   d. What specific assessment tools might you use in this frame of reference?

   e. Give an example of a group intervention using this frame of reference.

   f. Give an example of an individual intervention.

   g. Cite one study (research article) that supports this frame of reference.

   h. How might you apply this frame of reference to yourself or use it in your own life?

3. *Panel Discussion.* During class, share questions with the "experts" in each category and discuss how the

		Table 21-1						
			Frames of Reference Summary Template					
	Allen	**Toglia**	**Behavioral**	**Psycho-dynamic**	**Develop-mental**	**Sensory Integration**	**Motor Control**	**Motor Learning**
Focus								
Theorists, year(s)								
Basic assumptions								
Function-dysfunction								
Change								
Motivation (given as example)	Just-right challenge	Self-mastery	Reinforcement	Drive reduction	Resolve life tasks	Inner drive/ pleasure	Spontaneous CNS recovery	Task mastery
Assessment								
Intervention								

CNS = central nervous system

various theories may be "infused into practice." Groups will then revise their review documents and send them by e-mail to each other as an exam review and preparation for the comprehensive final exam.

Case Study 2: John

John, age 35 with a L5 spinal cord injury, has not made expected progress toward bathing and dress independently. The occupational therapist initially used a biomechanical-rehabilitative frame of reference, which focused on upper-body strengthening, practice in the use of adaptive equipment, and the application of specific movement strategies for bathing and dressing.

1. What do occupation-based models tell us about the nature of the disability as contributed by the person (client factors), environment (contextual factors), or the way the task is defined and structured? Which model is most helpful in understanding these factors, given your limited knowledge of the case?

2. What are some other options from the following frames of reference?

a. Cognitive behavioral

b. Psychodynamic

c. Motor control and learning

d. Dynamic interactional

e. Cognitive disabilities

f. Behavior modification

g. Developmental

For each explanation of the disability of dressing, choose one assessment tool and one intervention strategy based on the guidelines from your chosen frame of reference.

REFERENCES

American Occupational Therapy Association. (2002). Occupational therapy practice framework: Domain and process. *American Journal of Occupational Therapy, 56,* 609–639.

Cole, M. (1998). What, exactly, is a frame of reference? In K. Sladyk (Ed.), *The occupational therapy student primer: A guide to college success.* Thorofare, NJ: SLACK Incorporated.

Table 21-2

Consolidated Template of Frames of Reference Comparisons

Frames	Focus	Theorists/ Year(s)	Function/ Dysfunction	Motivation/ Change	Evaluations	Interventions
Allen Cognitive Levels (ACL)	Cognition, Mental illness, dementias, CNS damage	Allen, 1980s	ACL 1 to 6, 52 modes	Changes in brain, adapt task demand, cues, assistance, adapt environment	LCL, ACL, ADM, RTI, Cognitive Performance Test	ADL, crafts groups, caregiver education, adapt environment
Cognitive Rehab/Toglia's Dynamic Interactional	Brain injury, mental illness	Toglia, Abreu 1980s to 1990s; Toglia, 2005	Attention, visual perception, motor planning, problem-solving, occupations	Neuroplasticity, learning and practice of new strategies, multi-contexts, meta-cognition	Perceptual evaluation, dynamic assessment of task performance	Worksheets, task practice, strategy practice, use of technology, groups using graded games
Behavior Modification	Change in outward behaviors	Skinner, Pavlov, Lazarus, 1930s	Behavioral goals and objectives	External reinforcement, bio-feedback	Observation-based assessments	Shaping, chaining, extinction, rehearsal of specific behavior
Cognitive Behavioral	Changing thoughts, beliefs, emotions, and behaviors	Bandura, Beck, Ellis, 1970s	Behavioral goals and objectives, client priorities	Hierarchy of reinforcement, application of scientific method	Self-report, client-centered goal setting	Psycho-educational groups, use of strategies, self-management
Psycho-dynamic	Mental illness, emotional response to illness	Freud, 1900+; Fidler, 1950s; Mosey, Llorens, 1970s	Levels of personality development social (object) relationships	Drive reduction, pleasure principle, ego skill mastery	Projective tests, adaptive task performance	Creative arts, task-oriented groups, working through conflicts

(continued)

Table 21-2
Consolidated Template of Frames of Reference Comparisons *(continued)*

Frames	Focus	Theorists/ Year(s)	Function/ Dysfunction	Motivation/ Change	Evaluations	Interventions
Developmental	Ages and stages	Mosey, Piaget Erikson, Freud Kohlberg, Levinson, etc.	Stage of life, age, life structure, regression	Mastery of age-appropriate life tasks, resolution of conflicts	Age- and stage-specific skills	Groups focused on life stages, life tasks, transitions
Sensory Integration	Sensory development, handwriting, skilled movement, learning disability	Ayres, 1970s; Rood, King, Ross, Dunn, Wilbarger	Age-appropriate sensory integration, learning and daily functioning	Regulation of sensory input, graded activities, gross and fine motor activities	SCPT, SBC, SARIB, sensory profiles	Movement and cognition, five stage groups, games, use of equipment to give sensory input
Motor Control/ Motor Learning	Relearning skilled voluntary movement	Trombly, Rood, Brunnstrom, NDT, PNF, Carr and Shepherd	Degree of voluntary movement, ability to perform ADL	Client task choices and priorities, spontaneous relearning	Reflex testing, MMT, ROM	Movement-based therapies, reflex, sensation, PAMS, task-oriented OT approaches
Biomechanical and Rehabilitation	Physical disabilities and pain	Trombly, Anatomy and Physiology	Limitations in strength, endurance, ROM	Repetition, reinforcement, and successful task completion	MMT, ROM, increased independence in ADL, work	Exercise within context of client-chosen tasks

LCL = lower cognitive level; ADM = Allen Diagnostic Module; RTI = Response To Intervention; SCPT = ?; SBC = ?; SARIB = Smaga and Ross Integrative Battery; NDT = neurodevelopmental therapy; PNF = proprioceptive neuromuscular facilitation; MMT = manual muscle testing; ROM = range of motion; PAMS = patient assisted management of symptoms

(Courtesy of Marilyn B. Cole)

INDEX

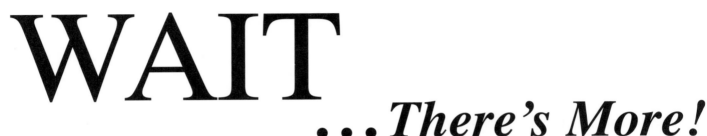

WAIT ...There's More!

SLACK Incorporated's Health Care Books and Journals offers a wide selection of products in the field of Occupational Therapy. We are dedicated to providing important works that educate, inform, and improve the knowledge of our customers. Don't miss out on our other informative titles that will enhance your collection.

Group Dynamics in Occupational Therapy: The Theoretical Basis and Practice Application of Group Intervention, Third Edition
Marilyn B. Cole, MS, OTR/L, FAOTA
432 pp, Soft Cover, 2005, ISBN 10: 1-55642-687-9,
ISBN 13: 978-1-55642-687-2, Order# 36879, **$46.95**

A core text for over 12 years, this revised third edition of *Group Dynamics in Occupational Therapy* incorporates the AOTA's *Occupational Therapy Practice Framework* and provides an updated perspective on the design and use of groups in emerging practice areas. Marilyn B. Cole explains how group activities can serve the needs of clients with similar physical disabilities and mental health issues by working on shared goals and providing a context of cultural and social support for engagement in occupation.

Quick Reference Dictionary for Occupational Therapy, Fourth Edition
Karen Jacobs, EdD, OTR/L, CPE, FAOTA; Laela Jacobs, OTR
600 pp, Soft Cover, 2004, ISBN 10: 1-55642-656-9,
ISBN 13: 978-1-55642-656-8, Order# 36569, **$31.95**

This definitive companion provides quick access to words, their definitions, and important resources used in everyday practice and the classroom. Incorporated within this user-friendly fourth edition are innovative and unique features that help you keep pace with the latest in occupational therapy. Over 3,600 terms are defined and 60 appendices are presented. Essential AOTA references are featured, including the *Occupational Therapy Code of Ethics–2000*, making *Quick Reference Dictionary for Occupational Therapy, Fourth Edition* ideal for students and professionals to enhance their knowledge base.

An Occupational Perspective of Health, Second Edition
Ann Wilcock, PhD, BAppScOT, GradDipPublic Health, FCOT
384 pp, Hard Cover, 2006, ISBN 10: 1-55642-754-9,
ISBN 13: 978-1-55642-754-1, Order# 37549, **$46.95**

Crafts and Creative Media in Therapy, Third Edition
Carol Tubbs, MA, OTR/L; Margaret Drake, PhD, OTR/L, ATR-BC, LPAT, FAOTA
304 pp, Soft Cover, 2007, ISBN 10: 1-55642-756-5,
ISBN 13: 978-1-55642-756-5, Order# 37565, **$41.95**

Vision, Perception, and Cognition: A Manual for the Evaluation and Treatment of the Adult With Acquired Brain Injury, Fourth Edition
Barbara Zoltan, MA, OTR/L
368 pp, Hard Cover, 2007, ISBN 10: 1-55642-738-7,
ISBN 13: 978-1-55642-738-1, Order# 37387, **$44.95**

Vision, Perception, and Cognition, Fourth Edition is a concisely structured text that expertly addresses clinical reasoning and decision making for the entire evaluation and treatment process of the adult with acquired brain injury. Provided are theoretical information, guidelines for both static and dynamic assessment, information on specific standardized evaluations, guidelines for adaptive and restorative treatment based on described theoretical and evidence-based information, and information on environmental impact of client performance.

Occupational Therapy: Performance, Participation, and Well-Being, Third Edition
Charles H. Christiansen, EdD, OTR, OT(C), FAOTA;
Carolyn Baum, PhD, OTR/L, FAOTA;
Julie Bass Haugen, PhD, OTR/L, FAOTA
680 pp, Hard Cover, 2005, ISBN 10: 1-55642-530-9,
ISBN 13: 978-1-55642-530-1, Order# 35309, **$72.95**

Applied Theories in Occupational Therapy: A Practical Approach
Marilyn B. Cole, MS, OTR/L, FAOTA;
Roseanna Tufano, LMFT, OTR/L
336 pp, Soft Cover, 2008, ISBN 10: 1-55642-573-2,
ISBN 13: 978-1-55642-573-8, Order# 35732, **$40.95**

Documentation Manual for Writing SOAP Notes in Occupational Therapy, Second Edition
Sherry Borcherding, MA, OTR/L
256 pp, Soft Cover, 2005, ISBN 10: 1-55642-719-0,
ISBN 13: 978-1-55642-719-0, Order# 37190, **$37.95**

Activity Analysis: Application to Occupation, Fifth Edition
Gayle I. Hersch, PhD, OTR; Nancy K. Lamport, MS, OTR;
Margaret S. Coffey, MA, COTA, ROH
192 pp, Soft Cover, 2005, ISBN 10: 1-55642-676-3,
ISBN 13: 978-1-55642-676-6, Order# 36763, **$43.95**

Please visit

www.slackbooks.com
to order any of these titles!
24 Hours a Day...7 Days a Week!

Attention Industry Partners!
Whether you are interested in buying multiple copies of a book, chapter reprints, or looking for something new and different — we are able to accommodate your needs.

Multiple Copies
At attractive discounts starting for purchases as low as 25 copies for a single title, SLACK Incorporated will be able to meet all of your needs.

Chapter Reprints
SLACK Incorporated is able to offer the chapters you want in a format that will lead to success. Bound with an attractive cover, use the chapters that are a fit specifically for your company. Available for quantities of 100 or more.

Customize
SLACK Incorporated is able to create a specialized custom version of any of our products specifically for your company.

Please contact the Marketing Communications Director of the Health Care Books and Journals for further details on multiple copy purchases, chapter reprints or custom printing at 1-800-257-8290 or 1-856-848-1000.

*Please note all conditions are subject to change.

CODE: 328

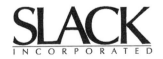

SLACK Incorporated • Health Care Books and Journals
6900 Grove Road • Thorofare, NJ 08086
1-800-257-8290 or 1-856-848-1000
Fax: 1-856-848-6091 • E-mail: orders@slackinc.com • Visit: www.slackbooks.com